WITHDRAWAL

Topics in Environmental Physiology and Medicine

edited by Karl E. Schaefer

Stress, Health, and the Social Environment

A Sociobiologic Approach to Medicine

J. P. Henry and P. M. Stephens

Springer-Verlag   New York Heidelberg Berlin

J. P. Henry
and
P. M. Stephens

Department of Physiology
University of Southern California School of Medicine
Los Angeles, California 90033

Library of Congress Cataloging in Publication Data
Henry, James Paget, 1914-
    Stress, health, and the social environment.
    (Topics in environmental physiology and medicine)
    Includes bibliographies.
    1. Medicine, Psychosomatic. 2. Human behavior. 3. Cerebral
dominance. 4. Social medicine. I. Stephens, Patricia M., 1930- joint
author. [DNLM: 1. Psychophysiologic disorders. 2. Social
environment. 3. Stress, Psychologicial. WM90 H522s]
RC49.H44   616.08   77-10500

© 1977 by Springer-Verlag New York Inc.

Printed in the United States of America.

9 8 7 6 5 4 3 2 1

ISBN 0-387-90293-7 Springer-Verlag New York Heidelberg Berlin
ISBN 3-540-90293-7 Springer-Verlag Berlin Heidelberg New York

"Vocatus atque non vocatus Deus aderit."

Deeply carved into the lintel of Carl Jung's home near Zurich is the Delphic Oracle's enigmatic reply to the Spartans who were planning a war against Athens; it translates as the foreboding, "Summoned and not summoned, God will be there" (Jung, 1961). Sociologist Peter L. Berger (1976) elaborates on the Twentieth Century's increasing secularization and disregard of oracles by commenting that the myths that guide life spring from the soil of religious faith. Their power comes from those realms of the mind in which the gods used to dwell, and the gods have always been relentless.

Preface

The mastery of a variety of biomedical techniques has led our society to the solution of the problems in environmental control imposed by space flight. By an unparalleled social cooperative effort, man has launched himself successfully on the path of interplanetary exploration and space travel. By a like synthesis of knowledge available to him, Stone Age man kept a foothold on tiny Pacific atolls for the better part of a thousand years, despite obliterating hurricanes and limited resources. By combining empiric navigational skills, such as the sighting of stars with intuitive feeling for ocean swells and other subtle cues, tiny populations were maintained in communication over vast distances. Atolls such as the Tokelaus, Bikini, Rongelap, or Puka Puka are scarcely larger than the one-mile diameter space stations being planned by today's technology.

Our Stone Age ancestors also developed cultural practices that permitted stable occupancy for centuries. In spite of violent perturbation following sickness, natural catastrophes, and competition for scarce resources, these primitive human societies found it possible to maintain an equilibrium. They avoided the self-destruction and disease that can so readily follow the escalation of social disorder in an isolated colony. By following a "code of civility" that may be as much a part of man's biologic inheritance as his speech, they established cultures in which power was exercised with sufficient respect to establish a consensus. They followed revered cultural canons, using an accumulation of rational empiric data from social experience to modify and control the inherited biogrammar. This we often fail to do. There is growing evidence that it is physiologically possible for the left hemisphere of the brain, which deals with logic and language, to be cut off from the right hemisphere and other realms of the mind, handling emotion, fantasy, and religious experience. Such alienation is fostered by today's secular technocracies that replace parental and filial care with institutions, govern by bureaucracy, and blur the identity of the sexes. Our health and well-being are endangered by a viewpoint overemphasizing left hemispheric function and distorting and suppressing traits inherited from our hunter–gatherer forefathers that normally speak to us through the archetypal patterns of symbols.

This book proposes why some societies remain relatively free from psychosomatic diseases that plague others; by a detailed observance of the normative patterns of their culture, they avoid a loss of values, thus following the preconditions for a healthy social life—thereby for health itself. Frequent confrontations and much emotional arousal occur from an extensive break up of the protective affiliative network which is man's basic social asset. The path is cleared for an excessive stimulation of the neuroendocrine apparatus by unconstrained fight–flight and withdrawal responses. The ensuing disturbed autonomic and hormonal levels in turn upset tissue regulatory balances, reducing their resistance to other influences and exposing the organism to the breakdown of disease.

We parallel Insel and Moos's (1974) anthology, *Health and the Social Environment*, which, from the clinical point of view, summarizes the evolutionary biologic approach of the Stanford medical group with which the Hamburgs have been associated. It shares our point of view and makes frequent references to the literature.

We have tried to show how the mechanisms controlling man's adaptation and resistance to certain diseases can be illuminated not merely by studies with primates, but also by work with colonies of tiny rodents. These social mammals are available in convenient genetic strains and live in accelerated biologic time. The preconditions for their health are clearly dependent on their social order.

This book has a dual authorship because of its dual origins. One of us is chiefly responsible for the collection of literature and its compilation; the other, for the fifteen years of social–ethologic study of rodent colonies on which our conclusions are based.

The authors wish, first, to thank Jo Kolsum for her sustained editorial craftsmanship and Dr. John P. Meehan, chairman of our physiology department, for his unfailing support of an esoteric approach to the study of disease.

The detailed and constructive criticisms by Dr. Daniel L. Ely and Dr. Peter H. Henry have been invaluable and most encouraging. The names of our other collaborators appear throughout the accounts of our experiments; they have given this work its momentum.

The authors to the best of their knowledge have obtained permissions for all copyright material; but if any required acknowledgements have been omitted, or any rights overlooked it is hoped they will be notified so that any omissions may be corrected for future editions.

It is a pleasure to acknowledge the support of the National Aeronautics and Space Administration-Ames Research Center Grant NGL 05-018-003 (NsG-433) and the National Institutes of Health Grants MH 19441 and HL 17706.

J. P. Henry
P. M. Stephens

Contents

1

A historical introduction and theoretical concept

Donnison's *Civilization and Disease*

As one of a series of books dealing with biomedical effects of the environment, this volume presents the thesis that more should be learned about the influence a social system has on the health of its members. Adequate experimental approaches are now available for studying the forces that can unleash the pathophysiologic influences latent in any social system, despite its current health. This holds true as much for rodent societies living in population cages as for modern man in his cities. Thus colonies of small laboratory mammals can be used in making controlled social–ethologic observations of the mechanism of disease, and data from such colonies will form a major part of this work. There have, however, been a number of similar viewpoints during the past 40 years, and reference must first be made to the observations of some men on whose work the present approach is based.

In 1938, Donnison wrote a foresighted book *Civilization and Disease,* arguing that the reaction of the organism to stimuli induced by life in a civilized community was responsible for much organic disease (Donnison, 1938). He had for years been a physi-

cian to a tribal reservation on the shores of Lake Victoria in Kenya. The observation that he could find no case of high blood pressure in the 1800 patients admitted to his hospital aroused his curiosity. He realized that their cultural patterns had not been seriously disturbed for generations and was struck by the difference between their time-honored methods of child rearing and those of his native England. In his book, he presented the hypothesis that the successful childhood integration of the inborn drives into socially acceptable patterns was the critical factor in their creation of a stable nonhypertensive society. Donnison could not at that time marshall sufficient evidence for his sociocultural theory, but it grows clear that he was correct that the successful care of its children is a society's most critical test.

Halliday's *Psychosocial Medicine: A Study of the Sick Society*

Writing 10 years later, the epidemiologist Halliday gave his book the title listed above, and in it he described the origins of illness due to defective social interaction

(Halliday, 1949). He recognized that the incidence of peptic ulcer, diabetes, high blood pressure, and coronary heart disease could be affected by a change in the milieu. He commented on Donnison's observation that such conditions were rare in primitive nonindustrialized communities. He also noted that their incidence was far less before the industrial revolution and attributed this to the radical changes in patterns of child care and adult life. To him, the earlier practices of rearing children were more favorable for emotional growth because the women handled their babies instinctively by maternal impulse. The new practices with the separation of the mother from her child at birth; the replacement of the breast by the bottle; the reduction of what he called "spiritual contact," i.e., effective communication between mother and child by such practices as the denial of the impulse to hold it when it cried; the loss of playmates due to the smaller families and separate houses; the constant admonitions to be orderly, tidy, punctual, dutiful, and toilet-trained—all in his opinion, had negative effects on emotional development.

In the adult, Halliday noted that changes in the environment introduced by the shift from a rural to an urban industrial life led to a loss of interaction with what he called the "time and tides of nature." There was also a loss of opportunity for free muscular exertion and an increasing neglect of seasonal and diurnal rhythms. Timetables and day and night shifts mean that working rhythms peculiar to the individual are increasingly disregarded.

Halliday was further concerned by the increasing frustration of manipulative creativity. Machine production of items, restrictions of output, and actual unemployment meant that a man's hands and ingenuity could no longer be used to fabricate items needed by him and by those significant to him. If the hunter–gatherer who makes his own weapons, shelter, and ornaments is acting out the inherited skills of man, the recently evolved tool maker, then to deny this activity is to frustrate an innate impulse pattern to work with his hands.

He discussed the increasing rapidity of change in the structure of society. Persons no longer knew where they stood or how long they would stand. English society before the mid 19th Century had stratified social classes and people "knew their place." He argued that they adjusted their goals to the possibilities of the position in life into which their parents had been born. He claimed that the breakup of this caste system led to many insecurities and frustrations as the society became increasingly unstable.

Halliday was also disturbed by the growth of examinations to judge fitness for jobs; this with the universal literacy led to an education mainly concerned with the acquisition of information from books. Schools and universities failed to recognize the need for educating the emotions, that is, of life training and the development of personality and character. He argued for teaching as a relationship based primarily on emotions and only secondarily on intellect. He accepted the importance of factual information, but argued it could not be a substitute for education in living. Finally, he came to the problem of motivation, of having an object to live for: the loss of an active religious faith, the failure of women to have and to raise children, and the craftsman denied the opportunity to watch the growth of the product of his manipulative activity. In short, he said there was a progressive restriction of emotional vision, of insight and movement toward a clearly envisaged goal.

Halliday summarized his view of the mechanisms underlying the growth of conditions such as hypertension and coronary disease as follows: A progressive increase of inner insecurity due to the altered early condition of the young and increasing insecurity of job, income, and status in the social setting led to emotional tensions. These could not be resolved due to progressive restriction in the creative activities of making and producing goods and because of increasing neglect of innate biologic rhythms. He said the tensions could not be canalized in the form of a drive to a goal either in this life or in a future one because of loss of inspiration. There was also a progressive recession of the sphere of the "divine" associated with an increase in the secularization of thought or rationalism. This withdrawal of "God," he said, is far from unimportant in its practical, psychologic, and social effects.

Halliday was writing over 25 years ago about the state of culture in England and its relation to the development of chronic disease. He concluded by stating that "the incidence of many incapacitating disorders and diseases that fall within the sphere of general medicine may be said, like the infectious diseases, to have an epidemiology. But unlike the infectious diseases, their etiology cannot be understood unless the environment is viewed in terms of its psychophysiological effects." At that time such a thesis could not be supported by facts. However, like those of Donnison, his intuitive insights helped to inspire research which has today provided a more convincing accumulation of data. The present review of new work in the areas of psychosomatic medicine, epidemiology, and the behavioral, social, and biosciences will indicate that both men came close to the mark.

Emotion as a driving force in evolutionary biology

In approaching the problem of how psychosocial stimulation can lead to chronic disease, a major question concerns the evolutionary reasons for emotional responses. Another is the mechanism by which an emotion many times repeated can lead to disease. With regard to the first, the psychiatrist Hamburg has presented an evolutionary argument (Hamburg et al., 1975). He proposes that emotions evolved as expressions of motivation which an animal must experience to meet the adaptive tasks necessary for survival. He must regularly seek food and water, avoid predators, mate, successfully care for the young, and train them to cope effectively with the demands of the environment. There is evidence of neurophysiologic machinery to accomplish this. In his text *The Brain and Reward,* Rolls (1975) has described the prime function of the amygdalar nuclear complex as that of attaching value to acts; thus it drives attachment behavior. It is important in the extensive reward system studied by the neurophysiologist Olds. The effect of the arousal of this system is to make the animal try harder to accomplish the particular task he perceives as connected with the reward. Olds showed that electrical stimuli given to reward areas in response to pressing levers could replace a normal sensory reward, such as a saccharine pellet (Olds, 1976). The animal would work to exhaustion if the system were effectively triggered. It is equally correct that avoidance is elicited by stimulation of the appropriate areas. Most of these, as in the case of reward, are in the limbic system and brain stem.

Hamburg et al. (1975) make the point that the normal animal finds species-preservative and self-preservative activities, such as the search for food and water, avoidance of predators, or care of the young, provide relevant feedback. They are intrinsically pleasant and result in activation of the rewarding areas of the brain.

Evidence that the limbic and striatal regions are the locus for the neuronal complexes mediating the emotions and behavior critical for self- and species-preservation has been presented by MacLean (1976). These complexes are wired by genetic determination in such a way that the organism will engage in territorial and attachment behavior appropriate for the occasion, as long as he has had certain socializing experience while maturing.

Tiger and Fox (1972) speak of a biogrammar. They say the human infant begins to smile at a predictable time and the adolescent boy loses his shrillness, yet becomes more annoying to his elders, because they are programmed to do so. They say that in just the same way that baboons growing up in captivity spontaneously produce a baboon social system, we have language and a complex culture because we are wired to produce them when given the right inputs at the right times. They and we behave in these ways because from an evolutionary point of view our biogrammar ensures that we find it rewarding to do what is needed to maintain the species. Tiger and Fox's term *biogrammar* is used because *instinct* is too strong a word, having become equated with the rigid performance of insects or fish. Just as grammar is concerned with only the rules or patterns underlying communication by speech, so biogrammar is concerned with only the patterns underlying flexible behavior that mammals, including man, use to attain desiderata, such as food or a mate. Grammar does not determine the specifics of what is spoken, nor does biogrammar precisely dictate behavior, but it does tell us the forms that are likely to be taken.

The archetype or emotional aptitude that Jung proposed is a related concept. In her study of complexes, archetypes, and symbols, Jacobi (1959) points to the archetype as an aspect of instinct. She cites Jung's early conclusions that a part of the central nervous system other than the cortex might be responsible for the behavior induced by archetypes. Jung saw that archetypes could exist in animals, and Jacobi equates this at the most basic level with Konrad Lorenz's theory of innate reactions to characteristic stimuli which are independent of experience in the sense that the tiny baby's smile releases innate reactions in the mother and the girl's smile, in the young man! The biogrammar or archetype can be seen as a vital but prerational element of behavior dependent on subcortical structures. It might be termed the language of psychologic programs that originate from the structures of the brain stem and limbic system.

In his recent book on *The Biology of Human Action*, Reynolds (1976) defines the extent to which inferences can be drawn about human behavior on the basis of evolutionary ancestry. He is concerned with the relation between biology, psychology, and sociology and questions whether the demands of man's culture and the urban society it has produced exceed the limits of his adjustability. Reynold's stance that what man has created, man can modify and improve is cogent, and his exception to arguments that life styles and societies are inevitable sequelae of man's biogrammatic wiring is well taken. The history of celibate social systems is adequate evidence of the power of culture over nature. Nevertheless, despite monastic achievements, the fact remains that female mammals are programmed by their biogrammar to care for their young and the latest research on the role of mother–infant interaction (see Chapter 2) indicates that the human female is no exception. It is the woman's biogrammar that induces her to respond to her infant by holding it face-to-face and releases the emotion binding her to that particular infant.

Without programmed motivation there will be no maternal behavior. It is not enough to have efficient sense organs and superb skeletal, circulatory, digestive, and effector systems. In order to attain desiderata they must be competently deployed; emotional arousal lies at the basis of this drive to act effectively.

So in addition to their subjective aspect, emotions inevitably have both behavioral action and physiologic or neuroendocrine components. When considering the evolutionary necessity that a mother mammal must be motivated to care for her baby, we are faced not only with the attachment behavior pattern, whose profound importance is detailed in Bowlby's ground-breaking treatise *Attachment and Loss*. We also find that there are neuroendocrine changes associated with her care of the young, and shifts abruptly occur in these patterns when the attachment bond is disrupted by removing the mother from her infant. These interindividual bonds with their related physiologic response patterns persist in healthy apes, and for years after the young have become self-sufficient, they return to be with their mother. In man this attachment behavior persists even more remarkably and with modifications by symbolism motivates a lifetime of socialized behavior (Bowlby, 1970).

Cannon and stress; Selye and distress

The above two names at once come to mind when the problem of connecting a social stimulus with physiologic changes is considered. It is a major theme of this book to show that the responses they discovered involved different autonomic and hormonal pathways and can be elicited separately. An animal that is pursuing a valued object and suddenly find himself obstructed in attaining that goal responds with an emotion. The average hungry dog eating a meaty bone will growl and show signs of fight if a stranger attempts to remove it by force. If, however, the stranger is big and aggressive, the dog may yield the bone and take off in flight. Physiologic measurements will show that his sympathetic nervous system has been thoroughly aroused and that adrenal medullary hormones have been released.

A continued observation of the bone loser may show further behavior which contrasts with the first observation. If day after day, the dog is offered the bone and then punished whenever he attempts to take it, if he is deprived of all rewards and positive reinforcement and meets with painful, capricious assaults he cannot predict or control, then he is likely to develop a different pattern of behavior. He may cringe, whine, and accept the beating, making no attempt to touch the proffered bone. The psychologist Seligman has recently described this behavior in detail (Seligman, 1975). He identifies it with a self-perception of helplessness and

the emotion of depression. It is more associated with activation of the adrenal cortex than with catecholamine excretion.

The pioneering studies of the first type of response were made by the physiologist Walter Cannon (1929). He used a barking dog to arouse a cat and demonstrated the role of the sympathetic nervous system and the adrenal medulla in determining the physiologic nature of this response to a challenge. His successful delineation of the release of catecholamines into the bloodstream during a reaction which prepares for fight, or primes for flight, led to the discovery of a broad series of neuroendocrine responses to psychosocial stimulation.

Starting in the 1930's, the other father of "stress" research, the endocrinologist Hans Selye (1950), concentrated on demonstrating the responses of rats to heat and cold, traumatic injury, and sometimes to just "nervous irritation." His measure was a newly found adrenal-cortical-driven general adaptation or alarm syndrome.

In his recent book *Stress Without Distress* Selye summarizes his psychologic insights after a lifetime of intensive endocrinologic study of this pattern. He points out that the Cannon response is associated with the arousal of an athlete competing hotly to stay ahead or of the parachutist keeping steady at the moment of jumping. He describes the critical contrast between such joyous excitements and those he defines as distress. The former, he argues, is what gives zest to life. It is associated with every sort of effort and is indeed nothing to be avoided. Distress, on the other hand, he associates with the unfulfilled need for achievement and with deprivation. It is distressing, he says, to have perceived oneself as having failed. Pride in excellence, he points out, is a "primeval biological feeling" shown by dogs, or seals, or man. The reverse leads to distress of frustration—a lack of purpose. A man, he says, must find a job he can do where his fellows appreciate his efforts. Constant censure is a stressor that more than any other makes work frustrating and harmful. His advice for achieving a sense of security is to pace your effort so as to avoid failure and frustration, generating aimlessness and insecurity.

If the preceding passages in which Selye discusses distress are reviewed in light of their context, and the words he uses to describe the condition are considered, the conclusion emerges that he is discussing a response differing from that of Cannon. Selye sees the condition as one connected with defeat and frustration. This loss of relevant feedback is characteristic of helplessness and depression described by Seligman in his dogs. It is also probable that the psychiatrist Engel and his associates, who have worked with humans, are describing a related mechanism in their conservation–withdrawal response (Engel and Schmale, 1972). It appears when Selye (1974) speaks of distress, he is describing the subjective behavioral aspect of arousal of the pituitary adrenal-cortical system as opposed to the sympathetic adrenal-medullary system of Cannon.

Although they are unpleasant, the moderate depressive responses associated with adrenocorticotropic hormone (ACTH) release and activation of the adrenal cortex have as much survival value as the fight–flight Cannon response. However, there is evidence if either system is driven too hard and too long, the arousal can become a health hazard. This makes a case for two sorts of stress with differing neuroendocrine responses and different ultimate disease states.

Helplessness → steroid
Arousal → Catechol

Wolff's *Stress and Disease*

Only four years after the epidemiologist Halliday completed his work, the psychosomatically oriented clinician Harold Wolff reviewed his experimental observations linking social stimulation with disease. This ground-breaking book was revised 15 years later by his friends and associates Wolf and Goodell (1968). It represents a clear summary of the mechanisms by which the nervous system can set the manifestations of disease in motion. The thesis was that the brain formulates physiologic patterns of adaptation to stress, evoking circumstances which may be inappropriate in kind, amount, and duration and hence may ultimately be disruptive and even destructive.

The authors believed that an understanding of the effects of environmental social change and of familial, social, and cultural demands was critical. They perceived circumstances that "a man sees to be dangerous, lonely, and hopeless may drain him not only of hope but also of health." On the other hand, given "self-esteem, hope, purpose, and belief in his fellows, he will endure great burdens and take cruel punishment."

Wolff illustrated his thesis with a 30-year series of experiments starting in 1932 (Wolf and Goodell, 1968). A major tool was his use of stress-inducing interviews, and he demonstrated that during migraine headaches there is arterial dilatation and that attacks could be induced by giving such interviews. He induced swelling and hypersecretion in the nose and asthmatic bronchoconstriction by discussing topics involving bitterness and helplessness. He used the same interviews to make his classic observations on Tom, the subject with a gastric fistula. There was an increase of acid secretion and hyperemia of the stomach when hostility and resentment were induced by unjust accusations. In another context, the stress interview induced an elevation of blood pressure and renal vasoconstriction. In further demonstrations, he showed that causing a certain patient to feel abused and angry, yet helpless, triggered vigorous urticarial reactions, and in eczematous patients, cutaneous vasodilation occurred during the interview.

The laboratory work of Wolff and his associates had established that by controlled experiments almost any organ system could be acutely disturbed by purely central nervous stimulation.

Hinkle's studies of sociocultural changes and health

Hinkle, originally one of Harold Wolff's associates, effectively extended the evidence from the acute laboratory experiment to the prolonged experiments of nature on groups of people at varying degrees of risk. His work has focussed on the question of how health is affected by changes in the cultural or social milieu or interpersonal relationships (Hinkle, 1974). By studying 1300 telephone operators over a 20-year period, he showed that the healthy ones liked their work better and found it easy and satisfying. They liked their friends and associates and were content and comfortable in their lives. Those who had many illnesses were more likely to find work confining and boring and were unhappy with their lot in life and in their families. Thus the personalities of the healthy insulated them. They could endure social change and personal deprivation without undue emotional response.

At first, by studying Chinese and later Hungarian refugees from Communist regimes and former American prisoners of war in Korea, he came to similar conclusions. Those who had experienced a greater amount of illness had perceived what could well have been the same environment as more threatening, challenging, demanding, and, frustrating than the healthier people. Indeed, people who remain free from illness in face of major life changes appear to him to have special characteristics that help insulate them from the effects of their life experiences. Those who could endure the loss of a husband or wife, isolation from friends and community, or failure to attain apparently important goals seemed to have a "sociopathic flavor." They lacked the normal

intensity of attachment to people, goals, and groups and too readily shifted to other relationships, behaving as if their own well-being was their primary concern.

Holmes–Rahe life change and illness susceptibility scale

The work of Hinkle showed that emotionally arousing situations occurring naturally will increase the incidence of disease. Another of Harold Wolff's former associates, Thomas Holmes, contributed much to the study of the relationship between psychophysiologic reactions induced by stressful life events and the natural history of a disease (Hawkins et al., 1957). Starting with tuberculosis, his group used a "life chart" to study clusters of events at the onset of symptoms. Typical events involved marriage, occupation, peer relationships, education, and so forth. Interviews showed them that various events elicited adaptive coping behavior. For years no allowance was made for the differing intensities of stimulation that might ensue from events as different as the death of a spouse and marriage. Then in collaboration with Richard Rahe, a list of standard events, called a Schedule of Recent Experience, was scored in an average sample of Seattle population based on the following instructions (Holmes and Rahe, 1967). The original list was accompanied by the following written instructions.

1. Social readjustment includes the amount and duration of change in one's accustomed pattern of life resulting from various events. As defined, social readjustment measures the intensity and length of time necessary to accommodate to a life event, *regardless of the desirability of this event.*
2. You are asked to rate a series of life events as to their relative degrees of necessary adjustment. In scoring, *use*

all of your experience in arriving at your answer. This means personal experience where it applies, as well as what you have learned to be the case for others. Some persons accommodate to change more readily than others; some persons adjust with particular ease or difficulty to only certain events. Therefore, strive to give your opinion of the average degree of readjustment necessary for each event rather than the extreme.

3. The mechanics of rating are these: Event 1, Marriage, has been given an arbitrary value of 500. As you complete each of the remaining events think to yourself, "Is this event indicative of more or less readjustment than marriage?" "Would the readjustment take longer or shorter to accomplish?" If you decide the readjustment is more intense and protracted, then choose a *proportionately larger* number and place it in the blank directly opposite the event in the column marked "Values." If you decide the event represents less and shorter readjustment than marriage, then indicate how much less by placing a *proportionately smaller* number in the opposite blank. (If an event requires intense readjustment over a short time span, it may approximate in value an event requiring less intense readjustment over a long period of time.) If the event is equal in social readjustment to marriage, record the number 500 opposite the event.

The scoring technique was based on a general principle already established by the psychophysicist Stevens (1966). Holmes and Rahe relied on the fact that subjective assessment plotted against physical dimension provides a remarkably reliable quantification scale. In subsequent studies, Holmes, Masuda, and Komaroff found that the scores assigned for various life events by Americans living in Seattle did not differ radically from those of Japanese (Masuda

and Holmes, 1967) and other groups, such as American Negroes and Mexican Americans (Komaroff et al., 1968). Table 1-1, which is taken from a review by Rahe (1972), presents the values attached to the original Life Change Events list by the Seattle sample. A somewhat more sophisticated version of the questionnaire appears in a 1976 report (Rahe, 1976) and Rahe and Arthur (1978) recently completed a valuable review discussing the future direction of this research.

Because the Life Change Score considers events inappropriate for young adults, such as a son or daughter leaving home, a *College Schedule of Recent Life Experience* has been developed by Anderson (1972) using Life Change Events relevant to students (Table 1-2). Marx et al. (1975) applied the Anderson scale to the freshmen class of the University of Kentucky and showed that men in a high life-change category had a significantly higher ($p > 0.02$) mean number of illness days (41) compared with the low life-change group (19). The corresponding figures for women were 55 and 23.

Ten years of studies by Holmes, by Rahe, and by others have established that when the total life change score was much increased, i.e., when changes had escalated in response to a life crisis, the probability of an onset of disease increased. Why does the list of life changes include events, such as marriage or promotion, which are usually regarded as positive? Because, according to Rahe (1974), these events, pleasant as they are, also challenge the individual's coping mechanisms and are frequently followed by illness.

The validity and reliability of the questionnaire have been challenged, but people rarely fabricate life events. As the time between the first and the second test increases from eight months to two years, the test–retest correlation drops from 0.90 to 0.26. Also, it is higher in psychology students (0.90) than in physicians (0.64–0.74). There is, however, as Masuda (1976) has shown, no question that with time people begin to

Table 1-1. *Holmes–Rahe Life Change Events for Seattle Adults* [a]

	LCU values
Family:	
Death of spouse	100
Divorce	73
Marital separation	65
Death of close family member	63
Marriage	50
Marital reconciliation	45
Major change in health of family	44
Pregnancy	40
Addition of new family member	39
Major change in arguments with wife	35
Son or daughter leaving home	29
In-law troubles	29
Wife starting or ending work	26
Major change in family get-togethers	15
Personal:	
Detention in jail	63
Major personal injury or illness	53
Sexual difficulties	39
Death of a close friend	37
Outstanding personal achievement	28
Start or end of formal schooling	26
Major change in living conditions	25
Major revision of personal habits	24
Changing to a new school	20
Change in residence	20
Major change in recreation	19
Major change in church activities	19
Major change in sleeping habits	16
Major change in eating habits	15
Vacation	13
Christmas	12
Minor violations of the law	11
Work:	
Being fired from work	47
Retirement from work	45
Major business adjustment	39
Changing to different line of work	36
Major change in work responsibilities	29
Trouble with boss	23
Major change in working conditions	20
Financial:	
Major change in financial state	38
Mortgage or loan over $10,000	31
Mortgage foreclosure	30
Mortgage or loan less than $10,000	17

[a]The now classic Holmes–Rahe Scale of Life Change Events showing the original Life Change Units (LCU) as determined by a representative group of Seattle adults. A reference value of 50 units was arbitrarily assigned to marriage, and each subject was then asked to assign proportional values to others (Rahe, 1972).

forget life changes and this affects the reliability of tests attempting to cover several years in retrospect.

Scoring life changes has become established as a successful method of measuring life events. It is challenged, however, by Hinkle (1974) who contends that individuals with more illness perceive life changes as more threatening. This problem is met to some extent by ensuring that events intrinsically the most disturbing are given higher scores and those less disturbing, lower ones. Thus, the death of a spouse ranks five times as high as a son leaving home which in turn is four times as high as a vacation at Christmas.

In two recent papers, Rahe et al. (1974a) describe the relationship between recent life changes and coronary death. In the first, they evaluated 279 survivors of myocardial infarction and 226 victims of abrupt coronary death. In separate interviews with spouses of all but one group of subjects, a significant increase of life changes was noted six months before infarction as compared to the same interval a year earlier. An increase in life changes was also observed in a second study by Theorell and Rahe (1975) in which 18 men and women with myocardial infarction who ultimately died from the disease were compared with 18 matched subjects alive six years later. Ballistocardiographic measurements of the force of systolic contraction had been made as well as retrospective evaluation of life changes. The authors demonstrated that those who died showed a build-up in both force and life changes which peaked approximately six months before death.

Despite these relatively successful observations, in a recent assessment of the value of life change measurements in predicting myocardial infarction, de Faire and Theorell (1976) point out how weak is the sum of life changes as a predictor when taken alone. But when life changes and an inverse measure of social support, which they describe as a "propensity to react," are used together, the power of the method

Table 1-2. *Life Change Unit Scores for Life Change Events Experienced by College Students*[a]

Area	Unit score
Family	
Death of spouse	87
Marriage	77
Death of close family member	77
Divorce	76
Marital separation	74
Pregnancy or fathered a pregnancy	68
Broke or had broken marital engagement or steady relationship	60
Marital reconciliation	58
Major change in health or behavior of family member	56
Engagement for marriage	54
Major change in number of arguments with spouse	50
Addition of new family member	50
In-law trouble	42
Spouse began or ceased work outside the home	41
Major change in number of family get-togethers	26
Personal	
Death of close friend	68
Major personal injury or illness	65
Sexual difficulties	58
Major change in self-concept or self-awareness	57
Major change in use of drugs	52
Major conflict or change in values	50
Major change in amount of independence and responsibility	49
Major change in use of alcohol	46
Revision of personal habits	45
Major change in social activities	43
Change in residence or living conditions	42
Change in dating habits	41
Outstanding personal achievement	40
Major change in type and/or amount of recreation	37
Major change in church activities	36
Major change in sleeping habits	34
Trip or vacation	33
Major change in eating habits	30
Minor violations of the law	22
Work	
Fired from work	62
Entered college	50
Changed to different line of work	50
Changed to new school	50
Major change in responsibilities at work	47
Trouble with school administration	44
Held job while attending school	43
Major change in working hours or conditions	42
Change in or choice of major field of study	41
Trouble with boss	38
Major change in participation in school activities	38
Financial	
Major change in financial state	53
Mortgage or loan of less than $10,000	52

[a]The Life Change Unit Scores for Life Change Events Experienced by College Students. Note that a score of 50 is given to college entry. This results in 77 for marriage and 76 for divorce. A large number of items relevant to students are to be found in this table, which is a modification by Marx et al. (1975) of the College Schedule of Recent Life Experience devised by Anderson (1972).

increases greatly. As de Faire and Theorell say, if the propensity to react is low (i.e., social support is high), the individual can experience many concomitant life changes without suffering pathophysiologic consequences. Rabkin and Struening (1976) come to the same conclusion in their review of life events, stress, and illness. Observations of life change taken alone have many weaknesses, although the original method is attractive for its simplicity and directness. The social support factor is critical in determining why health is sometimes affected and sometimes not. Rabkin and Struening point to the importance of meeting a life change with competence and experience and to the negative effects of social isolation and incongruence of status. This important addition of the parameter of perceived social support that changes the whole significance of the life change measurement technique is mentioned further in Chapter 11.

Mice, primates, and primitive man will be discussed in regard to their attachment and territorial behavior and its disturbance by changes in living conditions in the ensuing chapters. But how can this be related to a life change scoring based on modern technology? In Table 1-1 the sections Family and Personal are roughly concerned with events that affect attachment behavior, i.e., of bonding the individual to others; the sections Work and Financial are somewhat more concerned with the control that the individual exerts in relation to others, thus reflecting territoriality in its broadest sense, i.e., the capacity to hold one's own or to advance in a social hierarchy. These patterns, we show, are the warp and woof of the fabric of any mammalian society.

Theoretical mechanisms of psychosomatic disease

The principles by which social groups stay healthy can be explored in accelerated biologic time by studying colonies of mice who in two years run through the equivalent of a full human lifetime. Mammalian social systems, including monkeys as well as rodents, can be considered in context of three specializations of role and behavior held in common. (1) All have a social hierarchy in which some are dominant and others subordinated. (2) All have a functional subdivision into males and females with differing biologic roles which must nevertheless be knit into the framework of a unified group. (3) All progress from helpless vulnerable infancy through mature strength and activity to dependency or death.

We will examine these three aspects in normal and disturbed colonies of mice; in primate groups, such as the hamadryas baboon; and in man, the hunter–gatherer, living in the state for which his brain and body were evolved. The effect perturbation of social patterns controlling a healthy mammalian colony has on physiology and therefore on the pathophysiology of its individual members will be presented together with evidence as to the mechanism by which these disturbances can lead to chronic disease.

There has been skepticism that emotions aroused in a social context can so seriously affect the body as to lead to long-term disease or death. But work, such as that of Wolff, shows the machinery of the human body is very much at the disposal of the higher centers of the brain (Wolf and Goodell, 1968). Given the right circumstances, these higher controls can drive it mercilessly, often without awareness on the part of the individual of how close he is to the fine edge.

In the strenuously contested 1976 Winter Olympics a young, superbly trained, cross-country skier, who had already made his mark in two races, took off on the 50 kilometer marathon. Leading to the halfway point, he staggered across the finish line blinded by cerebral anemia due to acute heart failure. He was still a contestant finishing a respectable thirteenth. The stimuli driving his cardiovascular system to the brink of disaster arose at affective and cognitive levels above the hypothalamus. The intensity of his response to psychosocial stimuli may have been unusual, but the physiologic mechanisms his brain was driving respond to some degree in all of us.

With sufficient repetition even moderate stimuli can eventually have disastrous repercussions, and the theme we are pursuing is a detailed analysis of the chain of events leading from psychologic interaction between members of a social group to deleterious influences on their health. The whole of life from birth onward is involved. The patterns of behavior necessary to produce a successful, smoothly running society develop only when there is a proper sequence of interactions between the various members during their lifetime. The sequence must start with an effective bond between mother and infant and between mature siblings, if society is to provide for the individual's needs effectively in adult life.

Man's huge neocortex provides left and right hemispheric specializations that account for his unique language and technology. In effect, they are a twin sociocultural brain. But, in addition, he relies on the limbic system, which he shares with all mammals, and which lies at the root of attachments between individuals, provides for species' typical behavior, helps control the deference paid by one to the territory and desiderata preempted by another, and leads members of a group to support each other in reliable behavior patterns. The need for proper attachment and territorial behavior will not be fulfilled unless the experiences involved are rewarding to the individual. Members of a disturbed social system who do not feel rewarded will have aroused emotions as they compete with others in their disordered society, and these emotions will consistently elicit physiologic arousal. The ensuing fighting with its matching patterns of flight is an active response arousing the sympathetic nervous system and releasing the catecholamines, adrenaline and noradrenaline. An alternative pattern of passive withdrawal and social isolation may follow a failure to achieve successful control. The neuroendocrine pattern accompanying this depressive withdrawal involves the pituitary hormonal chain that arouses the immunologically debilitating hormones of the adrenal cortex.

The sympathetic adrenal-medullary and the pituitary adrenal-cortical systems that become aroused in states of psychosocial stimulation are only a part of a complex control of the organ systems that activate various emergency mechanisms, for instance, shutting down the pituitary hormones which control reproduction via the testes and ovaries. This shutdown is part of the total response pattern when a social system breaks down and the individual is left alone to struggle for survival.

If aggressive asocial behavior and associated emergency responses replacing normal nurturance and social patterning persist long enough, disease will occur. Blood vessels thicken with progressive loss of nutrition to tissues and immune responses become disturbed, rendering the organism susceptible to viruses and other parasites, neoplasms, and autoimmune diseases.

Thus the altered neuroendocrine function of disturbed social relationships eventually, by two pathways, leads to permanent pathologic changes, resulting in irreversible damage: in one case, arteriosclerosis, myocardial fibrosis, and interstitial nephritis and in the other, peptic ulcer, infections, and formation of tumors.

The mechanisms by which this chain of events can be reversed or blocked are currently being explored, especially in the context of human disease. We will discuss the role of social assets that counter the responses of rage, fear, and despair and group practices that specifically seek to control them. Practices such as meditation and relaxation, prayer, worship, and mutual encounter are associated with rules of behavior that counter social disorder. Their practice alleviates threats to the individual's goals of stable attachment and control of territory, and permits rewarding feedback with attainment of desiderata. When these procedures are a vital part of the culture of an organized group, they reduce the incidence of disease of psychosocial origin. These rules that determine social behavior by placing it in what is essentially a religious context have been termed the "cultural canon." The word *canon* refers to revered beliefs and values held by the group to be self-evident and of binding emotional significance.

The existence of such a canon holds the hunter-gatherers together in their mutually supportive groups. A viable cultural canon modulating the biogrammar of attachment and territorial instincts is vital for control of instinctual drives of members in a society. It patterns their individual urges for food, water, shelter, and reproduction into a socially harmonious set of activities. A breakdown of the canon heralds social disorder which, if unchecked, terminates the affected group by a combination of violence, disease, and reproductive failure.

Social environment as initiator of a chain of events

Our historical introduction sketched the development of a concept of the relation between dysfunction in the social sphere and disease. We have also carried the analysis a step further and briefly reviewed the argument of this book that a chain of events converts a psychosocial stimulus into nervous and then chemical changes, which in turn create a critical regulatory imbalance in the tissues. Recent surveys of the problem have shown a remarkable unanimity as to the sequence of events.

Cassel (1974) has argued that today's medicine has too simplistic a view. He says it has failed to recognize that psychosocial stimulation resulting from the arousal of an emotion is not directly pathogenic in the same way a microorganism, which causes a loss of fluid from the gut, could be. Rather, psychosocial factors act indirectly by serving as stimuli triggering neuroendocrine mechanisms, which if prolonged can lead to disease. The particular manifestation of a disease is determined by other factors acting in concert with the disturbed social process. Thus it is a common marginal status in society that triggers a high incidence of tuberculosis, schizophrenia, alcoholism, suicide, and multiple accidents. The particular breakdown suffered by a victim depends on his previous history and susceptibilities.

In his *Theoretical Principles of Psychosomatic Medicine,* Kurtsin (1976) clearly perceives the complex nature of chain reactions in producing pathology in an organ because of changes in neural and hormonal mediating components in response to what the Russians call corticovisceral disturbances. He believes they are based on disordered relationships between the neocortex and the nerve centers of the limbic system and thus presents the case for a hierarchy of control with the neocortical association areas influencing the visceral brain. Here the hippocampus and other limbic structures in turn affect the autonomic and the endocrine systems. Kurtsin's evidence from the operant conditioning and the conditioned reflex studies of animals convincingly describes their role in inducing corticovisceral disturbances which interfere with the function of the kidneys, stomach, and other organs.

Weiner's (1977) treatise on *Psychobiology and Human Disease* concentrates on diseases, such as hypertension, rheumatoid arthritis, and duodenal ulcers. He cogently presents evidence that all physiologic processes in the body are ultimately regulated by the brain which integrates the autonomic afferent inflow and the response to external stimuli by complex regulating mechanisms. He has woven the social, familial, and physiologic factors into one piece: pharmacopathophysiology and the clinician's story. Weiner's (1975) approach is succinctly presented in a recent editorial in *Psychosomatic Medicine* in which he observes that psychosomatic diseases are increasingly regarded as disorders of regulation in which the necessary complex feedbacks for homeostasis are somehow disturbed. More than anyone else, Page (1949) should be credited with originating this approach with his mosaic theory of the classic psychosomatic disease: hypertension.

He broke ground in 1949 because he did not seek to define a single cause, but perceived that a steady state exists in the circulation in which important regulatory factors are in equilibrium, maintaining blood pressure and tissue perfusion at a relative constancy adapted to tissue needs. The number of variables that could be changed in an independent manner to produce high blood pressure was arbitrarily placed at eight, and a mosaic was drawn to show how several causes act together to produce a multifactorial process of disease (Figure 1-1). He further saw that the development of such a regulatory disease is a long one. Large changes do not have to occur at any one time because years, not hours or days, are concerned (Page and McCubbin, 1965).

Page conceived of the problem as primarily in the physiologic sphere and concen-

trated on factors operating "below the hypothalamus." Twenty years later, matters had advanced to the point that the physician–psychologist team of Harris and Singer (1968) suggested various psychologic factors were critical in the etiology of essential hypertension. Starting with a person's interaction with the environment, they argued that this impinges on the patterns of personality and behavior and thus results in stimuli to the neuroendocrine system and eventually to the cardiovascular system. They suggested that ensuing episodic increases in blood pressure eventually lead to a consistent rise in blood pressure relative to the normal value. They too recognized the factor of time as a second major influence. In a disease such as high blood pressure this could extend from childhood throughout adult life or the impact of social stimuli could be deferred and only strike with full force after half a lifetime.

Social psychologists Kiritz and Moos (1974) have argued along similar lines. Social stimuli do not act directly on an individual. It is his perception of the social environment as mediated by personality variables, role, and status relationships and his behavior within the environment which affects him, influencing his personality and behavior.

Seeking to illustrate the nature of these perceptions, they point out that two individuals within the same social group might be treated differently because of their differing behavior. A suspicious, contentious person might find the office in which he works nonsupportive, whereas someone who is more friendly and cooperative will perceive the same place in a different light.

Even given similar perceptions, two persons working in the same nonsupportive environment might respond differently because they have very different social assets. The one may have a loving wife and children, many friends, and a history of interpersonal successes. The other may be recently divorced and may have long regarded himself as an interpersonal failure. The two would be likely to differ in their emo-

Fig. 1-1. Page's mosaic theory is diagrammed here. It draws attention to the multifactorial nature of hypertension as a disease of regulation. Many factors play a part in controlling pressure and resistance which determine the extent of the vital variable—tissue perfusion. He chose the eight shown as examples of the interlocking process *(Page and McCubbin, 1965).*

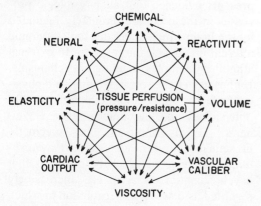

tional responses to the same environment because their resources for defending against emotional arousal would differ so greatly. The result could be that while one sent out repeated stimuli initiating the fight–flight response, the other might remain tranquil and relaxed in precisely the same circumstances.

Commenting on this idiosyncratic effect of a stimulus affecting each person differently, depending on his personality and interpretation of the situation, Cassel (1974) cites the ancient folk wisdom that "one man's meat is another man's poison," while Hinkle (1973) points out that "In view of the fact that people respond to their 'life situation' or social conditions in terms of the meaning of these situations to them, it is difficult to accept the hypothesis that certain kinds of situations or relationships are inherently stressful and certain others are not." In other words, the life change units to be assigned to any particular event differ according to the background of the individual. For example, one patient may deny the significance of a moderate anginal pain that immobilizes another.

Rahe is another person who has presented a model of the pathway along which environmental stresses must "travel" and the transformations that occur before they stimulate the subject's reports of illness (Rahe, 1976). His conceptualization is presented in Figure 1-2. It uses optical lenses and filters to illustrate the various steps along the pathway from nervous excitation to pathophysiology. Light rays of various intensities are drawn at the left edge to symbolize the environmental input. They represent various life events of different unit intensity (LCU). The solid black lines represent high LCU exposures; the thinner lines, more moderate ones; and the thin dotted lines, the least significant ones.

He sees the first filter as representing past experience, showing how in its light various LCU's may alter their values— some increasing and others diminishing. The concave lens represents the individual's psychologic defenses; some LCU's are deflected, others pass through without being affected by rationalization and other unconscious defense processes. The ensuing physiologic reactions are presented in the next step. This, he says, involves the entire discipline of psychophysiology. Many studies have shown that life change events perceived by a subject result in physiologic activation of various regulatory systems (Wolf and Goodell, 1968). After this step, the solid and dotted lines change in meaning and now represent various intensities of physiologic

Fig. 1-2. Rahe has presented this model of the pathway between a subject's exposure to recent life change and behavior during illness. It is depicted as a series of rays of varying strength and schematizes the transformations undergone by these stimuli and the route they must travel from recent life change to reports of near future illness. The diagram draws attention to the filters of experience and the psychosocial defenses that must be passed before the stimulus becomes a physiologic reaction. Depending on the coping and adaptation responses, any particular life change may or may not get through to contribute to the load that eventuates in a report of illness *(From Rahe et al., 1974. © 1974, American Medical Association. Reprinted by permission.)*

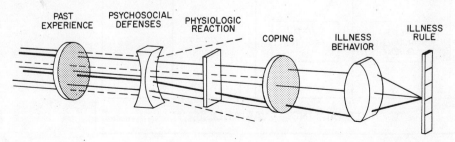

activation instead of life events. The filter represents coping mechanisms that Rahe sees as specifically affecting this physiologic activation, rather than the psychologic variables cited previously. Examples would be the reduction of blood pressure or pulse rate by biofeedback and the relaxation response of Benson et al. (1976). The final stage indicates that although physiologic activation occurs despite the coping activities of the previous step, there is still no guarantee that the subject will develop body symptoms and perceive himself as sick. Furthermore, even after having developed and acknowledged the illness, he must still report body symptoms to a medical authority. The doctor in turn must diagnose them along with possible pathologic tissue changes as illness.

Rahe thus sees a subject's recent life change experience as passing through several stages of perception and defense before body symptoms are perceived and reported as pathology or illness.

Kagan and Levi (1974) of the World Health Organization, International Research and Training Centre, Stockholm are a fourth group who have used a similar sequential view of the psychosocial processes involved in the development of chronic disease. In a recent review of the role of psychosocial stimuli in relation to society, stress, and disease, they presented the theoretical model shown in Figure 1-3. They define the terms in each of a series of interacting boxes as follows. *Psychosocial stimuli* originate in social relationships and act through higher nervous processes. The *psychobiologic program* is the propensity to act in certain ways when adapting to the challenge of the stimulus. Determinants are *genetic factors* and *earlier environmental influences*. *Mechanisms* are physiologic reactions resulting from the action of psychosocial stimuli. *Precursors of disease* are malfunctions in mental or physical systems developing from physiologic reactions, which if sustained will result in disease. *Disease* they define as disability caused by men-

Fig. 1-3. Kagan and Levi's model for psychosocially mediated disease recognizes the combined effect of psychosocial stimuli and the psychobiologic program. Together these determine the psychologic and physiologic reaction mechanisms, e.g., stress, of each individual. These may under certain circumstances lead to the precursors of disease and to the disease itself. They saw the sequence as being promoted or counteracted by interacting variables; for it is not a one-way process, but part of a cybernetic system with a continuous feedback *(Kagan and Levi, 1974).*

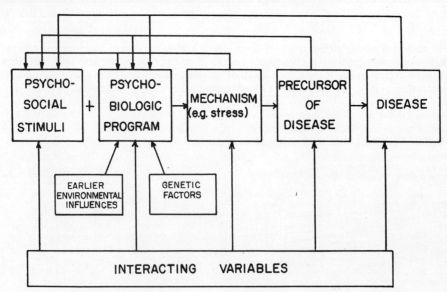

tal or physical malfunction. The feedback of interacting variables either promotes or prevents this series of events. Kagan and Levi present an impressive array of evidence suspicioning psychosocial stimuli in causing disease.

Our format: from stimulus to pathology

The format of our book also follows the chain of events theme already outlined, beginning with psychosocial perception and concluding with chronic disease. An ethologic approach is taken, citing the role of attachment and territorial instincts and, whenever possible, parallels are drawn between ordered and disordered societies of rodents, subhuman primates, and human hunter-gatherers as steps in a continuum of increasing complexity, ending with our modern society.

As the legend to Figure 1-4 indicates, the chapter sequence has been set up to follow the model of psychologically induced states of disease that has evolved from the preceding discussion. For simplicity the diagram is confined to the concept of a progressive chain of events.

Chapters 2 to 5 referred to in the first two boxes on the left are concerned with psychosocial stimuli plus the psychobiologic program. The initiating stimulus is the product of environmental interaction with the behavioral patterns we inherit as a genetical-ly determined biogrammar, modified by the effects of early experience. The mixture determines the response of the individual as he operates within a network of the young and old, males and females, and the social hierarchy. An analysis of behavior patterns and hormone levels permits a differentiation between various role players.

Chapter 6 discusses the role of the neocortex and the limbic system in social interactions. The corpus callosum may be related to a control of information transfer between the hemispheres, and rapid eye movement (REM) sleep appears to be involved in translating the biogrammar of the limbic system into the cognitive sphere and behavior that deals appropriately with environmental challenges.

Chapter 7 compares the behavioral significance of arousal of the sympathetic adrenal-medullary and the pituitary adrenal-cortical systems. These are seen as different response mechanisms leading to different pathophysiologic breakdowns. In Chapter 8, the functional and structural changes occurring in response to repeated arousal of either or both of these systems are presented. The evidence that structural autoregulation of the vascular bed is critical in the etiology of essential hypertension is reviewed as an example that bridges the gap from function to pathology. The chronic disease that ends this chain of events is arteriosclerosis and organ failure.

Evidence that psychosocial stimulation can induce states of chronic disease is discussed in Chapter 9 for animals and in Chap-

Fig. 1-4.   In this book the sequence of chapters from 2 to 10 follows the chain of events involved in the psychologically mediated disease, as shown in the Kagan–Levi model (Fig. 1-3). A final chapter discusses the control of psychosocial stimulation in man by biofeedback, small groups, and a revered cultural canon.

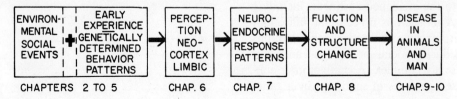

ter 10 for men. Chapter 11 reviews the growing bulk of data indicating that chronic disease is less prevalent in individuals and groups with an organized cultural canon giving them attitudes and social assets that control the intensity of arousal in response to psychosocial stimulation.

Summary

A generation ago, Halliday and Donnison both perceived that the growth of technocracy was depriving us of critical early learning experiences needed to consolidate patterns of behavior essential for continuing smooth social cooperation. The result of this inadequate learning is a chronic disturbance of emotional responses. Yet emotions are the crucial drive mechanisms for species-specific behavior patterns. Each basic emotion has a background of nervous and hormonal changes peculiar to it.

By using the stress interview technique, Wolff showed that emotions could elicit manifestations of a wide variety of diseases, including migraine and eczema. His associate, Hinkle, moved the investigation from the laboratory to the human ecologic scene. He demonstrated that in a group of normal persons, those who had the most illness over a course of 20 years were likely to have been more discontented with their lives at work, home, and play than those who had the fewest. Thus he linked emotion-producing personality characteristics with disease. Holmes and Rahe have shown that in addition to personality, the frequency and severity of social events play a part in the disease process. The sum of life changes experienced in a year, with allowance for readjustment that each change has demanded, is related to the incidence of illness, including lethal events such as myocardial infarction.

The mechanisms by which emotions induced during social interaction can result in disease are complex. A chain of interlocking causes operates in sequence over time.

To start: A basic inherited biogrammar interacts with the social environment. Certain patterns are predictable because all mammalian societies are differentiated into males and females, young and old, and all have a hierarchy of those with more control, i.e., dominants, and those, who in that particular social context, are subordinated. Two major pathways have been identified by which the ensuing emotions progress through neural and chemical regulatory processes to influence the tissues. The pathophysiologic mechanisms of the ensuing chronic disturbances of regulation vary according to the tissue being affected. The above consensus of opinion regarding steps in the development of psychosomatic disease is used as a basis for the chapter format of this book.

2

Basic patterns of social interaction

The basic patterns

Natural selection imposes behavioral patterns on us in order to ensure that certain crucial adaptive tasks will be carried out effectively. Intrinsic mechanisms arouse emotions urging the individual to accomplish these tasks. This inborn biogrammar is at the subjective roots of the organism's behavior and neuroendocrine state (Tiger and Fox, 1972). Three such major patterns can be discerned in all mammals. The first is the recognition of leadership. It is not only in the human social system that distinctions between individuals and between their control of access to desiderata, such as food, water, and shelter, are found. Even in the simple rodent society, an order of precedence usually permits discrimination of dominants from subordinates. When such precedence is accepted by various members of a mammalian group, a stable social order ensues. When each knows his place, role competition wasteful to the species is avoided.

Another differentiation is gender. The differences between the role of the male and the female, so fundamental in rodent or in subhuman primate societies, is also clear in societies of hunter–gatherers. Whether this sharp role discrimination must persist in contemporary society is under challenge. However, the evidence of Tiger and Shepher (1975) indicates that when given the freedom to choose their area of work, young women will select family and child care. Shepher, a kibbutz member himself, suggests they are being driven to it as an expression of the biologic determinants of gender. The authors see the engagement of men in economic and political activity as a counterbalancing expression of the same biogrammar. Their thesis, which is based on the statistics of a half century of social experimentation with the equality of sex roles in the kibbutz movement in Israel, shows quite an unexpected bias toward a growing male–female differentiation of tasks in the community.

A third biologically based distinction between the behavior patterns of any mammalian social group discriminates the young from the old. The young must be fed, protected, and given the chance to learn adult skills. At the other end of the scale, the more complex the society, the more chance the aged have to survive by trading strength and speed of response for skill and experience. Although the apex of this development is reached in our technocracy, the trend is clear in primitive food-gatherers among whom strength is not everything. Indeed, the Australian aborigines celebrated a formal graduation at the time the oldest child of a couple was declared marriageable. It was comparable to the initiation ceremony on entering manhood and represented recognition of a third degree of seniority. The ritual gave notice that the individual's experience and ripening wisdom were available to the community in place of lost fertility or hunter–fighter ability (Wynne-Edwards, 1962). Thus this chapter is concerned with dominants and subordinates, males and females, and young and old.

Territory in relation to dominance and subordination

The anatomy of an animal, his behavior, and his way of life form an integrated unity (Ewer, 1968), whose significance is best understood in light of his evolutionary history and relationships with other species as well as the habitat. The behavior of mice, for example, can be viewed in terms of interactions always going on between members of the group as they compete for environmental and social goals (Crook, 1970). High ranking animals feel free to initiate interactions and thus suppress activity in others by outright conflict if necessary. The less successful learn to avoid confrontations, and this avoidance-learning leads to a free hand on the part of the high rankers to move about in competition for commodities in short supply and to initiate various types of behavior interactions with others.

The territory available to an animal is thus determined by his relationship with his fellows. It can be far less extensive than the home range or the familiar region because it represents that core from which he excludes fellow members of his species. It includes places of importance such as areas for feeding and drinking and resting. Thus we use territoriality as a broad term, including life space, home range, and hierarchy: In an ethologic context, all have important differences in meaning, but in the present more general context, all are seen as expressions of the same basic biogrammar.

The first approach to a new territory is by investigation as the topography is learned; Ewer (1968) notes that this type of activity is marked by extreme caution. The strange area is approached slowly with much sniffing. At the slightest sound or odor, there is a hasty retreat followed by a fresh advance. By contrast, in the reconnaisance of familiar territory, the occupant patrols his range fully alerted, using all his sense organs to keep check on the area (Crowcroft, 1966) (Fig. 2-1).

Fig. 2-1. The movements of an alerted dominant mouse in a large room equipped with 15 nesting boxes and a number of feeding areas as he moves toward shelter in his home nesting box. A direct route is avoided, and the sequence by which he touches base at a large number of places in his territory is similar to the patrols he makes when not alarmed *(Crowcroft, 1966).*

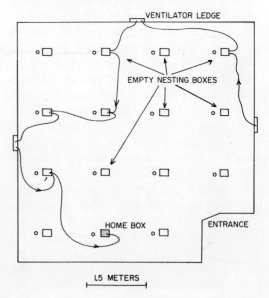

Mice live in mixed groups of about 10 to 20 members, called *demes* by ethologists and derived from the Greek word *dēmos* meaning: a people. Within its territory the group reproduces and builds up population density (Reimer and Petras, 1967). At a certain point, the deme breaks up and some go off to set up their own. In each deme there is usually a dominant male, along with others who share the area and are thoroughly familiar with it, but who are subordinate. The dominant covers the limits of his territory which he frequently inspects; he attacks and chases other males who venture within its boundaries (Fig. 2-2). Pregnant and lactating females will also fight to keep males out of their communal nurseries (Noirot et al., 1975).

Once a mouse has learned his area, he ceases his hesitant, investigative activity. It is now harder to get him to retreat. This assurance is basic to true territorial behavior. The mouse to whom the area belongs will have a confidence based on familiarity, whereas interlopers will be hesitant and cautious. The result is a sliding scale, adjusting the boundaries to permit establishment of a stable territory without costly fighting.

The primary function of territory is to ensure that the holders have sufficient area for their needs and for those of their young in terms of food and shelter. The strongest, most alert, and most able mice in a population will be able to hold the best parts of the habitat; the weaker ones are pushed into the less desirable areas. Thus there is a spacing out which ensures that the available habitat is fully exploited. The interpenetration of territories is accomplished by deliberately ignoring other individuals when their paths cross, as on the way to and from the same water hole (Ewer, 1968). Each animal in a series of adjacent demes will periodically meet neighbors at borders. Known neighbors are recognized and treated with a degree of tolerance that would not be permitted strangers.

Territory has the added importance, in addition to spacing out the individuals and ensuring an adequate area for rearing each family, of ensuring that whereas all females breed, only the strongest and ablest males

Fig. 2-2.   A healthy dominant will immediately attack an intruder, usually biting at the tail or rump where injury is trivial.

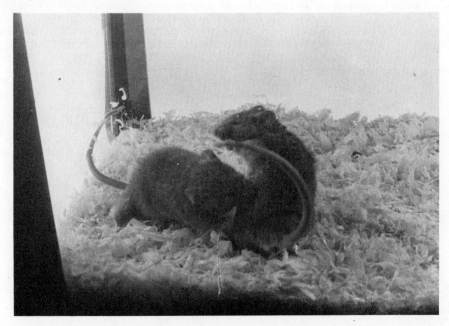

will father the largest number of offspring. In social species, such as mice or baboons, it is usual for the group to form a community in which aggression is reduced, but animals of the same species which do not belong to the group are treated as enemies. Ewer points out that without some such system for differentiating group members from strangers, the social unit would have no coherence and holding territory would be impossible (Ewer, 1968).

Dominance and subordination in monkeys

These principles apply throughout Mammalia in species differing as greatly as mice, wolves, and primates, including man. It is believed that man represents a branch of the ape line which ventured out of the forests to become a hunter on the open grasslands several million years ago. This brought them into competition with efficient predators and forced the protohominids to adopt a highly organized hierarchy (Maclay and Knipe, 1972; Alcock, 1975).

The baboon, also a savannah-living primate, gives some impression of the likely organization of early humans. A baboon troop consists of 20 to 30 individuals with a dominance hierarchy among the adult males. They may run the troop single-handed or more often by a small coalition consisting of two or three large individuals. Young males are peripheral to this group. Mating is not exclusive, but the dominant males have access during estrus. They defend the group from real danger, while the young males form an advance screen to give early warning, especially when the troop is on the move. At this time, the females and the young are in the center with the dominant males, the subordinate males on the periphery (Fig. 2-3). Aggression between the males within the group is kept down by intervention of the dominants (Eimerl et al., 1965; Bernstein and Gordon, 1974).

Members of the troop show deference to their superiors by presenting the rump; by doing so, they avoid punishment of being bitten for infractions of status. The order in which baboons present themselves gives some idea of their relative rank. On the other hand, peacefully grooming one another gives

Fig. 2-3. A troop of baboons on the march through open country. The adult males are distinguished by their large size and well-developed manes. Females with babies move in the center. Two females in estrus (dark hind parts) move in consortship with the most dominant males. A group of young juveniles are shown below center and the old juveniles above. Other adult males and females precede and follow the group's center (see Fig. 3-7) *(From DeVore, 1965. © 1965, Holt, Rinehart and Winston. Reprinted by permission.)*

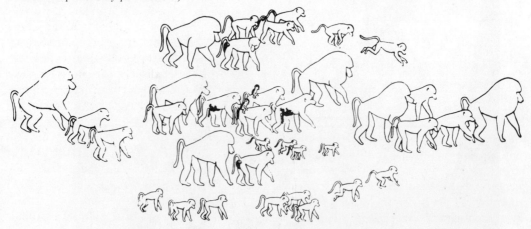

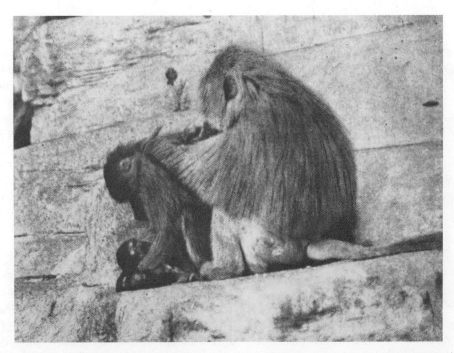

Fig. 2-4.   The dominant is usually the one to be groomed. However, in this photograph of disturbed hamadryas baboons at the London Zoological Gardens, a female baboon with her dead baby in her arms is being groomed by her overlord *(Zuckerman, 1932).*

them a means of expressing mutual attachment (Fig. 2-4). Dominant animals receive the most grooming but give the least. These social grooming periods are found not only in baboons, but also in chimpanzees and serve to reaffirm the troop's rank-order relations in the emotional context of affection and contentment (Eimerl et al., 1965; Van Lawick-Goodall, 1973).

Conflict behavior in rhesus monkeys

In an important review of the function of aggression in primate societies, Bernstein and Gordon (1974) note Southwick's discovery that competition for resources does not necessarily increase aggressive interactions (Southwick, 1967). On the other hand, they have studied the effects of introducing ani-

mals to one another either singly or in groups and found that fighting between rhesus males is limited to their use of incisors and not their formidable canines (see Fig. 5-7). The vulnerable throat and abdomen are avoided in favor of biting the back or tail (see Fig. 5-8). Animals that give up defending themselves by crouching and turning away are soon left alone. Thus there is a ritualization of fighting. Further, the dominant animals would intervene to break up a fight between two or more members of lower rank by a brief display of aggression. The authors conclude that the major function of dominance hierarchies is the control of aggressive competition. The dominant can be recognized from his stance with tail and head erect (Fig. 2-5). The difference between the dominant and the hunched up, subordinated, depressed animal is striking (Fig. 2-6).

The further apart two animals are on the

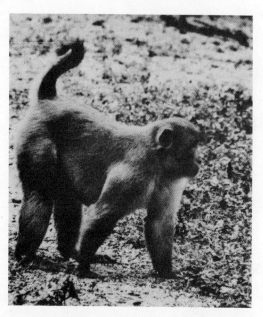

Fig. 2-5. The characteristic pose of a dominant male with head erect, a direct gaze, and tail high *(DeVore, 1965)*.

social scale, the less likely they are to be involved in fighting each other. For example, a control animal rarely directs aggression toward juveniles in the group. Aggression, on the other hand, acts to curb upward social mobility. The male fighting potential is released only in response to a serious threat to survival, and aggression is a primary mechanism. As Bernstein and Gordon (1974) state: "The most potent cause of

Fig. 2-6. A typical subordinate pose in flexion with rounded back and lowered head and tail *(From Hinde, 1974. © 1974, McGraw-Hill Book Company. Reprinted by permission.)*

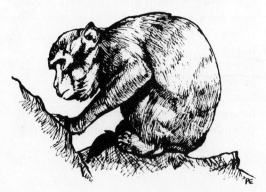

aggression is the threat of disruption of an established social organization." A social order once established serves to maintain itself, and any threat to the integrity of that organization is met by using all the resources at its command. Thus aggression is the primary response of group members, regardless of their status in the hierarchy, to any challenge of the social system.

Dominance and subordination in man

Understanding the human aspects of territoriality and the dominance–subordination hierarchy forces a reconsideration of the bases of human society itself. Traditionally, they are thought of as the product of man's unique cognitive capacities, his logic and rationality. Maclay and Knipe (1972) point out that the discovery of sophisticated social systems in apparently irrational lower animals changes this. It is now known that an unbroken continuum of cooperative social life stretches back to the early primates and beyond. Human social structures are gradual developments of a hierarchic system, and they raise the question as to what extent man is still a dominance-order animal.

The most obvious example of institutionalized rank order is that of the military. In all societies soldiers wear uniforms to reduce their individual appearance to the common base of group solidarity; badges and decorations are added to give measures of rank. Epaulets are piled on the shoulders of high ranking members to make them appear more formidable (Fig. 2-7). Tight discipline keeps everyone in his proper place, creating an almost perfect animal dominance order with greater privileges accorded to the higher ranks.

The hierarchy principle applies throughout most societies, as witnessed by universally used concepts implying rank: "insolence," "disrespect," "being put in one's place." Anthropologist Tiger (1969),

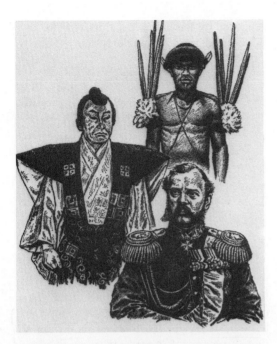

Fig. 2-7. In a broad range of cultures, the human male has a tendency to emphasize his shoulders so as to look more formidable. In this photograph a Waika Indian, a Kabuki actor from Japan, and a European high official show this same trait *(From Eibl-Eibesfeldt, 1972. © 1972, R. Piper & Co. Verlag. Reprinted by permission.)*

in his basic text on the male bond, points to dominance order as the backbone of a human community and sees patterns of dominance and submission as being of crucial significance. One reason is that in a group where order and rank are clear, social unrest is not as marked; the secret of a successful social response to emergencies is that social rank be well defined. This, he says, is clearly demonstrated in a police unit, especially in one used for emergencies such as for riot control. It may be generalized that all social vertebrates have status roles with high ranking control animals and subordinates that check their own ambitions and accommodate to demands on them.

The capacity to switch from an aggressive self-confident demeanor of one in a control position to that of a modest deferential subordinate is particularly necessary in human society where activities fall into different categories. A leader in a game or sport, such as chess or skiing, may have far lower status at work or at home. This dominant–submissive shift as various behavioral roles are assumed means that a man must be able to submit rapidly and obey without question when suddenly confronted by an authority in a field in which he has low status.

Maclay and Knipe (1972) list a number of characteristics of human society that appear to be homologous with those in animal society. They equate the greater personal space given a dominant animal with that claimed by a dominant man, and the motivation of a grooming cluster around a baboon troop leader or a wolf pack leader is equated with that of persons gathering around a successful man. They comment on efforts made to avoid bumping into people in a crowd; on the submissive posture suggestive of the subordinate animal; on the bared and bowed head of a man in a holy place or before a tribal ruler (Fig. 2-8). They also comment on the institution of private property and locked doors; on the kitchen as territory for the woman of the house, or the den for the man; on owner's rights signaled by "knocking before entering;" on the deference shown in approaching the desk of a superior—all of these point to the sensitivity of man toward personal space.

A further point of analogy between humans and social mammals is staring. This is a characteristic of the dominant primate or wolf. In human society the concept of the evil eye and the shifty gaze of guilt and fear is contrasted with the direct gaze of honesty, self-confidence, and self-esteem. The monk's hood which prevents eye contact and the penetrating, unselfconscious stare of royalty are contrasts in status behavior. Maclay and Knipe (1972) contrast the swagger or strut of the dominant monkey (see Fig. 2-5) with the arrogant walk of the matador or the movie gunslinger. They point out that in Pacific island cultures the chief stands erect, but the commoners must stoop or squat. The essence of military bearing is erect posture; it reflects optimism, confi-

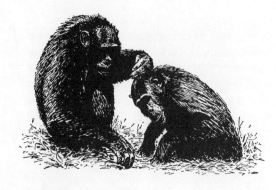

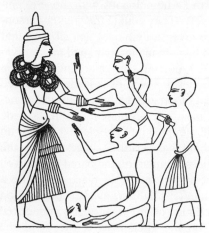

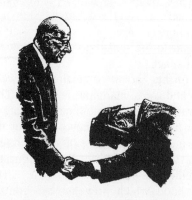

Fig. 2-8. The female chimpanzee greeting a male assumes a deferential posture, which is probably a ritualized invitation to groom. The same bowing is seen in an ancient painting of a group greeting an Egyptian dignitary and in a contemporary news photo of a German policeman greeting the late French President, Charles De Gaulle *(From Eibl-Eibesfeldt, 1972. © 1972, R. Piper & Co. Verlag. Reprinted by permission.)*

dence, and assertion as opposed to the slouch and round shoulders seen in pessimistic depression.

Depression and loss of status

The reactions of society to the individual's fluctuating sense of his own worth are exquisitely sensitive, including support for those who feel diminished self-confidence after a "put down" or defeat and subtle denigration of those who boast and attempt to "step out of line."

The significance of this hierarchy in terms of our topic on the relation of health to the social environment becomes clear when considered in light of Price's important hypothesis (Price, 1967, 1969). He proposed that the mood of depression evolved as an adaptive mechanism helping to stabilize changes in rank. The perception of self as gaining status and overcoming opposition is associated with elation and its extra self-confidence and energy. On the other hand, the loser in a dominance–subordination conflict becomes depressed. The latter, Price points out, is calculated to lead to the idea of adjustment to a lower level in the hierarchy. The depressed man sees himself as inferior and unworthy. He withdraws, he forgets positive memories that might create self-esteem, he loses appetite and libido. All these responses have the effect of perpetuating loss of status, thus giving the winner in the contest freedom from expending effort in further competition. (The neuroendocrine mechanisms underlying these changes are discussed in Chapter 6.)

Male and female patterns of behavior

The differences between the male and the female master roles are another critical distinction running through the structure of mammalian society. These gender differences vary independently of status. High and low status females are found in societies of mice and primates as well as in those of man. Just as there are neuroendocrine concomitants for depressive and elated behavior, so does gender identity depend on hormonal and phylogenetically determined characteristics as well as acquired behavioral ones.

Men and women differ in muscular strength which first develops at adolescence and is shown by the simple hand grip test. The average man enjoys nearly a 2 to 1 advantage (Beach, 1974; Hamburg, 1975). Along with this strength goes the capacity for powerful overarm throwing due to differences in the pectoral girdle. In general, it can be said that the secondary sex characteristics of the female function as a social signal in those primate species, such as man, whose sexual difference in size is not great. Women, says Hamburg (1977), show a lack of structures and minimize behavior that would elicit aggression or threat signals in men; children also have this quality, for example, both lack a heavy chin and beard. The residual hairiness of the chest and shoulders in man may be related to the primate pattern of piloerection, making the animal seem bigger during a display of threat. Women also show differences in quality of voice, facial and jaw structures, neck muscles, shoulder breadth, pelvic configuration, and hair patterns of the scalp. These characteristics help to make the woman and the child immediately recognizable and hence less likely to be attacked when fighting breaks out among men in the group (Eibl-Eibesfeldt, 1972; Hamburg, 1975) (Fig. 2-9).

Certain differences between masculine and feminine behavior patterns are virtually universal regardless of the culture of the group. Thus, D'Andrade (1966) reviewed cross-cultural data from several hundred societies. He concluded that although the precise behavior is not the same in all cases, modal patterns of sex role typing and behavior are strikingly widespread. The prevalent

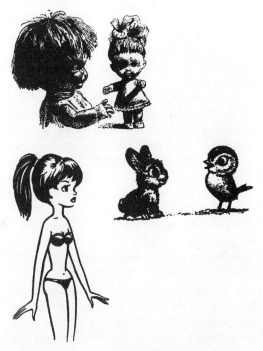

Fig. 2-9. The infant schema involves a large head in relation to the body, a high prominent forehead, chubby cheeks, and short rounded limbs. These characteristics are given to dolls and to animal toys to increase their attractiveness, for they inhibit male aggressiveness and release the protectiveness of both males and females (*From Eibl-Eibesfeldt, 1972.* © *1972, R. Piper & Co. Verlag. Reprinted by permission.*)

findings were: Men are more sexually active, more dominant, more deferred to, less responsible (in the sense of being adventurous and achievement oriented), less nurturant, and less emotionally expressive than women. Women almost universally were given child-rearing roles.

Society has played on the gender role differences given by nature and has encouraged their exercise, including exploitation of the male–female differences in strength, agility, physical endurance, and other biologic variables. In many societies boys are trained to throw at targets, run races, catch balls, climb trees, and in general are encouraged in activities for which most men are better suited physically than most women, by virtue of their superior control over large muscle groups and eye–hand coordination. But the differences which are exploited in this way by the culture arise early in development.

Ethologist Blurton Jones's scholarly study of English two to four year-old nursery school children showed there was no difference between boys and girls in the overall frequency of aggressive behavior where this referred to disputes over property. Boys did, however, engage in more rough and tumble play than girls, and during this time displayed more wrestling and hitting activities. Indeed, the mock fighting that little boys enjoy so much is a characteristic of all male primates (Blurton Jones, 1972).

Throughtout mankind, the division of labor by sexes differs surprisingly little in principle from that found in primitive hunter–gatherers such as the Bushmen of the Kalahari Desert. Women stay in relatively restricted areas, caring for the young, gathering fuel and water and food from roots and berries, and hunting for insects and small animals. They also make and repair clothing. On their hunts, men operate at a considerable strain over the huge area of 1600 odd square kilometers (Lee, 1972; Silberbauer, 1972). In the chimpanzee it is the male who throws sticks and stones, but the female more often hunts for termites (Eimerl et al., 1965). In man the dichotomy sharpens with the strenuous role of hunting which demands teamwork and long periods of absence on travel. This is the task of men together with the job-related roles of tool and weapon making, as opposed to the manufacture or repair of clothing. Finally, warfare is assigned exclusively to adult men.

The roles of the mammalian male emphasize patrol of territory and involve protection of females and young from predators and other intruders. To this extent masculinity, dependent as it is on testosterone for its full development, has the same significance in terms of the master behavior pattern of dominance and the defense of territory in man, as in other primates and social mammals, including mice (Rose et al., 1975).

Male–female differentiation in the kibbutz

There has been a failure to appreciate the importance of the biology of gender in determining social behavior. Tiger and Shepher's (1975) important work on *Women in the Kibbutz* demonstrates the differences in a quantitative study of the generations-long experiment in the kibbutz as their laboratory. Although no biologic reason exists why men and women should not do the same things and experience the same emotions while doing them, nevertheless, a statistical bias of skills and enthusiasms discriminates between them. The kibbutz, they point out, gets rid of the basic social problem of women by providing collective meals, laundry service, and nursery care. Thus they may have the independence permitting them a career as well as children. Furthermore, the egalitarian principles of the kibbutz allow a freedom of choice, so should men wish it, they could also be involved in child care.

In practice, a sexual division of labor exists whereby men work in production, and women in service areas of child care, food, and clothing. Originally more than half the women worked in production, now the sexual division of labor is 80 percent of the maximum possible and is indeed higher than in Israel in general. Despite the formal equality of political rights, women confine themselves to social, educational, and cultural problems, leaving men to work in economics, general policy making, and security. Indeed, the higher the authority of a kibbutz committee, the fewer women there are who participate in it. Despite precisely equal education, women are overrepresented in elementary school teaching and medical nursing; men go into agriculture, engineering, economics, and management. In the army into which they are drafted, women do secretarial and service jobs, leaving the combat and command jobs to men.

The family, which scarcely existed in the original kibbutz, has become a basic unit, fulfilling important functions in consumption and education. The increase in birth and marriage rates is further evidence of family growth. Tiger and Shepher ask why the kibbutz has not lived up to its goal of abolishing the sexual division of labor even though it has successfully maintained its communal, economic, social, democratic, and educational thrust. They propose that the young mothers in the kibbutz are following their own ethologically determined drives. They have acted against the principles of their own socialization as well as against the wishes of the men in their communities. Instead they have devoted more and more time and energy, as the generations have passed, to the traditional female roles. In seeking an association with their own offspring, women in the kibbutz are following the same drive that induces the Bushman woman to carry her four-year-old child while gathering food (Lee, 1972).

Tiger and Shepher believe that the idea of severing the mothers from their children in the original kibbutz was a product of male thinking. Most of the new generation of sabra girls who were born and grew up in the kibbutz have had the experience of mothering youngsters in communal nurseries while still adolescents themselves. The result is they more actively seek attachment to their own children and avoid male roles. They are returning to a pattern typical of women of our hunter–gatherer-evolved species with its inherited need for intensive socialization. They argue that this pattern of sexual differentiation of behavior may have been vital for the survival of human species in the past. They suggest that the high cost of children in terms of energy and time for attachment behavior has been borne by the female, while the male was involved in work, inventive play, politics, and war. They question why men everywhere should give so much of their time and energy to support women and children and maintain family life if not to have specialists in birth, love, and child care. In summary, the kibbutz evidence points to an innate biogrammar driving the young woman, whose hormonal mechanisms have initiated her into the reproductive period, to act this way, despite every cultural opportunity to continue in the same undifferentiated role she enjoyed while growing up in the bisexual children's group.

Attachment behavior in female mice

The master pattern at work in the female is the vital cement of society—attachment behavior. First clearly brought to attention by Bowlby (1970, 1973), and differentiated from dependence, its work in the mother–infant dyad is described most vividly in his masterly treatise on *Attachment and Loss.*

In rodents such as the mouse, parturition is accompanied by a striking display of maternal behavior which starts as soon as females begin licking their newborn. This is in contrast to their earlier response when not pregnant or during early pregnancy. A naive virgin mouse, which has not previously encountered pups except for littermates, will commonly show avoidance at first, followed by aggression. This aggression, switching over now and then to sniffing or licking, coincides with attempts to bury the newborn in bedding material. After repeated brief presentations of the newborn, the naive female will begin to build a nest, to retrieve and lick pups, and to assume the crouching–nursing position over them.

By contrast, naive newly delivered females display immediate and adequate maternal behavior toward their newborn (Noirot and Goyens, 1971). The farther along in pregnancy the female, the less exposure to pups is needed to induce maternal reactions. This reactivation of maternal behavior patterns may depend on hormonal changes occurring at termination of pregnancy, combined with stimuli from the pups, including their olfactory and ultrasonic signals. The intensity of the fully developed pattern of retrieval in rodents can be remarkable, as is shown in Muul's (1970) report on the flying squirrel. A wild squirrel will climb the observer's pant leg to retrieve the young, accidentally fallen from their nest, which had been placed in his pocket! The attraction appears to be the ultrasonic distress cries of the infant.

As time passes, the maternal care given to pups will gradually decrease in intensity as the mother takes longer and longer periods away from the nest. As the tenth day is passed, and the pups' eyes open, they begin exploring their environment vigorously. Their return to the nest is first determined by the mother's retrieving activity; later, pups make their own way back, returning to the mother to sleep in what is often a communal nursery until they are about six weeks old. Since they can be weaned at 14–21 days, this represents continuing maternal–infant attachment to a stage of considerable maturity.

Maternal attachment in primates

The attachment bond between the primate mother and infant is of dramatic intensity. The baby monkey expresses its need for physical attachment and constantly demands contact–comfort for the first few months, clinging to the mother for safety and security (Harlow et al., 1971; Hinde, 1974). For the first few weeks, the baby is oblivious to its surroundings, but from the second to the seventh month, it wanders away from the mother (Fig. 2-10). At first the mother is always watchful and the sorties are brief. Encountering any strange object is occasion for the infant's immediate return to her. But after the seventh month, the mother encourages more separation, and the infant's attachment extends to age-mates and to other members of the group. Evidence is gradually accumulating about the factors controlling attachment bonds formed between the mother and young and between siblings. In the chimpanzee it lasts for many years, and related animals will form a group organized for mutual help (van Lawick-Goodall, 1973).

Mother–infant attachment in man

The development of attachment between the human mother and her young has recently received intensive study with startling results. Klaus and his associates were intrigued by the well-known importance of mother–infant contact in goats, cows, and sheep shortly after birth. They, therefore, initiated a study to see whether the weeks of separation from her premature infant experienced by the mother before finally gaining care of the baby affects the formation of attachment bonds, and perhaps changes her mothering behavior for months and years after the delivery (Klaus et al., 1972, 1975; Kennel et al., 1975).

To determine this, 28 *primiparous* women who had just delivered normal full-term infants were divided into two groups. For four days, the control group of 14 had the usual physical contact with their infants. The extended contact group had an additional 16 hours; some of this time was spent fondling the baby during the immediate postpartum period. A mother who is quite free to act in privacy at the time of delivery immediately picks up the baby, and after a few minutes of looking at the baby face-to-face, she touches its head and body with the palms of her hands (Fig. 2-11). The mothers' backgrounds and the infants' characteristics were similar in both groups. About a month later, each mother was given the same standardized interview; her baby was examined and its behavior during bottle feeding was filmed. Mothers were not told the purpose of the study, and the nurses giving the extended contact test spent equal time with the controls. The mean age of mothers was 18 years and all but one in both groups were Negro. The length of hospitalization was the same, i.e., four days, and as many male as female infants were examined in both groups. Films were made with consent, but through a one-way mirror. The time spent face-to-face with mother and infant aligned in the same vertical plane and the time spent

Fig. 2-10. These histograms schematize the work of Spencer-Booth and Hinde on the mother–infant interaction of rhesus monkeys. They show that the frequency of the infant's distress "whoos" increased sharply when the mother was removed from the infant for six days (ordinate is "whoos"/unit time). In addition, locomotor activity in terms of boxes explored per unit time decreases while the percent of time the infant is held by the mother increases for some time after she returns. It takes several weeks for these effects to revert to control levels *(Spencer-Booth and Hinde, 1971).* C, control.

TEMPORARY MOTHER-INFANT SEPARATION

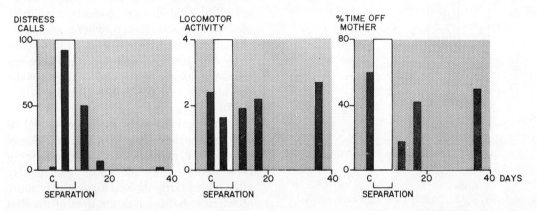

fondling, i.e., stroking, kissing, bouncing, and cuddling, were measured. At one month there was a highly significant difference between the two groups of mothers (Fig. 2-12). The mothers having extended contact with their infants could also not so readily tolerate letting the baby "cry it out" instead of picking it up. They did not feel easy about going out and leaving the baby with someone else and could not sit quietly relaxed

Fig. 2-11. A mother reacting to her newborn full-term infant during the first hours after birth will lie *en face;* the position is defined as one in which the mother places her face so that her eyes and those of the infant meet in the same vertical plane of rotation *(Klaus et al., 1975).*

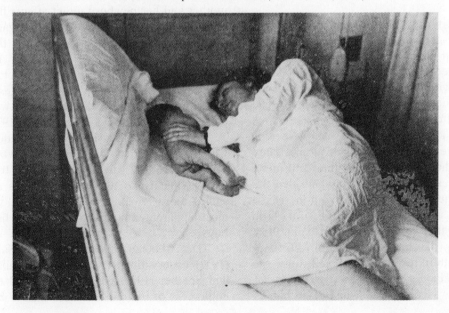

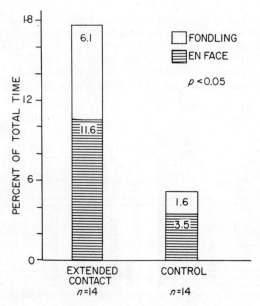

Fig. 2-12. Analysis of film on maternal behavior while feeding infants at one month contrasts mothers who have had early extended contact with their infants with control mothers who have not. Mothers having early extended contact with infants spend more time *en face* and fondling them *(From Klaus et al., 1972. Reprinted by permission from the New England Journal of Medicine.)*

while the baby was examined. They were impelled to soothe the baby when it was crying.

These studies were followed up one and two years later. After one year, the mother was again interviewed and her baby examined. She was separated briefly and her reunion with her one-year-old was observed and the normal feeding was watched. The extended contact mothers spent more time *en face,* i.e., looking at the baby—seeking eye-to-eye contact, with heads in line. They fondled their babies and continued to nurse them, despite employment outside the home. There was no doubt about increased maternal attentiveness, and, in turn, little question that this encouraged exploratory activity by the child (Kennell et al., 1974).

In a third recently completed study, the speech behavior of the same two groups of mothers was compared when their babies were two years old. Those who had been given extra contact with their infants during the neonatal period used fewer commands and content words, but their conversation contained more appropriate forms for imparting information or eliciting a response or elaborating on simple concepts. They asked their babies more questions and modeled better "what, when, where, and who" sentences. The authors believed this sensitivity and increased attention could have significant influence on the child's language and bearing far into the future (Ringler et al., 1975).

In a recent review of this work, Klaus and his associates comment that in a Guatemalan study, mothers who had 45 minutes of early contact with the infant immediately after giving birth showed significantly more attachment behavior at the time of the first breast feeding (see Figs. 4-6 and 4-7). They conclude that there is a sensitive period for the development of preprogrammed patterns in the human shortly after birth which has long-lasting effects on maternal attachment and may affect the development of the child (Kennell et al., 1975).

In a recent comprehensive discussion of neonatal care De Chateau (1976) describes how the intensity of interaction between a mother and her newborn infant affects their relationship later in life. Investigators arranged for 20 mothers to receive their babies immediately after delivery and encouraged each mother to fondle and closely cradle her own for 15 to 20 minutes of intimate skin-to-skin contact. This work confirmed the results of Klaus et al. (1975). Tests at three months showed that a mother who has had extra contact with her newborn spends more time later looking at her baby and kissing it and the baby cries less and smiles more ($p < 0.02$). This behavior was most apparent among mothers with baby boys.

De Chateau also confirmed Salk's (1973) observations and those of Weiland and Sperber (1970) who demonstrated that 80 percent of the mothers hold their babies on the left side of their body regardless of their own left- or right-handedness. Whether this mechanism is related to a soothing effect the baby receives from its perception of the maternal heart beat is not known. It appears that babies more often turn their heads to the right, and De Chateau suggests that the sensitive mother may follow this cue.

De Chateau showed that the 15 to 20 minutes of immediate postpartum interaction between mother and infant eliminated the occasional clumsy pattern of a mother carrying her baby in outstretched arms in front of her body. He also showed that separating a mother and her baby for 24 hours or more was associated with an increased preference for holding it on the right side. Three years later, a follow-up study showed that mothers who held their babies on the right side requested almost twice as many home visits by nurses from the Child Health Care Center than those who held them on the left. Thus De Chateau's work also points to a biogrammar that determines attachment behavior between mother and infant. This innate behavior pattern is significantly affected by what transpires between mother and infant during a sensitive learning period which, as in other animals, appears to be at its peak during the first hour after delivery.

Generalization of attachment during maturation

If the master role of male behavior is territoriality, exploration, and control, that of the female is attachment. As times goes on, this bonding behavior in the mammal extends from the mother–child dyad to include the male and siblings. This behavior is most powerfully developed in the primates. The ties formed between siblings will determine later coalitions between males forming the controlling establishment of a primate social group (Kummer, 1968, 1971; Washburn and Hamburg, 1968). Jane van La-

wick-Goodall (1971) also observed that the aging female chimpanzee remains associated with her grown young. In man the master social phenomenon of the family is an extension of this attachment behavior. Beatrix Hamburg (1975) has further developed Beach's (1974) conception of the critical importance of male–female attachment behavior, or to adopt Harlow's provocative synonym *love* (Harlow et al., 1971). The love of mother for child, brother for brother, man for woman, and the devotion of a man or a woman to the institutions, beliefs, and patterns of the culture in which they were reared are all modifications of attachment behavior.

The attachment between siblings is discussed by Harlow et al. (1971) as peer love and play. He points out that following effective mother–infant bonding, the proper value is placed on body contact and a basic trust and a sense of security develop. Once these responses mature, the infant feels secure enough to wander away from the mother, and a period of vigorous peer interaction follows from the fourth month to three years. At first this play is presocial and one infant monkey will merely follow another as they walk across a high rod or use a swinging ring in sequence. But social play soon follows with wrestling, rolling, and sham biting. The chaser and the chased alternate; there is much rough-and-tumble play. Evidence points to noncontact play forms as more female, and the rough-and-tumble as male (Harlow et al., 1971).

Blurton Jones has described similar patterns of rough-and-tumble play in young children. This vigorous play is a social activity in which the child learns dominance–submission rules as well as exploring the environment and developing skills. Peer play goes on to discover the social and cultural patterns of the group and hence the route to social acceptance. Formation of bonds between members of the same sex constitute friendships leading to stable social sets that may form viable cliques in the baboon or human context (Blurton Jones, 1972).

The wish to be held and the need for attachment

Tiger's text on *Men in Groups* is a massive ethologically oriented study of the male bond and human aggressive behavior. He follows the story of attachment behavior as it starts with the mother and child, extends through the love between children, and reaches up to the bonding between adult men that renders human society effective (Tiger, 1969). Tactile aspects of this bonding have been brought to attention by Hollender in his discussion of the wish to be held (Hollender, 1970; Hollender and McGehee, 1974). Although he describes this as primarily demonstrated by women, he recognizes that it may also represent a significant element of male attachment behavior. He found that the need or wish to be held or cuddled is found not only in the infant but also in the adult. The meaning to the person of being held was security, protection, comfort, and a feeling of being "together" which assuaged loneliness. Hollender's point is that although frequently mistaken by the male partner as seductive behavior, in practice it is an important nonverbal, nonsexual gesture having a variety of meanings according to its social context. However, it is primarily an expression of the attachment behavioral pattern in the human adult.

In his illuminating discussion of the uniquely supportive nature of certain types of friendship, Weiss described a relationship particularly important in preventing loneliness. Simple sociability and friendly interaction, no matter how frequent, do not lift the depression created by a severe event, such as bereavement. But intimacy defined as a relationship in which a person can express his or her feelings freely without self-consciousness and usually with an accompanying expression of intimate body contact does assuage grief (Weiss, 1969). In an illustration to his article, he shows a girl embracing a boy on whose knees she is sitting. Thus, to Weiss intimacy appears to involve the mutual embrace of Hollender's wish to be held. One would suspect it is an important aspect of the attachment behavior so important in all mammals, but especially important in the higher primates.

Weiss's observations were supported by the quantitative studies of Brown et al. (1975). Their research into defenses against depression following severe life events and long-term difficulties in a series of London housewives showed that intimacy, defined in Weiss's terms, was a powerful social asset. If a woman had a boyfriend or, better yet, a husband who regularly gave her such mental and physical support, she was almost completely protected from depression despite severe events. A control group of women who lacked such confidants were significantly more vulnerable despite having friends and acquaintances.

It is interesting that depression which accompanies bereavement commonly elicits the desire to be held, but that anger does not. Thus the feeling of insecurity and uncertainty elicits the desire. The brief embrace among both men and women as a sign of companionship—the *abrazo* of the Mediterreanean peoples and the Arabs—is an aspect of this response pattern (Fig. 2-13).

The wish to be held merits further study as an expression of an inherited biogrammar related to continued attachment behavior. Those persons who have ready access to one or more intimates with whom they can talk freely and with whom they can express attachment nonverbally by touching and holding each other enjoy an important social asset, protecting them against depression.

Montagu (1971) summarizes his book-length inquiry into the importance of tactile experience in the development of personality as follows.

It is not words so much as acts communicating affection and involvement that children, and, indeed, adults require. Tactile sensations become tactile perceptions according to the meanings with which they have been invested by experience. When affection and

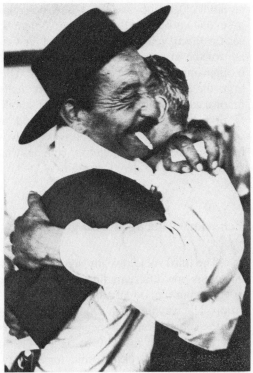

Rene Burri/Magnum

Fig. 2-13. A brief embrace occurs between both males and females as a sign of companionship. It appears to be a spontaneous mark of the desire to extend sympathy and counter depression as well as to express shared elation *(Thomson, 1975).*

involvement are conveyed through touch, it is those meanings as well as the security-giving satisfactions, with which touch will become associated. Inadequate tactile experience will result in a lack of such associations and consequent inability to relate to others in many fundamental ways. Hence, the human significance of touching (Montagu, 1971).

Human sexuality as a behavioral reward system

The attachment between the human male and the female of which the wish to be held is a symbol, in the opinion of Beach (1974), is due to the peculiar human need to co-opt the male into the primary social group of mother plus young. Human young are very slow in attaining maturity and it takes even longer for them to acquire mastery of their environment. It takes many years of experience for the food-gatherer's child to learn all about the local flora and fauna, their flowering, their seed ripening time, their locations, and other characteristics. The details of tool making, hunting, food handling, and all the technology of the primitive human takes still longer to acquire.

A central feature of social maturation is successfully learning tasks peculiar to the respective gender roles. The social organization of the hunter-gatherer society into male hunters and female gatherers represents an important, perhaps genetically determined, division of labor. The campfire site to which all returned was the locus where the sick and wounded could recover and from which males and females moved out into their specialized roles. Beach suggests that one important behavioral reward system tying them together and stabilizing the male–female bond is the capacity of the female to experience an orgasm comparable to that of the male and her relative, though not absolute, freedom from the endocrine determination of sexual behavior. He further suggests that the absence of estrus and this potential for sexual arousal at all stages of the menstrual cycle, and during pregnancy and lactation helped to stabilize human male–female pair bonding.

The kibbutz experiment was an important study of gender behavior untrammeled by social prejudices. The results of the study by Tiger and Shepher (1975) cited earlier show that young women actively choose a role in life permitting them to care for children. Equally compelling are the observations of Shepher (1971) in his study of marriage in the various kibbutzim. Out of 3700 marriages not one heterosexual partnership or marriage occurred when both persons had been socialized in the same peer group for more than three years up to the age of six years. Further, the frequency of interpeer-group marriages varied inversely with emphasis on group solidarity in the ideology of the particular kibbutz. Where there is more familism, hence less solidarity between peers, interpeer-group marriage is more common. Also males excelling in leadership in the army tend to marry interpeer-group partners.

Shepher explains this avoidance of heterosexual relationships between peers by the ethologic theory of imprinting during a sensitive learning period. He points out that youngsters are encouraged by nursery attendants to live together in the utmost familiarity and with frequent body contact. They establish a feeling of warm solidarity which is confirmed and reassured by the significant adults around them. The result is a group with strong attachment bonds that loves and cherishes one another. He cites evidence that, even as adults, when the group loses a member, the rest react with typical grief and bereavement. However, when these children mature, they are not interested in each other in a sexual way. Thus, despite the lack of social barriers against their having an affair or of being married, he could find no such evidence from examining several thousand cases.

This raises the question about the mechanism of falling in love as it exists between human beings. Perhaps it is a further example of the attachments binding infant to mother and mother to infant, both of which have a sensitive period, i.e., six–18 months of age for the infant and the few hours immediately after delivery for the mother. It has been suggested that the hormonal status of a parturient woman with its fall in progesterone may sensitize the nervous system so that she becomes attached to the infant at hand. It may be that falling in love with its periods of intense erotic arousal alternating with periods of depression during absence from the attachment figure also has a neuroendocrine-facilitating mechanism involving the adrenocorticotropic hormone (ACTH) and the androgens. When a young adult is effectively stimulated by an unfamiliar adult of the opposite sex, whose behavior is sexually arousing, the stage would then be set for the development of yet another variant of the attachment behavior seen in the mother–infant/infant–mother bonding. This time the bond would be between sexually mature adults, and it is critical for the stability of human society that once formed, it persists for many years. Perhaps it involves neuroendocrinologic regulatory changes that eventually will be demonstrated.

Behavior of the aged food gatherer

The third sociologically significant master role is one differentiating the very young or the aging individual from the rest of the group. The way in which a child is integrated into the social group has been outlined. It is described for the monkey by Hinde (1974) and Harlow et al. (1971), and for man by Bowlby (1970, 1973).

Thanks to his experience, the aging primate past the reproductive period may still maintain status as a codominant. Thus Kummer (1968) described aging baboons that still influenced the directions followed by the troop. Even at the rodent's simplistic level of behavior, the dominant may be able to sustain his position until quite a late stage of enfeeblement, provided the hierarchy is stable.

In man, the patterns of behavior shift with age, a change which Gutmann (1977) attributes to innate developmental rather than extrinsic social environmental causes. His own studies of the Maya of Mexico, the Navajo of the United States, and the Druze of Israel together with reports on societies in Asia, the Middle East, and Africa have led him to conclude that transcultural universals, i.e., biogrammar, rather than rules and norms of the culture push people into different behavioral patterns at various stages in life. In their younger and middle years, men have an urge to be competitive, active, and independent, but, in later life, a reversal of these priorities occurs. Familism takes priority over exploratory activity; a cooperative attitude toward women tends to replace independence; and a passive affiliation with a supernatural power replaces the control and deployment of individual strength.

Women have a reverse behavioral shift with age in comparison to men. Although adult men begin with active mastery and proceed toward passive mastery, women begin with passive mastery, characterized by dependence on and deference to their husbands, but, in later life, move to active mastery. Across the cultures, as women age, they seem to Gutmann to become more domineering, more active in outside pursuits, and less willing to trade submission for security. Looking across cultures, he finds a mid and late life "women's liberation" even where this development is not formally recognized or acknowledged.

Gutmann sees the sharp sexual distinction of early parenthood as based on the vital needs of children for physical and emotional security, which induces members of one sex to surrender to the other sex those qualities that would interfere with their special role. Men, as providers of physical security, give up dependency to develop courage and endurance; women provide emotional security, but give up aggression which could alienate the men and harm the children. Thus men and women sublimate those aspects of their nature which could interefere with their parental role. But with the maturation of children, men tend to slip into a more feminine type of behavioral pattern, and women generally become more independent. The older man in a traditional society puts aside temporal power and the acquisition of possessions and becomes more sensitive to emotional relationships. The older women in turn assumes more power in the household; she manages the daily affairs and rules by the force of personality.

The aging man's more nurturant pattern of behavior means that he willingly takes care of the grandchildren at the campsite, while the parents are away hunting and gathering food. Men as well as women pass on their fund of long-accumulated experience to youngsters: knowledge about the best places to set traps, plant crops, and collect flint and food. More importantly, because attachment to the young extends from the mother to grandparents, they can assume a socializing as well as a pure knowledge-transmitting function. Over the years, the young acquire the manners and morals that make up the cultural beliefs or canon of the hunter–gatherer group. These are held with reverence and constitute a set of values that must be followed with ceremonials whose celebration is critical to the continuation of their society.

Wynne-Edwards (1962) argues that the white discolored hair of an aging animal is a significant indicator that he is not a threat to the controlling group. This, he says, is highly developed in man and is a distinction of great social significance, devoid of any connection with reproduction. Despite the loss of physical powers and reproductive capacity after some 25 years of maturity, humans remain valuable to the community because of their experience and wisdom. This is especially true in nonliterate communities where memories of rare events can be of critical importance for group survival. Since baldness is very localized and does not affect the eyebrows, for example, he argues that white hair and selective loss of hair from the top of the head are positive and functional adaptations. They dignify the individual with an aura of vulnerability which in its proper sphere commands the respect and deference of juniors. Thus chiefs and matriarchs are often drawn from this postreproductive caste.

In his fascinating book, Guthrie (1976) discusses the social signals given off by man's various physical characteristics and devotes a chapter to the signs of age and the status that goes with it. He arrives at the same conclusions as Wynne-Edwards, and points out that some of the changes occurring in the aging man or woman are part of the paraphernalia for social signalling. Balding, graying, voice changes, and coarsening of the skin are not simply symptoms of deterioration, they seem to be an important part of age-related status shifts, and Guthrie speculates that there has been selection for these traits. He shows the continuum of signals expressed along an age gradient from puberty to old age: An important aspect is the color and distribution of the hair on the head (Fig. 2-14).

Status in man, he says, is not simply a product of fighting ability, nor is net reproductive performance based simply on one's early sexual vigor.

> Rather, it includes providing for family welfare, correct decision-making based on experience, and continuing to reproduce throughout one's later years. Perhaps in early societies, and surely today, elders have high positions not only because of their accumulated information and experience, but also as a result of longer periods to collect the paraphernalia that symbolize status, and hence privilege. Seniority systems and forms of gerontocracy probably stretch well back into our simian ancestry. Physical changes reinforce a social position that is based directly or indirectly on seniority. If this is so, having organic symbols of age past maturity could increase the total effect of status signalling, resulting on one's likelihood of maintaining a dominant position and an increase in lifespan. A longer life in turn would increase the likelihood of a greater

genetic contribution to the next generation (more wives, greater possibility for remarriage in a monogamous situation, prolonged care for offspring and their offspring, and so forth). (Guthrie, 1976).

Eventually the aged become ill and so weak and frail that they cannot survive environmental stress in times of crisis. In *The Heart of the Hunter,* Van der Post (1961) describes how he observed a food-gathering group who had to leave an aged couple behind when they were under great pressure to find water by trekking to a new water hole. His moving description of their immediate return with water-filled ostrich eggs to search for the parents is evidence that in a healthy society the attachment behavior which starts with the mother and the newborn child and spreads to include the entire group can persist as a social force for as long as life itself.

Summary

The role of aggression in maintaining social order within the group and in defense of territory from outside threat explains the great importance of this trait in the human primate. The role of attachment behavior as a cement uniting the primate group is seen at work in the human mother. Recent experimental work with women points to a rela-

Fig. 2-14. A continuum of human physical status signals can be expressed along the age gradient in humans from puberty to old age. A number of such signal combinations are portrayed here: for example, changes in size of neck, nose, beard, and eyebrows, degree of balding, graying, and wrinkling. The signs of age do not exclude high status; indeed, deference is paid to their possessors *(From Guthrie, 1976. © 1976, Litton Educational Publishing, Inc. Reprinted by permission of Van Nostrand Reinhold Company.)*

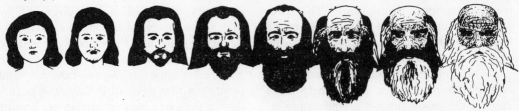

'tively brief postpartum sensitive–learning period when important attachment to the newborn develops. Male–female gender behavior patterns show consistencies throughout the mammals and appear to depend on the action of inborn patterns of behavior. The importance of these patterns in human evolution may be their contribution to the unique permanent male–female attachment bonds and the like bonding of the male to the young. The ensuing social cohesion is unique, and it brings the male into a full partnership in the task of feeding and raising the young and caring for the sick and aged.

3
Inherited behavioral patterns as social assets

The preceding chapter described critically important master roles or behavioral patterns by which individuals of a society are integrated into a viable system, presenting a more or less united front to the environment. But the health of a society will be at risk and the biochemical and physiologic precursors of disease will be set in motion unless its members can act out the behavioral demands imposed by these patterns.

In general, healthy animals have social assets of attachment to others and protective maneuvers or coping mechanisms for meeting these demands. This is the plus side of the equation; the minus includes such elements as life changes, which strain adaptive mechanisms by inducing emotional disturbances and promise to disrupt the individual's role in the social order.

In the final analysis: Despite the great complexity of man's social behavior, the variety of neuroendocrine responses resulting from psychosocial stimulation are limited. These changes are at a basic level in the central nervous system and involve release of the same catecholamines or corticoids or both, which are found in all mammals. They

Freuds Libido & Aggression

are, in fact, expressions of the basic emotions of anger, fear, and depression, and are triggered by the perception of a threat to the desired expression of territorial and attachment behavior. The social assets that protect against excessive neuroendocrine response are detectable in rudimentary form, even in the mouse. They are determined by the efficiency and reliability of the individual's social system, by the bounty of the ecologic niche it occupies, and by the extent to which it occupies a position of strength and favor in the society.

Normal behavior patterns of mice

Normal mice live in an organized community, as described by Crowcroft (1966) in his excellent and delightfully written book *Mice All Over*.

He introduces his observations with the wry comment: "The more I observed mice, the more I came to recognize elements of the behavior of my fellowmen, and the more I began to understand both species." He and his collaborator Rowe watched the interactions of wild mice and found that a clear-cut hierarchy developed with a dominant controlling a certain territory by constantly patrolling and exploring its limits. He had set up a number of nest boxes in a large room with plenty of food and water and found that the mice settled down into an organized social structure. Figure 3-1 is a diagram of the five-meter circular pen used for his first study. The male occupants defended the stippled areas against all intruders. No other mice were tolerated in the area, except the attached females and their young. The following excerpts are from their description of typical behavior.

Male No. 31 was the most active and most aggressive mouse. He lived in a large nest-box (*d*) with two wives, and he also owned two adjacent boxes (*c* and *e*), which he could not make use of himself, but which he would not allow any other mouse to use. He was the most aggressive mouse I had yet met. Most of his waking hours were spent in patrolling his territory, or in mounting guard over it from a vantage point at one corner of the roof of box *d*. Here he would crouch, sniffing the air, and peering about below, and if a strange mouse entered his territory, he would hurl himself through the air like a tiger on to the intruder and drive it away. I have seen him spring across a distance of two feet, land with precision upon his victim's back and deliver a bite on its rump as he landed.

After expelling an intruder, and these attacks were invariably successful, No. 31 always "went the rounds" of his territory. This patrol included a visit to boxes *c* and *e*, I always, perhaps unfeelingly, looked forward to this, for box *c* was a regular refuge for a whole crowd of mice from box *b*, and up to half a dozen would sneak into it unobserved between patrols. This visit by No. 31 always provided a diversion as well as some information.

When he entered, a short tense silence was followed by pandemonium. Mice erupted from the box's two entrances, or rather exits, tumbling over one another in their rush to escape the fury inside. Then No. 31 appeared at one entrance, ran around quickly to the other, inspected the interior and the roof, either returned to his sentry duty or had a brief snack, a drink, a short stroll and went to bed. . . .

This male appeared to be so preoccupied with his territory that he showed little curiosity about the rest of the pen. He knew his way about it however, and the location of the food and water containers made it necessary for him to take short excursions outside, except when he ate food stored in the nest. He avoided aggressive contacts with other territorial males by keeping outside their territories. His demeanour was strikingly changed when walking abroad; he would retreat at once from a mouse which he would savagely attack if encountered within his territory a few feet away. I never saw him receive a beating, but he came close to it when he chased Male No. 41 away and followed him into his territory. They crossed the neutral zone into the territory around box *r* (the narrow end of No. 41's domain near box *q*). Suddenly No. 31 was forced to

Fig. 3-1. Plan of a circular pen in which territorial defense was observed between different dominant male mice. Each dominant became defensive when outside the boundaries of his particular territory (*Crowcroft, 1966*).

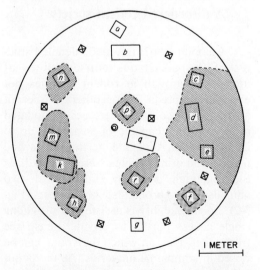

⊠ FOOD   ◎ WATER   ⌧ NEST BOX   ▓ TERRITORY

retreat from a mouse miraculously changed from a craven victim into a savage attacker. . . .

Four of the males, those occupying boxes *f, n, p,* and *r,* may be considered together, as they behaved in the same manner and each played the same part in preserving the social order. The male living in box *r,* resembled the ferocious No. 31, in that he acquired two mates, but he lost one, due, I think, to my interference at censusing.

In any bout of activity each of these four males spent most of his time sniffing about or sitting on top of his nest box or on the floor close by. He fed at the nearest food tray and took a quick excursion to the centre for a drink. If a mouse approached his nest box, he attacked it, but the chase was short and ended less than a foot away.

Occasionally each went for a cautious trot around the enclosure, sniffed around some of the other nest boxes, and in this way, apparently, kept himself informed about the whereabouts of the other males. The direct paths taken when attacked showed that all of these mice knew their way about all of the pen.

The eight males living in box *a* were the weak and down trodden of the colony. They seemed to stay together for the very good reason that none was allowed to remain in peace for long anywhere else. Harking back to work on the conditioning effects on aggressive behaviour of success or failure . . . we might say that each of these males had been chased down the scale of aggressiveness to zero, and was being kept at that level by the frequent attacks of the territorial males.

By huddling together in box *a,* which contained no nest material whatever, they not only conserved heat, but also obtained some degree of security from attack. Although their individual attempts at defense were feeble, their combined protests were enough to keep an intruder out. An inquisitive mouse poking his head in the door of box *a* was greeted by a chorus of plaintive squeaks and was apparently sufficiently deterred or disgusted to abandon exploring further.

Box *b* contained 30 mice, of which 13 were males. These formed a dominance–subordination group, in which one male completely tyrannized most of the others and exerted an uneasy dominance over the rest. These attacked their subordinates and occasionally attacked the dominant, probably by mistake. . . .

The movements of these males resembled those of the miserable males in box *a;* they loitered in the open at their end of the pen and trespassed in box *c;* they often moved about during the day; and their wanderings about the rest of the enclosure provoked many attacks by the territorial males. None of them was conspicuously damaged but the fur tended to appear dull and scruffy compared with the sleek glossy fur of the property owning plutocrats.

The various acts and attitudes of fighting seen in [these mice]. . . could now be . . . seen as behaviour which imposed a social structure similar to that known in populations of territorial birds (Crowcroft, 1966).

Crowcroft has accurately delineated the behavior of mice in a large population cage as we have also observed them. The events he described in this pen showed that mice are capable of organizing themselves into a stable society under appropriate conditions.

A disordered rodent society

Calhoun (1962) has made detailed studies of the disastrous consequences of unchecked growth in rodent colonies not exposed to predation or other sources of attrition. His colonies were accommodated in large rooms capable of sustaining up to 2000 animals. Adequate nesting areas and feeding and drinking sites were provided. At the beginning, a colony starting with two animals had no problems with numbers (Fig. 3-2). Social stability is assisted by providing single access portals to private areas, free from other mice, in which the young can be raised in communal nurseries. As the population grows, older residents retain these

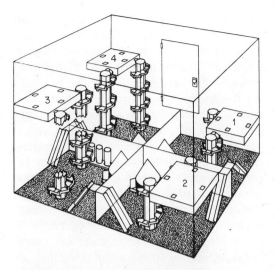

Fig. 3-2.   A room used by Calhoun to observe the deterioration of social behavior in a rodent colony whose members had increased to the point of overpopulation. Numbers 1 to 4 represent nesting boxes, each served by two spiral staircases. Food and water were available *ad lib* in one location in each quarter of the room. Ramps permit passage from one quarter to another *(Calhoun, 1962).*

by a few nips on the rump, the nature of the fighting now changes; severe wounds are inflicted and the aggression becomes lethal. The young are fought over at birth and cannibalized by the females and the normal behavioral sequences are disrupted.

Starting life without adequate attachment bonds and with all their attempts at social interaction broken down by constant interruption, the normal sequences of social behavior fail. Without bonding of the young there is no behavioral training, and nest building and patrol activity are abandoned. The survivors in such systems are unable to reestablish a healthy social system, even if placed with healthy mice in adequate harborage (Ely and Henry, 1974; Watson et al., 1974). Their social assets have been destroyed at the roots of their behavior, and they can no longer adapt to the demands of a hierarchy. Later it will be shown that they die prematurely, physiologically as well as psychologically destroyed by the loss of social assets needed for the development and support of territorial and attachment drives.

desirable harborages and new generations of adults are forced out into the open spaces, these the mice avoid, for they always seek structured enclosed areas (Snyder, 1968). The ousted animals seek such nooks, but are fought off by the territorially dominant males and nursing females until they are overwhelmed by sheer numbers. Despite their subordination, the mass of dispossessed mice eventually overruns the desirable harborages. Thus the tiring, aging, territorial males fail to maintain their privacy. As for females, once they have delivered their young, they are unduly aggressive; experiencing a constant invasion of privacy themselves, they force the young out prematurely, thus depriving them of socialization. As a result, when they mature, these poorly socialized animals will not respect territory and the social system breaks down. Whereas, in a stable colony, the ejection of a subordinate from the territory is accomplished

Normal primate behavior patterns

The advantages of cooperation in the primate social system are lucidly discussed by Hamburg and others in recent comprehensive reports (Jay, 1965; Hamburg, 1968; Kummer, 1971; Alcock, 1975). By shifting from the forest canopy to the ground, the assets and the ecologic range of social species, such as the baboon, greatly increased, but only after the society had significantly changed in its organization. The groups became larger and their cohesion more intense. The males' body size increased, creating a sharp sexual dimorphism as they developed large canines and acquired very aggressive behavior. Thus the primates' increased vulnerability to predators resulting from their emergence into the savannah was compensated for by organizational changes and sexual specialization. In this way they gained the assets of greater variety of terrain and more sources of food, while retaining an effective defense (Eimerl et al., 1965).

In the case of the baboon, whose social life is probably similar to the protohominids, the basic dyad of mother and infant has the male added to it in making the successful change into this new environment. The infant's black color makes him readily recognizable, for adult males and females are brown. Both will rescue an infant straying into a dangerous situation, such as when a predator is nearby. The new social system is designed to protect females although they are only occasionally sexually available. Other bonds must be at work because for most of her life the female is either a juvenile, pregnant, or lactating. Yet she is in the protected core of society enjoying the maximum assets the group can offer (see Fig. 2-3).

The mother–infant relationship is the key; it is on this pivot that the survival of the young, and hence of the whole group, is dependent (Harlow and Harlow, 1965). The relationship lasts beyond infancy extending into maturity. This long period of protection is a vital social asset which permits the infant to adapt to a diversified environment while still flexible and able to learn. Success depends on emotional attachment motivating the mother to protect her young and attaching them to her. In addition, the dominant group of powerful aggressive males must be emotionally attached to the females and young; hamadryas males can even be seen with small infants riding on their backs (Kummer, 1971) (Fig. 3-3). The juvenile female bonnet macaque is highly motivated to care for infants, so that she is experienced in handling them by the time she has one of her own, and so strong is the drive that on occasion she will adopt motherless infants (Fig. 3-4). At the same time, the young male learns to associate with females and infants and becomes paternally protective.

The great asset conferred by the group is that the young learn complex behavior patterns with a resultant combined knowledge and experience of the group which is greater than that of the individual. Juveniles spend but little time feeding; most of their day is involved in practicing adult behavior, learning the skills of running,

Fig. 3-3.   This young adult hamadryas male baboon demonstrates nurturant attachment behavior by carrying a motherless infant that he has adopted *(From Kummer, 1971.* © *1971, Hans Kummer. Reprinted by permission.)*

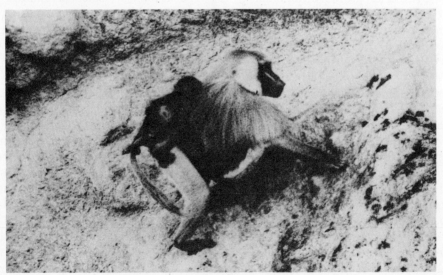

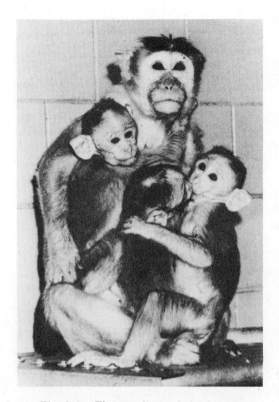

Fig. 3-4. The attachment behavior of bonnet macaque monkeys extends to all young in the group. Here, a female holds not only her own, but two separated infants that she adopted. She nursed, carried, and protected them throughout their separation *(DeVore and Konner, 1974).*

climbing, charging, and wrestling. Their social life and their extensive explorations, says Hamburg, are not directly utilitarian. They are responses to the motivation to build up knowledge and skills so that later the rich environmental resources of the savannah can be used skillfully. Often this is by locally learned adaptations leading to differences between the culture of their own group and one nearby. The potato washing culture of the Japanese monkeys is one example. Started by one bright female who washed them in a stream (Fig. 3-5), the entire group gradually got the idea of washing the sand away and flavoring the sweet potatoes they were given on the beach with seawater (Fig. 3-6) (Jay, 1965). Interestingly, the old dominant male was conservative, resisting the new behavior longer than the others.

Another example was the alert behavior of a baboon troop, who for years after two of their members had been shot, consistently avoided man. They did this in an adaptive fashion: climbing trees to avoid predators, but descending from them to avoid becoming a target for men with their guns (Zuckerman, 1932).

The prolonged infantile growing period

Fig. 3-5. Learned behavioral patterns differ in different rhesus monkey groups. Here, a member of the Koshima group in Japan washes potatoes in the sea. This is a newly invented behavioral pattern which was eventually adopted by the entire group. *(From Kummer, 1971. © 1971, Hans Kummer. Reprinted by permission.)*

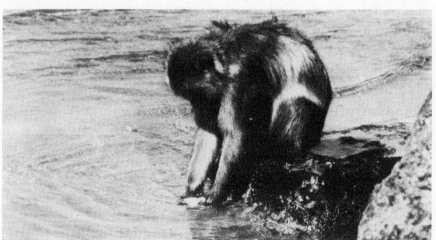

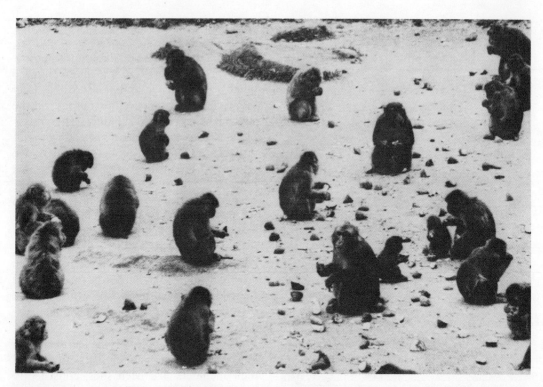

Fig. 3-6. Potato washing (Fig. 3-5) originated spontaneously among a large group of Japanese macaques, part of which is shown above. They regularly assembled at a permanent provisioning spot on the beach to eat the sweet potatoes put out for them. The original intent for this provisioning was to bring this forest dwelling group out into the open for observation *(Jay, 1965)*.

of the higher primates permits a gradual transfer of the traditions and social skills from the group to the young, including learned behavior, such as using twigs to gather termites out of a small hole in the wall of their nest. Young chimpanzees can be seen paying careful attention and then practicing for hours to consolidate their skills. The mutual protection provided by members of the social group permits the growing young to spend years watching adult behavior. Finally the animal acquires a full repertoire of adult skills, including those of sex, feeding, and aggression, together with gestures by which members of the group communicate (van Lawick-Goodall, 1973).

A well-adjusted primate society has an advantage over the individual. The territory and the more vulnerable members are protected against predators by strong, aggres-sive dominant males; they use aggression successfully against smaller predatory leopards or cheetahs. Lions are another problem! Mothers use aggression to protect their infants within the group, and adult males use it to settle disputes. The group sleep together sitting in a large tree (indeed, chimpanzees sleep in tree nests they learn to build). Individual survival depends upon group survival. The group selects the sleeping place and shares the knowledge of local foods, paths, and dangers. Members interact with each other in play and mutual grooming. The individual does not go alone to the water hole but waits for others to accompany him; upon arrival, some drink, some watch, and vice versa (Jay, 1965; Kummer, 1971).

Thus the social system endures the disadvantages of a long period of immaturity and overcomes the dangers of exposing pregnant females or females with young infants to predators due to their slow, hampered movements. It accepts the need for their protection by the males in exchange for the enormous asset of the combined skills of the group. By living together and by learning for a period of years, members of a healthy community build up a knowledge of coping with hot or cold, wet or arid weather. They come to know where to find food and water during all seasons. These diverse environments are automatically learned and mastered by the infant as he remains attached to and interested in the adults: The females associating with females and the young males, apparently more fascinated by adult males, learn their skills in fighting. When enmeshed in such a smoothly working social system and a member of its establishment, the individual enjoys a large number of social assets that assure his survival under conditions in which the isolated animal would necessarily succumb (Kummer, 1968, 1971).

An excellent description of the working of a healthy primate social order is given by Eaton (1976) in his account of a troop of Japanese macaques living on a grassy two-acre corral at the Oregon Regional Primate Research Center. He illustrates their class structure with the diagram shown in Fig. 3-7 and describes this in the following excerpts.

The most striking feature of social behavior in the troop is the fact that a few males dominate all the other animals. Next one notices several old females that attack other females without retaliation, and many adult females that threaten and chase males. It soon becomes apparent that there is a rigid dominance hierarchy, analogous to a pecking order. The top position, that of the "leader," or "alpha" monkey, is almost always occupied by a mature adult male that sometimes does not attain this rank until he is 18 or 19 years old. . . . Immediately below the alpha male are typically five or six "subleader" males, followed by most of the adult females, which reach puberty at three years and full body size at six to eight and together with their infant and juvenile offspring form the middle of the hierarchy. The remainder of the adult males are at the bottom of the hierarchy, and in the wild they live on the periphery of the troop. . . . High rank does not necessarily entail a high frequency of aggressive behavior. Our second and third-

Fig. 3-7. The class structure of a 200-member Japanese macaque social group living at the Oregon Regional Primate Research Center on a two-acre corral. The order is determined by age, sex, and dominance rank. Each class has specific roles to perform. The bars show the relative proportions in each group (see also Fig. 2-3) *(Eaton, 1976).*

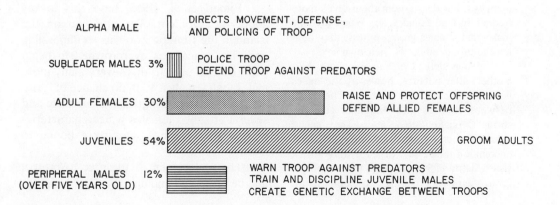

SOCIAL ROLES IN A GROUP OF RHESUS MONKEYS

ALPHA MALE — DIRECTS MOVEMENT, DEFENSE, AND POLICING OF TROOP

SUBLEADER MALES 3% — POLICE TROOP / DEFEND TROOP AGAINST PREDATORS

ADULT FEMALES 30% — RAISE AND PROTECT OFFSPRING / DEFEND ALLIED FEMALES

JUVENILES 54% — GROOM ADULTS

PERIPHERAL MALES (OVER FIVE YEARS OLD) 12% — WARN TROOP AGAINST PREDATORS / TRAIN AND DISCIPLINE JUVENILE MALES / CREATE GENETIC EXCHANGE BETWEEN TROOPS ranking males . . . are both more aggressive than the alpha male . . . because, among other reasons, *Arrowhead* receives more "respect" from the other troop members and therefore does not need to maintain his position by constantly attacking other animals or even threatening them. . . . The dominance rank of an animal is closely correlated with the rank of its mother. . . . only the sons of very high-ranking females are allowed to stay in the center of the troop: the other males are driven to the periphery when they are about five years old, about a year after they have reached puberty. . . . The role of the alpha male appears to be one of directing the movement of the troop and defending it. . . . The principal role of the subleader males is to stop fights. This they usually do by chasing away the more aggressive of the combatants. . . .

The role of the adult females is to raise their offspring and protect them. After birth and for the first few days, the mother supports the infant with one hand as she moves about. . . . When the infant is about two weeks old, the mother appears to teach it to walk by placing it on the ground and then backing away, encouraging it by smacking her lips. . . . Sex differences in behavior develop as the infants begin to venture away from their mothers. Juvenile males tend to spend more of their time roughhousing in play groups consisting of their peers and an occasional adult male than juvenile females do; the females are most occupied in grooming activities with their mothers and sisters. Occasionally a female joins a male play group, but she usually does not stay long before she returns to less strenuous activities. Juvenile males seldom groom other monkeys, but they groom themselves more frequently than females do. When juvenile males and females groom others, they both tend to groom adults of their own sex.

Siblings defend one another and their mother; after puberty, however, the males no longer defend the mother. The bond between mother and daughter remains strong throughout their lives. They spend much time grooming each other; it is not uncommon to see two or three fully grown sisters deftly picking through their mother's fur as their own offspring play beside them.

A disordered primate society

In his excellent account of the *Social Organization of Hamadryas Baboons,* Kummer (1968) describes the smoothly working baboon social system in the wild mountain country of Ethiopia. The effect of gross disorder is clearly seen in an equally brilliant study by Zuckerman (1932) of the hamadryas colony of Monkey Hill in the London Zoological Gardens toward the end of the 1920's. An important feature of the hamadryas as opposed to the anubis baboons is the formation of attachment between the male and his group of females. Kummer (1968) demonstrated that the normal animals are programmed to respect each other's harems; they will not encroach upon each other's prerogatives in this matter, despite the olfactory and visual stimuli of estrus. One problem with Monkey Hill was its small size and lack of resources in comparison with the population. The separation of groups and the formation of territory was not feasible. Figure 3-8 shows a good part of one of the two bare concrete "hills" that constituted the tiny 30-meter-long, 18-meter-wide oval enclosure. Each hill has electrically heated cave shelters built in. Thus the baboons lived in what is more or less a reproduction of the cliff sleeping quarters that wild troops occupy. But they lacked the 60 square kilometers of bush in which to roam and gather food during the day, essentially they were imprisoned.

Eimerl et al. (1965) have this to say about the problem. The situation on the island in the London Zoo was an impossible one. The place was overcrowded to begin with, but worse still, there were many more males than females. With no chance of forming the persistent subgroup of one male and several attached females which characterizes this species, the males were bound to fight.

The real cement is the urge to protect and be protected and also to enjoy the sense

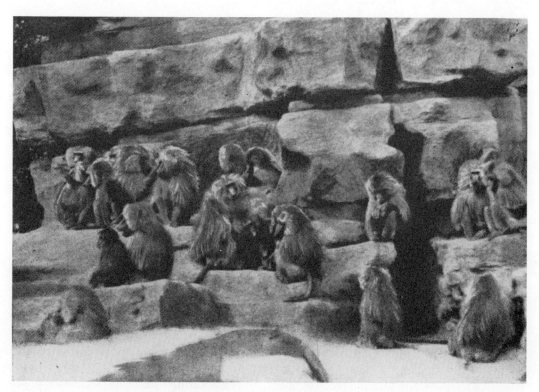

Fig. 3-8.   Members of the ill-fated hamadryas baboon colony of Monkey Hill in the London Zoological Gardens. The photograph shows a good part of one of the two bare concrete hills located in a 30 × 18 meter oval enclosure *(Zuckerman, 1932).*

of ease that comes from living among familiar faces. To monkeys as to most men and women, old friends are the best friends. Most important of all, the group provides a secure environment in which young monkeys can grow up in safety until they have learned enough and are strong enough to assume their own places in the group. However put upon it may be, a baboon or a macaque is absolutely loyal to its group, and with few exceptions passes its life with the one into which it was born. Actually it doesn't suffer much. Firm though group discipline may be, the existence of a subordinate baboon or a macaque is far from intolerable. Living together from birth, the members of a group learn how to get along. Those who cannot stand each other keep at a distance, and when tensions do arise, the monkeys involved usually stay apart until

tempers have cooled. Only the attempts of one male to displace another in the hierarchy precipitate really vicious fighting, but such occasions are rare. They crop up perhaps once every few months inside even a large group. Because each monkey knows its place, daily life is fairly peaceful. For it is uncertainty that creates conflict; the hamadryas baboons in the London Zoo fought with such savagery largely because they were all strangers, trapped and brought together from different groups and were too closely confined to avoid each other (Eimerl et al., 1965).

About 100 adult hamadryas males were released on the island in the spring of 1925. Unfortunately six females were accidentally included in the intended all-male group. By December of that year, 27 males had died from various organic diseases, but only one death was directly attributable to the trauma of chronic fighting. Of great importance from the viewpoint of this book is that, at post mortem, atheroma, pericarditis, pneumonia, emphysema, ulcerative colitis, pancreatitis, and nephritis were found. Infestation with worms was a minor problem and there was no tuberculosis (Zuckerman, 1932).

The greatest number of deaths occurred after the baboons had been assembled and an abnormally ferocious and long drawn-out struggle for dominance ensued. As is seen in the evidence in Chapter 7, the mechanism by which disease can develop during such a long period of intense psychosocial stimulation is becoming clear.

By early 1927 the population was down to 56, following 24 months of intense social interaction among the almost exclusively male colony. The successful survivors had established some sort of social stability, but the entire system was again thrown into disorder by introducing 30 new females of which 15 were literally torn to pieces by the males in fighting for their possession during the first month. Eventually some 30 females died in the fighting. By 1930 only 39 males and nine females were left. That year three males sickened and died, and four more females were killed. The extent of the social disorder may be judged from the fact that even a dominant hamadryas will normally respect the male–female attachment bond.

Final peace was imposed when the five surviving females were separated with utmost difficulty from the dominants who were attached to them, and the colony was stabilized as an all-male group of approximately 30. Only eight males died as a direct result of fights, but 53 died from disease during these years of intense turmoil.

Zuckerman concluded that the number of fatal fights over females that followed the death of males on the Hill was too great to be without significance. He saw that the equilibrium of the social group was dependent upon the mutual reactions of all its members. When a male died, his female was then freed for other males to fight over. For even in this disordered society, bonding was generally respected. However, with the death of her overlord, the now unbonded female became fair game for all males, including dominants who already had females. There was no possibility of escape from others on the tiny island, and no male with a new female remained unchallenged long enough to establish the necessary firm bonding for the relationship to be respected. The consequence was that the female died because of repeated fights for her possession. Zuckerman concluded that an enormous number of nonfatal as well as fatal fights were occurring in a social system in constant turmoil. Of 15 babies born in a five-year period all but one died. He noted one cause of infant death was accidental injury. When a nursing mother became embroiled in the melee of a fight, she tightened her hold on the clinging infant and it suffocated (Fig. 5-8) (Zuckerman, 1932).

Zuckerman made an additional observation which became the forerunner of the important Harlow studies of subhuman primate maternal care (Harlow and Harlow, 1965). He noted that some of the mothers appeared to be ''inexperienced'' and extremely ''careless'' with the baby. Instead of holding it gently, a mother would clasp it roughly or place the newborn beside her on the rocks. This behavior is reminiscent of that described by Harlow et al., (1971) in socially deprived mothers.

In addition to their inadequacy as parents, such disturbed animals fail to establish a position in the social system. Anecdotal observations of the fate of socially deprived rhesus monkeys that were released into a half–tame group living on an island reservation show they were rapidly destroyed. The assets of these animals are minimal because of their deficient early experience; when confronted with the resident established males, they react inappropriately, failing, for example, to make the proper submissive gestures.

Normal behavior patterns of hunter–gatherers

In human social systems it is even more apparent that the social assets of an individual are crucial for his survival. If the system is disordered, the chance for members to succeed individually is astonishingly small. The Bushmen of Botswana are an example of a healthy and well-organized group whose Stone Age hunter–gatherer culture has survived relatively unchanged (Fig. 3-9). They have been the subject of a number of careful anthropologic and medical surveys during past decades; their way of life and health, including their remarkable freedom from cardiovascular disease, is well documented (Kaminer and Lutz, 1960; Truswell et al., 1972).

The significance of such studies is that man has lived as a hunter–gatherer for 99 percent of the 2,000,000 or more years since the first recognizable human beings emerged. It is thus a lifestyle for which he is singularly well adapted. Further, this lifestyle can be observed without the complexities caused by the agricultural life that started only a few thousand years ago, or those caused by the industrial age into which we have catapulted the past two hundred years. The way that hunter–gatherers handle aggression, territory, social control, and leadership represents patterns that fit closely to man's inherited patterns of behavior. One point is quite clear: The food gathering societies did not live in constant fear of starvation, expending much labor for meager returns. Rather it is the agricultural and industrial revolutions that have imperilled man's individual adaptation and some of his social assets.

Bushmen used to occupy most of South Africa until about 200 years ago when, except for Botswana in South-West Africa, they were exterminated by the pastoral Bantu and the Caucasians, who clashed with them over the use of their former hunting grounds for cattle grazing. They are probably indigenous to the region and thus represent a direct line of culture reaching back to the Stone Age. They live in a loose confederation of small communities, or bands, each of which is autonomous. Each group of bands may total 1000–2000 persons who share a common language. Different groups occupy different areas and speak different languages. Eibl-Eibesfeldt (1974) has recently noted that these people are strongly territorial insofar as a group speaking a particular dialect is concerned. Individual bands are free to move about within the group, subject to the courtesy of asking the permission of an adjacent band before crossing their territory.

Eibl-Eibesfeldt also demonstrated that Bushmen children display quite normal patterns of aggressive behavior and rivalry. His photographs show they have the same threat gestures, stares, and the same patterns of

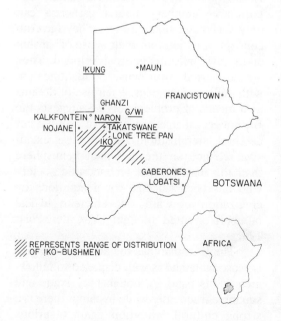

Fig. 3-9. Map showing the range of distribution of the !Kung Bushmen of the Kalahari Desert *(Eibl-Eibesfeldt, 1974).*

submission, i.e., pouting, lowering the head, avoiding eye contact, as do children of other cultures. He did note, however, that in keeping with their balanced and healthy disposition, Bushmen have efficient ways of coping with aggression when it is aroused. Friendly attachment behavior predominates in the interaction of adults, and many hours per day are spent in mutual grooming, chatting, and playing with children. He comments on their capacity to be "human" in a friendly way.

Their pure Stone Age culture gives Bushmen quite a formidable technologic control over an apparently inhospitable environment. Living in the Kalahari Desert where the annual rainfall is only 10 centimeters, the Bushmen's knowledge about the two dozen-odd food plants they gather and the same number of animals they hunt constitutes an impressive body of information which they effectively master beyond the point of mere survival. Expertise in field botany is passed on from women to girls while out together gathering plants. They are taught to identify edible and poisonous species and to learn the seasonal availability and locations. All persons, including men on the hunt, moving about in the territory belonging to their own community pass on such information to the group at the campsite. Thus they have a system for constantly updating their knowledge of where plants are ripening and when they are likely to become available. The same holds true for their observations of animal life.

Bushmen camps hum with the sound of constant conversation. Much of it deals with information vital for effective hunting and gathering and involves weather conditions and the state and distribution of their shared food supplies. Their efficiency is such that it is estimated that Bushmen spend less than half of their days hunting and gathering and the rest of the time interacting socially in their own camps and in those belonging to others in their group. Older men continue to work snaring small mammals, but abandon the demanding tasks of bow and arrow hunting. Bushmen must constantly migrate to seek different sources of food. There is no ownership of property except that which can be carried, and their simple huts and shelters are erected in the matter of a morning or a day (Lee, 1972; Silberbauer, 1972).

Although they are aggressive and courageous fighters, members of the various bands avoid conflict. Women contribute a large part of the subsistence calories and are treated on egalitarian terms with men. Marriage may be within the band or outside of it, i.e., exogamous. When drought and food shortage strike, the bands break up into small family units of 10 or so, making a rigid tribal hierarchy impossible. Territory is owned by the group, and individual power and authority are confined to the power of persuasion and example (Eibl-Eibesfeldt, 1974).

The South African poet–writer Van der Post spent much time studying the Bushmen. He was fascinated by the people's relaxed adaptation to life which he attributed to their intimacy with the natural ecology. It remains more positive and less ambivalent in Bushmen that in most primitive people in these days of worldwide cultural changes. He points out that their culture cannot support large numbers; hunter–gatherers can only survive in small groups. They have no concept of nation, but their sense of kinship and individualism is finely developed. They are supported by a sense of identification with their environment. Their use of dreams as a means of problem solving suggests the Bushman is at an earlier stage of evolution of cerebral lateralization, and puts less exclusive reliance on the dominant hemisphere than the man from a technocratic society who has been selected for generations by civilization's rewards for efficient, logical numbers-oriented thought (Van der Post, 1961).

The Bushman has the attitude that man is reasonable and is well disposed to fellowmen of his band. Although they argue and squabble frequently while in camp, there is a strong cultural inhibition against serious conflict. Their constant gossip and humor work to bring in others and help to keep tensions from rising too high. Babies are carried everywhere. They are breast fed up to the age of 3 years and sleep in their mother's arms (Fig. 3-10). Not only do the women and girls show a fondness for babies, men and boys do also (Fig. 3-11). Punishment of older children is rarely more than a reprimand or a slap; nor are they thrashed. Children in the camp are under the supervision of a camp-keeper. This person is commonly an older man or woman who conducts a sort of school in which advice and instruction are imparted to the young on every topic that

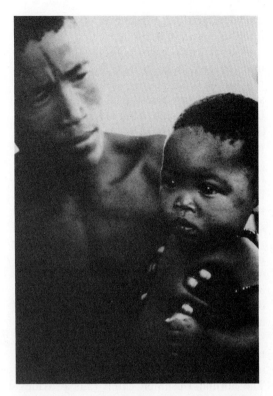

Fig. 3-11. Illustration of the interaction between a Bushman father and his child. Men exhibit fondness and tolerance for babies, but have a secondary role in their care *(DeVore and Konner, 1974)*.

Fig. 3-10. This photograph of a mother teaching peer relations was taken in a !Kung Bushmen camp. These people are believed to have followed an unbroken hunter–gatherer tradition in this same territory in the Kalahari Desert since prehistoric times. If so, they represent ancestral man as he evolved prior to the agricultural revolution *(DeVore and Konner, 1974)*.

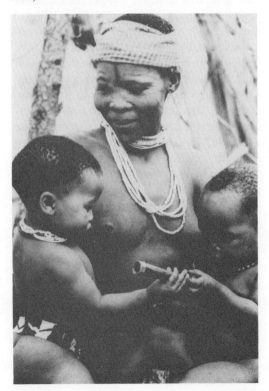

crops up. Their games are imitations of adult activities and constitute effective training for adult life. Girls join their mothers as soon as they can manage long walks (DeVore and Konner, 1974).

The picture is one of a well-integrated social system with strong social assets. The aged are respected leaders of the camps and are collective owners of the water holes by virtue of their long tenure. They embody a repository of medical skills, rituals, and dream interpretations. They are supported long after their productivity as hunters or even gatherers has fallen off; abandoning the aged is done only under pressure.

Draper (1973) has discussed the close proximity in which these people choose to live. Like the Eskimos, they share very crowded quarters; a group of 30–40 will fit into the center of a circular camp not more than 40 meters across, including the individual center-facing storage huts. Children remain in camp under continuous adult supervision, since only half of the group is foraging at any time. Men always return for the night. The group seem to enjoy close physical contact, leaning against each other while talking and chattering. Children cluster informally with adults, girls more so than boys. Since the available space is 20 square meters per person, children are always in close association with adults.

One secret of tolerance for this crowding, Draper concludes, is the enormous space available outside the camp; it may be 30 kilometers to the next one in this lonely desert. Further, the group is closely related and everyone knows everyone else. If tensions do arise which group discussion cannot resolve, they are dissipated because the aggravated persons move to another camp. The normal Bushmen camp thus provides the physical proximity that a closely interlocked social group requires for communication; the result is a mutually supportive system which is a strong social asset to individual members.

The interesting work of social psychologist Freedman (1975) on crowding and behavior, in his book of the same title, should be mentioned at this point. His research involving the City of New York demonstrated that density, as measured by the number of people per square mile and the number of people per room in housing, was not related to crime rates if other related factors were controlled, such as income, education, and ethnic background. He cites Mitchell who found the same results in the extraordinarily crowded city of Hong Kong. Mitchell (1971) found when income level was controlled, crowding was not related to health.

According to Freedman, the crucial issue is: The organization of the city should be such that the patterns of social interaction are appropriate to human needs. He also stresses a need for the sense of a community which is fostered by appropriate architectural design of living space. He points out that man has always lived in crowded groups and quotes Draper's observations of the crowded Bushmen campsites (Draper, 1973) to support his contention. The future, he argues, will probably continue to demand crowding. However, despite Freedman's optimism, when population density exceeds certain levels and the total population attains the vast numbers found in a contemporary city, it becomes difficult to arrange enough room for all persons to pursue their individual goals. If life under intensely crowded conditions, such as on a submarine, is to be comfortable, a high degree of tightly disciplined social organization is demanded.

Only a very well-ordered society can impose this demand on young male primates who need to be able to explore, to run and play, and to play–fight. If the ensuing social interaction involves too many confrontations, their escalating frustration leads to high levels of arousal. Unless an excellent social hierarchy with established cultural norms exists, the constant struggle for control eventually leads to a social breakdown. Once this occurs, the individual maturing in such a society becomes psychopathic and sustained social disorder follows. But if psychopathy has developed, the disorder persists, regardless of how much space is made available. Individuals who cannot tolerate each other because of a deficient attachment and a lack of respect for the subtleties of territory and hierarchy, lack the required elements for a stable social order.

A disordered primitive human society

The contrast between the mutually supportive, socially adjusted Bushmen and a group of former hunter–gatherers in northern Uganda, recently described by anthropologist Turnbull (1972), throws light on the mechanics of social disintegration. In the 1930's, the Ik roamed a 40,000-square-kilometer area ranging from Lake Rudolf in Kenya to the Didinga Mountains in the Sudan. Mobility was as crucial for them as it was for the Bushmen. They were nomads, also, thoroughly familiar with their environment, living in sympathy with it, rather than trying to dominate it. But World War II led to the emergence of intense nationalism with conflicts on the common frontiers between Uganda, the Sudan, and Kenya. Not only were the Ik forced to stop their organized exploitation of the huge area, but they were excluded from a large-game producing valley that was converted into a National Game Reserve. Their pattern of living had been the same as that of the Bushmen, with women doing much of the gathering, while men hunted. Similarly, the basic unit was not the family but the band. The children, according to Turnbull, regarded any adult living in the same camp as a parent and any age-mate as a sibling. The central theme holding their lives together was the environment.

A generation ago, when the Ik were forced to abandon their nomadic hunting–gathering way of life, they struggled to survive as farmers in their old mountainous headquarters, but the climate and terrain were unsuitable. In three years out of four, there is just enough rainfall, but crops fail completely in the fourth year, and life can be sustained only by illicit hunting or raiding cattle. When Turnbull arrived 30 years later, the ancient Ik society was on the course of dissolution as a viable system. He found a completely demoralized people suffering from two years of famine and drought. Their situation was as impossible as that experienced by the hamadryas baboons on Monkey Hill.

The description of these baboons as ruthlessly selfish and aggressive also applies to Turnbull's view of this gravely disordered human society. He says he found no evidence of family life, and no sign of love with its willingness to sacrifice and to accept the need of one for another. He saw little affec-

tion and few tears. He concluded that these starving people had no room for family life, for sentiment, love, and cooperative sociality. The clue to the problem appears in the lack of parental care with which the !Kung are so lavish. The new family structure required by village life into which the Ik hunter–gatherers had been forced, lacked the traditions necessary for survival. Mistrust began between husband and wife; the next phase was a weakening of maternal care. Dependent children were neglected. As soon as they were capable of surviving on their own, they were left to forage in bands, while parents took care of their own affairs. The design of their villages strikingly illustrates the inhabitants' difficulties in adjusting to cooperative living. Each house has its own corridor to the outside of the stockade, so its occupants had no need to see their fellow villagers or to share any common ground with them (Fig. 3-12).

This is in sharp contrast to the healthy Bushmen social system in which training persists to adulthood together with active bonds of affection. The ensuing disastrous social disintegration of the Ik had had 30 years to pursue its course. Thus when Turnbull arrived, most of the adults of child-rearing age probably had inadequate socialization in their own lives because of parental neglect. As Bowlby has pointed out, attachment behavior is dependent upon proper parenting, and parents of battered children or of those suffering from growth deprivation have frequently been victims of child neglect themselves. Turnbull was observing the same consequences of social breakdown that Calhoun (1962) reports in mouse populations exceeding the available harborage.

A hunter–gatherer band forced to abandon their traditional life-style and hereditary territory to eke out an existence in only a fraction of the former area by using vastly different techniques must inevitably change standards. With the destruction of maternal and paternal care systems, the group became anomic and psychopathic (Harlow and Harlow, 1965; Bowlby, 1973). As will be

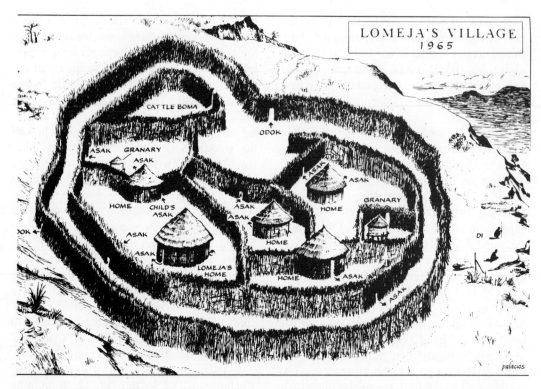

Fig. 3-12. This village of the formerly nomadic Ik tribe in Uganda has an arrangement of separate entrances and an absence of common areas for social interaction, bespeaking of their social alienation. Contrast this design with that of the famous man-made island of Sulu Vou of the Lau Tribe, off Malaita in the Solomon Islands (Fig. 10-13) and of the village of the Yąnomamö Indians in South America (Fig. 10-14) *(Turnbull, 1972).*

pointed out, such groups are subject to degenerative diseases, such as hypertension and arteriosclerosis. It is suspected that Turnbull would have established a high prevalence of these diseases had he looked for them.

Summary

Examples of socially healthy systems with a great reservoir of assets have been cited in murine, primate, and human societies. They have been contrasted with systems in which parental care is deficient and in which the subtler cooperative aspects of social relations and territoriality are disordered or absent. Victims of such disturbed social systems who already lack the most vital social assets will become exposed to gross and sustained stimulation of the motivational systems arousing the neuroendocrine defense and alarm responses. A healthy society protects its members against such undue and prolonged arousal, despite the inevitable losses and changes occurring in their lifetime. Crises are met by social support, food is shared when little can be foraged, and the loss of a close relative is met by foster parenting.

4

the critical role of early experience and the programming of behavior

The critical role of early experience

Ethologists have described the sensitive adjustments in behavior patterns characteristic of mammalian social groups. Maternal and paternal care of the young, hunting, gathering food, seeking shelter, the behavior of the dominant animal and the meshing support of subordinates do not develop spontaneously. Nor are they purely learned behavior, even in man. Rather they are a mixture of experience and prior programming and require the proper experience at the right time to develop appropriately.

This chapter describes how mammals at birth begin to acquire the facility of making appropriate emotional and behavioral adjustments to the intricate network of their social system. The human infant is also primed by innate patterns to initiate this crucial sequence of learning, and the program must be fleshed out by appropriate experiences during the sensitive learning period. The process begins when the newborn interacts with his mother and continues until early adult life; there is evidence of a sensitive learning period that helps the recently delivered mother to display attachment behavior toward her infant. Shepher (1971) has described how kibbutz siblings during the first six years become attached to one another despite the differentiation of gender behavior. Yet the powerful bonds holding brothers and sisters together are subtly different in men and women from love bonds which are exclusively outside the sibling group.

This attachment bonding that has started with the mother and infant gradually, by appropriate stages, comes to enfold the father, and then extends in larger and larger orbits until it encloses the extended family, the class, and the society. Neumann (1954) has discussed this increasing range and complexity as this bonding comes to include loyalty to the leaders of the sovereign tribe and to the territory it controls. With the development of civilizations, it incorporates devotion to craft and to professional groups, church, army, or business enterprise. An individual who lacks the appropriate parental and sibling attachment as a part of his early experiences will have difficulties later in transmuting this quality into loyalty to these more remote groups.

Socialization in mice and early experience

Crowcroft (1966) points out that in a healthy colony of mice females form communal nurseries. In this way, the young have access to suckling at all times, even when a particular female must be away foraging (Fig. 4-1). This expression of social solidarity is a valuable asset for the mouse whose young are born blind and helpless and need sustained care for several days.

The dominant mouse respects the communal nursery but includes it in his patrols to check on the territory. If an intruder is found, not only the dominant but also his females and their young will give pursuit. The nursing female defends her nesting area against all comers (Fig. 4-2). Failing this, as with a disturbance by a predator or if the nest loses its security because of disrupted cover or harborage, the female or females will move the young to another area as far away as possible from the intruding element (Fig. 4-3).

Reimer and Petras (1967), who have used complex population cages to study the behavior of mice observed that the dominant male has not only two to five females with him in his territory, but subordinated males as well. They called this grouping a family or a deme. The size of the group may be up to 10, and, once formed, the deme remains stable and defends its territory against intruders for several generations. Infants grow up with special privileges and are safe from interference as long as they stay in parental territory.

Brown (1966), who has studied field mice in their natural habitat, agrees that these small mammals live in an organized

Fig. 4-1. Mice form communal nurseries where several litters will share the milk and attention of as many as five mothers. Animals ranging in age from neonates to weanlings will thus grow up together as siblings.

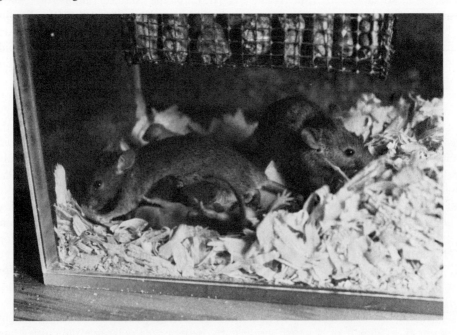

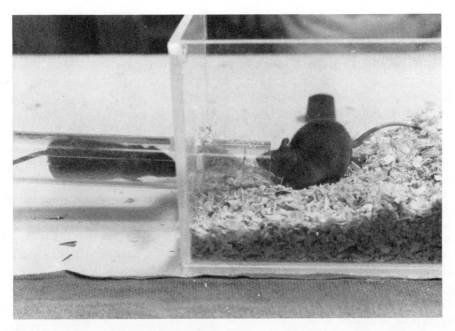

Fig. 4-2. A female with young will vigorously defend the nursery territory against intruders. Males not belonging to the deme are especially unwelcome.

Fig. 4-3. A pup that strays from the nest is retrieved by the females and occasionally by a male. Fully furred weanlings are unceremoniously dumped in a new nesting area if the mothers decide to shift in response to environmental threats.

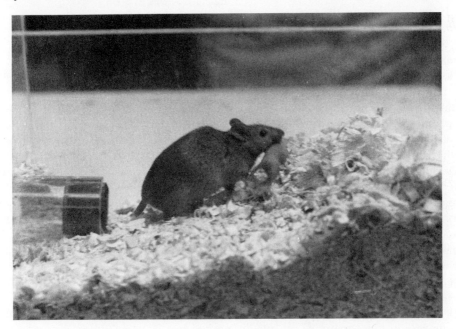

community. Using a tracking system, he showed that a dominant male ranges far more widely within a specific area than the subordinates. He explores the areas of his range, which may cover several acres, section by section. Subordinates will postpone visits to desired areas until the dominant has moved on, but as members fitting into the society they are free to move about. A strong dominant and subordinates who defer to him result in a stable society.

The picture is one of a stable social system which occupies a prime region and uses it to give protection to its favored members. Less fortunate males are excluded by vigorous defense. Indeed, the dominant male reminded Crowcroft of a successful businessman protecting his assests. Mice unable to maintain territory withdraw. They live on the periphery huddling for warmth (Fig. 4-4), and avoid the dominant by sleeping in less desirable locations. At a disadvantage because they are excluded from the safest shelter from predators, the best access to food, and the best protection from the weather, they will be forced to seek new space where they will try to organize hitherto unclaimed territory and to attract females (Brown, 1966; Christian, 1970).

There are physiologic and behavioral sequelae to these social adjustments. Hofer (1976) has demonstrated such changes in two-week-old infant rats who experience 24 hours of maternal absence. An increase in time spent awake and a reduction in time spent in paradoxical or rapid eye movement (REM) sleep were observed, also an increased frequency of transition from the one sleep state to the other. Body movements were increased and nonnutritive sucking decreased during paradoxical sleep after separation. It is possible that if these disturbances of state persist, they are associated with social inadequacy.

For if they have not lived in a communal nursery and have not had an adequate social interaction with siblings and adults, mice lack the perception of normal cues. In the extreme case of those maturing in isola-

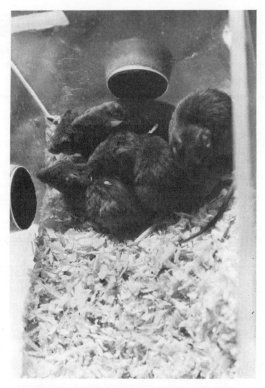

Fig. 4-4. Subordinated mice with disarrayed fur and nicks and bites on the tail and rump will huddle for warmth in a peripheral location. In a population cage, this less desirable area also serves as a latrine box.

tion, it can be shown that they fail to achieve stable dominance, yet are too aggressive to survive as subordinates. Apparently they do not recognize social gestures and thus fail to perceive communications that are critical for a stable hierarchy. Colonies made up of such mice have no cohesion. Females fail to maintain communal nurseries and vicious fighting develops, as temporary dominance shifts from mouse to mouse (Ely and Henry, 1974; Watson et al., 1974). This instability, the consequence of deficient early experience, vividly demonstrates the importance of having the right inputs during the critical learning period.

Well-fed and warm and not having to waste growth metabolites for calories, a mouse born into a stable system will grow larger. He even receives some training. Crowcroft observed a mother and a male together shepherding the young around the territory. As in the larger mammals, young mice have the asset of being socialized by their parents. They will, for example, continue to sleep with the mother until six weeks old. They learn to respect the dominant, and, by associating with him, get to know the various rewarding and dangerous aspects of the territory. Thus in even so small a mammal as a mouse, the social assets enjoyed by those born into a stable, successful group are significant compared with those in a system that has broken down.

Socialization in subhuman primates and early experience

There is new evidence that early experience is important in determining the later behavior of primates. The studies of Jane van Lawick-Goodall in Africa (1971, 1973) showed that among normal socially supported chimpanzees in the wild, a young animal experiences acute distress at separation from its mother. She did not see an unaccompanied young animal less than four and one-half years old. When in difficulty and unable to return quickly to its mother, the young chimpanzee emits a "whoo" whimper to which the mother normally responds by fetching it at once; she reciprocates with the same sound when attempting to retrieve the young animal from potential danger. The second signal for reestablishment of the mother–infant contact is a scream which leads to an immediate attempt at rescue. The proximity of the young to the mother is maintained until preadolescence; separations are rare and are rectified by these vocal signals and by mutual search (van Lawick-Goodall, 1971, 1973).

The consequences of forced separation in rhesus monkeys have been studied in

detail by Hinde (1974), and the results have been reviewed by Bowlby (1970). A brief separation is followed by the mother's ferocious attempts to regain her infant (Kaufman, 1974). After being reunited, the infant's screams are immediately stilled by close ventral body contact. Five minutes of separation is followed by 15–40 minutes of mutual clasping (Fig. 4-5). When an infant is separated for longer periods, i.e., weeks, the initial violent screeching and scampering about in the cage dies out within a few hours. It is followed by five to six days of inactivity, no play, and occasional whimpering. The infant sits hunched over, rolled almost into a ball, with its head between its legs and will move only to eat or in response to agression. Indeed, little food is eaten during the first 24 hours (Fig. 4-5). The infant is disinterested in the environment and play ceases. A slower pulse and loss of rapid eye movement (REM) sleep point to underlying neuroendocrine changes. Gradually the symptoms wear off and by 30 days the infant appears alert and active (Reite et al., 1974).

Behavioral disturbances ensue even if the mothers are reintroduced after a week. Infants cling to their mothers much more than before (Fig. 2-10), and they now have intense temper tantrums when rejected. Their behavior may remain normal during an uneventful day, but if the environment is disturbed, they revert to their clinging behavior, revealing more timidity and anxiety. Previously separated animals show less locomotor activity and less social play than the controls. Hinde (1974) maintains that several six-day separations at the age of six months will have measurable effects two years later.

In his treatise on attachment, Bowlby, a child psychiatrist, concludes that most of the symptoms developing in the human infant after separation are also to be seen in the infants of subhuman primates. Lewis et al. (1976) have reviewed this question and agree that Bowlby's protest–despair response can be reproduced by separating rhesus monkeys from their mothers. They warn that the

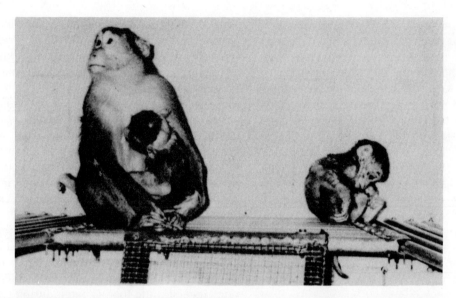

Fig. 4-5. The contrast between the depressed, separated, infant pigtail rhesus monkey, on the right, and the mother and infant in intimate ventral contact, on the left, is sharp. The depressed animal shows a characteristically flexed, hunched-over posture *(Kaufman and Rosenblum, 1967).*

results are variable and propose peer separation as an alternative model. All in all, however, they agree that isolation from peers and parents has the same disastrous effects on social adaptation in subhuman primates as it does in man. This indicates the response to separation involves emotional processes and the distress entailed is not confined to man.

What then are the effects of removing a primate, such as a rhesus monkey, from his maternal and peer attachment figures and permanently isolating him? As the Harlows have shown, although the effects become progressively more and more disastrous with prolonged social deprivation, the animals remain physically healthy, but their behavior is grossly disturbed (Harlow and Harlow, 1970). After six months of isolation, they are dominated by fear and do not join in activities or develop social ties. This social dysfunction is even more severe after one year of isolation, and they are attacked by the more normal animals. At the age of three years, their behavior was compared with that of older normal adults, normal adults their own age, and younger animals (Harlow and Harlow, 1970). Although terrified by strangers, the isolates would attack even dominant adult males. This extraordinary aggression could result in their deaths. The isolates were also agressive against juveniles, again contravening normal social behavior (Sackett, 1968; Kaufman, 1974).

In human terms, according to the Harlows, these unloved delinquent animals were disturbed and were unable to form affectional bonds. They failed to acquire sexual partners and were grossly inadequate parents, ignoring their young. Although careful testing showed their cognitive function to be unimpaired and their learning response to be normal, they failed to develop the mature social patterns that restrain and modulate behavior, such as aggression, which can be socially disruptive. In other words, normal animals learn to check in-group aggressive behavior when it is inappropriate but it remains available, and they use it vigorously against intruders.

Programming of behavior in man and early experience

The frequency of social deprivation with its unfortunate consequence of the defective development of man is becoming vividly apparent. Work with the newborn shows that most infants can be consoled by speaking to them softly, picking them up, and rhythmically rocking them. They have the innate capacity to respond to these stimuli in addition to their own adaptive responses, such as sucking when hungry or crying when in pain (Freedman, 1974). Infants have a visual acuity of at least 20/150; they perceive objects not merely in terms of their retinal correlates but also in terms of an innate ability to gauge size, distance, and solidity. In addition, their heart rate changes in response to synthetic speech sounds, lending support to the speculation that speechlike sounds may be processed in the higher centers of the brain by genetically determined patterns (Freedman, 1974).

From an evolutionary point of view, research into human development shows that a newborn is programmed to respond to a parental figure and vice versa in such a way that a woman becomes socially attached to her child, thus assuring its survival. One aspect of this is the intense anxiety aroused in the parent or parental figure when the baby cries, few sounds are more disturbing to the human. The outcome is body contact, with the mother cradling the baby in her arms (Freedman, 1974). In the human, as in most social animals, some form of physical contact, for example, the embrace of those with a need to be held, remains an important means of relating to others throughout life (Hollender, 1970; Hollender and McGehee, 1974).

What causes an infant to respond? A sense of hearing induces the infant to respond to the parent, and the higher-pitched female voice is the preferred stimulus. Another is the degree of "faceness" of a stimulus, i.e., the presence of eyes, nose, and mouth in correct numbers, and juxtaposition is important even to the newborn (Fig. 4-6A, B). Finally it was shown that the new-

Fig. 4-6. Exposing a newborn infant to a model of a face elicits an inborn preprogrammed response. The more scrambled the face, the less the response. The figure (A) shows the stimuli of differing "faceness" used in the study; (B) contrasts the response in terms of average head-turning versus degree of "faceness." (The maximal score is 90° to each side, i.e., 180° total.) The comparisons were significant ($p < 0.005$) *(Reprinted with the permission of the author and publisher. From Freedman, D. G. Human Infancy: An Evolutionary Perspective. Hillsdale, N.Y.: Lawrence Erlbaum Associates, Inc., 1974.)*

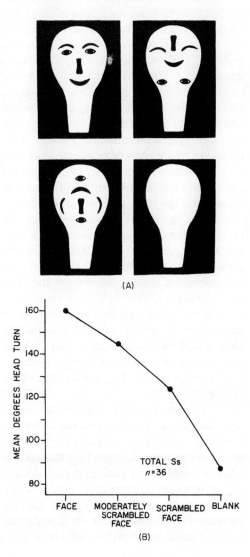

(A)

(B)

born is most responsive to the combined effect of the human face and voice and being held on the lap; all this supports the concept that the preparedness of the nervous system is genetically determined (Freedman, 1974). The smile of an infant has the strongest effect on the person taking care of it. The newborn smiles with eyes open and has a smile reflex when dozing after being fed. This can be elicited by a rocking motion or the sound of a gentle high-pitched voice. Even blind and deaf infants smile fully and normally, indicating that smiling is an inherent phenomenon (Freedman, 1974).

Hinde (1974) has discussed the possibility that the phylogenetic origin of this facial gesture is from the fear grin of the primate; in other words, that its function is to soothe and pacify. The smile accompanied by a direct gaze is a means by which mother and child are united as a social unit. Throughout life it remains a major means of establishing and reestablishing the oneness of people who feel close to one another. Further, it is a reflection of a feeling of personal adequacy.

There is evidence that infants only a month old can make remarkably fine discrimination in the perception of speech sounds. The rapid development of the uniquely human linguistic mode with its universal phonemes and organization of words across cultures indicates that infants are tuned into the spoken word from the start. This supports Chomsky's long held thesis that inherited brain structures determine the acquisition of syntax; it also accounts for such speech peculiarities as a child's correct use of pronouns in spite of hearing grammatical errors made by its parents (Harlow et al., 1971).

Laughter, a further mechanism fostering attachment, is an important means by which one partner can evaluate the emotional state of another. Laughter implies an invitation to continue interplay; crying, to stop it. The inherent programming of infants enables them to read these signals expertly (Hinde, 1974). Playfulness is a necessary trait for exploration and hence for learning

about the world; it is also programmed and occurs during the early phases of development when a child has its basic needs taken care of by adults and has the time to play (Freedman, 1974). Other innate response patterns are seen in vigilance, in reluctance to touch new objects, and in the fear of unknown persons shown by an infant six to 18 months old. It appears that the looming stranger poses a threat, thus fear prevents dilution of a primary relationship with the parental figure as the child begins to explore (Freedman, 1974).

By the end of the first year, an infant imitates others and displays assertive anger in addition to his desire for physical proximity, watching others, sucking, cooing, and laughing and playing with his mother or other parental person. Any breakdown of bonding behavior between infant and mother which may occur when the latter is depressed or shows rejection can be as damaging to the infant's social adaptation as physical isolation.

Bowlby concludes that is is essential for attachment to occur by the age of seven months. This approximates Harlow's critical six months for the monkey. Young orphaned children will show little exploratory behavior, preferring to remain in one spot. This lack of mobility is typical of depression (Bowlby, 1973).

Innate facial expressions and body gestures in man

As already noted in Chapter 2, a human mother free to act in privacy at the time of delivery immediately picks up her baby and within a few minutes spontaneously touches its head and body with the palms of her hands. Later efforts to breast feed her baby, to initiate close body contact, and to exchange eye contact and speak to it will be maximized if she has had this exposure during the sensitive period starting immediately after the delivery (Klaus et al., 1975) (Fig. 4-7). Thus innate programming of the newly

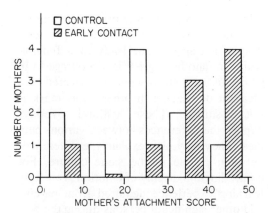

Fig. 4-7. These data point to a sensitive period for the human mother. Twelve hours after delivery, the attachment scores of nine mothers who had had immediate contact with their newborns differed significantly ($p < 0.06$) from the scores of 10 who had been separated from their babies at birth *(Kennell et al., 1975)*.

possible facial muscular configurations, only a fraction of these are universal expressions. Regardless of language or of whether the culture is Western or Eastern, industrialized or preliterate, Ekman finds that happiness, sadness, anger, fear, disgust, and surprise elicit the same facial expressions (Fig. 4-8). The same muscular movements of the face occur in both Japanese and Americans watching a motion picture showing a terrible accident.

In a special effort to find people who

Fig. 4-8. A series of facial expressions that have been successfully used by a number of workers in cross-cultural research in various countries. From above, downward, they read: (left) happiness, fear, and disgust; (right) anger, surprise, and sadness *(Ekman, 1972)*.

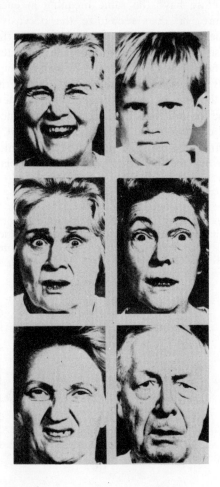

delivered woman causes her to respond appropriately to signals coming from her baby and to interact with them. On the other hand, a newborn has a programmed expectancy for this face-to-face interaction initiated by the mother, and the research of Brazelton et al. (1975) shows that when this expectancy is violated by a mother's immobile unresponsive face, her infant becomes disturbed and interrupts the cycle of interaction between the two.

Since even the newborn recognizes a human facial expression, this is evidence of a basic set of universal facial expressions of emotion. Such a common facial language will not vary from one country to another. It should be possible to show that one does not need to be taught a totally new set of muscular movements plus a new set of rules for interpreting facial expressions if one travels from one culture to another. Ekman (1972) has carried out a detailed and extensive series of studies disentangling the role of culture in determining facial expressions. There are both universal and culture-specific expressions, and the same facial response is associated with the same basic emotion for all peoples. Despite the many anatomically had no prior contact with our culture, a group of recently discovered New Guineans were tested. When asked to show what their faces would look like if a child had died or if they were angry or were about to fight, they too made the same facial muscle movements as Euro-Americans.

Ekman concludes that facial expressions do not represent a learned language by which arbitrary muscle movements have a different meaning for each culture. He postulates a neurocultural theory by which facial expressions of affect depend on programs located in the nervous system (Fig. 4-9A) (Ekman and Friesen, 1969). These programs link particular facial muscle movements with specific emotions (Ekman, 1972). However, while he postulates a biogrammar whereby facial expressions are inherited and therefore have the same meaning in each culture, he does recognize the pervasive influence of the environment as well; the possiblity of cultural variation is indicated by the words *amplify, mask,* or *blend* in Fig. 4-9B. While the basic responses are inherited, the rules of emotional display that determine the affects shown are socially learned and can vary with the culture (Fig. 4-9C). Further, the consequences of aroused emotion may be interfered with by the display

rules. Thus, weeping and other signs of sorrow may be prohibited in one society, despite a tragedy that leads to a funeral; while in another, grief is encouraged. In some cultures, anger would be covered by a pleasant demeanor; in others, this mask is not assumed. These cultural overlays explain the differences between various peoples. They may also explain the differences between people in the same culture. For controlling the display of emotion is an early learning experience acquired from parents and other significant persons during the sensitive period of socialization.

Eibl-Eibesfeldt has demonstrated other subtle gestures, which, like Ekman, he concludes are innate. These include the eyebrow flash of recognition (Fig. 4-10), threat displays, subordinate-to-dominant respect rituals, and adult consort embraces. These appear to be inherited patterns. For despite the intervention of learned variations, he found these basic role gestures in men and women all over the world. Humans are programmed to communicate emotional responses by a complex body language in addition to their basic facial responses. These are a vital part of the means by which members of a social group communicate emotions, express their attachment for one

Fig. 4-9. Diagram illustrating Ekman's proposal, suggesting that the inherited biogrammar for spontaneous facial expressions is modified by locally culturally determined rules of expression to yield a display that induces a culturally acceptable expression of affect. See text for details. *(From Ekman and Friesen, 1969. Reprinted by permission of Mouton & Co., Publishers.)*

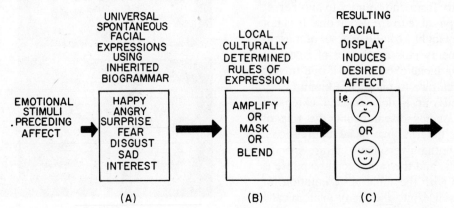

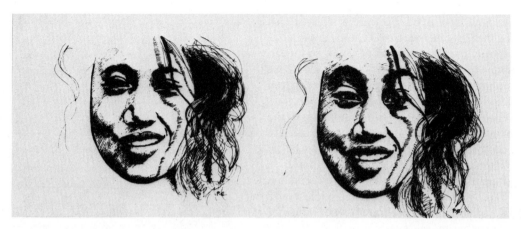

Fig. 4-10. The eyebrow flash of recognition appears to be innate and is one of a number of gestures uniformly found throughout the world. *(From Hinde, 1974. © 1974, the McGraw-Hill Book Company. Reprinted by permission.)*

another, and keep others who are less attractive at a distance (Eibl-Eibesfeldt, 1972, 1975).

In her work with chimpanzees, Jane van Lawick-Goodall (1973) points to the important calming effect on an excited subordinate of a touch, a pat, or an embrace by a dominant animal. The clinging of a frightened adult male to one of his companions has been described by Kummer (1971) in baboons. The reverse is seen in the accompanying figure where a male hamadryas embraces his attached female (Fig. 4-11). Bowlby (1970) argues that this attachment behavior, whose origins are found in the mother–infant bond, is in fact the cement of human society. The reliable patterns insisted on by a culture are crucial for conveying a sense of mutual support and for preventing the feeling of isolation that causes anxiety levels to rise, not just in the infant but in the adult also.

During adolescence the child's continuing attachment to its parents comes to be shared with other figures. Indeed, Bowlby sees the intense attachment behavior of man to woman as an extension of the parental bond.

In his studies of the kibbutz, Shepher (1971) has shown that when attachment develops between persons of the opposite

Fig. 4-11. Attachment behavior finding its direct expression in the wish to be held is found in subhuman primates, as well as in man, as is vividly portrayed in this photograph of an adult male hamadryas baboon with his consort (see also Figs. 2-4 and 2-13) *(Zuckerman, 1932).*

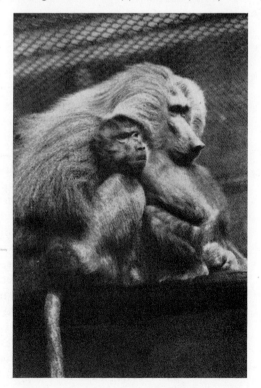

sex who have lived together as siblings during the first few years of life, they are inhibited from the phenomenon of falling in love in spite of the development of an intense mutual attachment. The fact that children who shared parental care throughout their sensitive learning period from infancy to the point of becoming aware of gender do not become sexually bonded appears to be an example of the role of early experience influencing later adult behavior. Neumann (1954) points out that during adolescence and adult life, this programming of behavior is caught up by symbolism and directed toward institutions and groups, i.e., school, college, religious or political groups. Often the actual attachment is facilitated by a direct transfer to a person holding a prominent position within the group. Bowlby (1973) comments, as does Neumann (1954), that for many a citizen's attachment to his state is a derivative of and dependent on his continued attachment to its sovereign or president. Attachment thus plays a vital role in shaping man's life from birth to old age.

Summary

If an infant mammal does not have the right sequence of experiences with parents, siblings, and members of the same species during the sensitive learning period, he will be at risk. As an adult he may miss vital signals dictating appropriate behavior. His failure to give the right gesture to a dominant or to hide from a predator, ever ready to strike an exposed member lacking protection, may prove fatal. The importance of mother–infant bonds leading to effective socialization is indicative of the intense attachment of young to mother and vice versa. The human newborn is programmed to attract the mother during the first hours postpartum and so initiates attachment. This is done by innate facial and bodily gestures whose significance in infants as well as in adults has only recently been appreciated.

5

Monitoring behavioral disturbances in experimental social systems

Concepts and reasons for monitoring

Although clinicians and epidemiologists in their work with humans first perceived the details of a relationship between emotional disturbance and physical illness, we make the point in preceding chapters that man is not unique: The life changes confronting him are, in fact, responsible for stimulating or straining the instinctually determined male–female bonding, parental attachment, and territorial behavior that he experiences just like other mammals. Human society also has dominants who control access to desiderata and are high in the social hierarchy (Maclay and Knipe, 1972). All mammals continuously pass down the stream of time—the aged eventually vanish, but the young are trained and incorporated into the establishment to preserve the species. Dramatic crises arising when these life changes suddenly occur are clearly intensely arousing to humans as well as to other mammals. The final breakup of a marriage bond when one partner walks out slamming a door or dies suddenly because of

an accident or from natural causes often results in an acute episode of depressive bereavement (Parkes et al., 1969). The fury of a quarrel between men competing for the same woman, the terror of being trapped under water in a car at night have their less dramatic equivalents in the steady attrition of day-to-day social interaction. The marriage bond may be strained by lack of money, inadequate, crowded housing, and difficulties with children (Brown et al., 1975). The stimuli received from inconsiderate neighbors, from petty criminals and sociopaths, and from crowded, inadequate mass transportation can lead to repeated daily stimulation of the emotions of anger or fear or depression, or a mixture of these.

The question arises as to whether these daily repetitions of emotional arousal can be reproduced in colonies of animals, such as monkeys and mice. What is the effect on a male baboon that is strongly attached to a female if she is assigned to a rival in an adjacent cage (Lapin and Cherkovich, 1971)? What happens to a young monkey that is removed for one week from his mother (Hinde and Spencer-Booth, 1971)? What behavioral and physiologic changes ensue? Do they differ when the animal is enraged as opposed to depressed? What are the biochemical changes? How does chronic high blood pressure develop? Is it a fact that chronic disease follows sustained and repeated emotional interaction? These are all questions that cannot be answered as readily for humans as for animals in which heredity and early experience and salt intake, cholesterol, and fat in the diet can all be controlled. The possibility of examining the tissues at various stages during chronic social interaction is largely confined to experiments with animals.

Basic types of behavioral monitoring

Attachment and territorial behavior as well as the role of the male and female and of the young and aged within a social hierarchy of a normal animal community are critically dependent on emotional stability. Only recently has a concerted effort been made to observe the alteration in behavioral patterns and in the nervous and hormonal consequences resulting from a disturbance of equilibrium in such a hierarchy.

Ethologists, following in the tradition of naturalists, laid the foundation. The work of Jane van Lawick-Goodall (1971, 1973) with chimpanzees and of Kummer (1968) and Eimerl et al. (1965) with baboons in their natural habitat has illustrated beautifully the mechanisms of attachment behavior as cement binding the primate social group. Bowlby (1970) has presented the evolutionary explanation that the mother–infant attachment is so strong because without it the young would be exposed to predators from the air and on the ground; these are always ready to strike those who stray from cover beyond adult protection. On the other hand, an excellent explanation of the role of aggression in holding a baboon troop together is found in a recent article by Bernstein and Gordon (1974). For similar observations

in societies of mice one has only to turn to Crowcroft's (1966) inimitable *Mice All Over.*

The method used by these pioneers was to watch animals as unobtrusively as possible, for months at a time, relying on their gradually becoming habituated to a human intruder in their midst. This technique, however, is both time consuming and arduous. Jane van Lawick-Goodall spent 4000 hours distributed over a period of five years, with most of the critical information becoming available in the fourth year. During the first year, she saw only little black blobs at a distance of about 500 yards. Not only is the habituation of animals critical, but also the ability of the observer to recognize individual animals.

A simplified approach is to track animals by making them project a signal that can be detected at a distance. Thus large birds with tiny transmitters attached to their bodies can be successfully tracked even during migration. Much information of great value to ecologists is being gathered by this method (Craighead and Craighead, 1972). Small transmitters in sterile cases can be implanted in the abdomen of animals to transmit body temperature, blood pressure, and blood flow in major arteries (Rader et al., 1974), but these have a short range and can be used only when animals are confined to a limited area.

Narrow vivarium cages, which merely suffice for the support of life, are inadequate for studying the normal behavioral interaction of social groups. Some freedom of movement and the stimulation of variability in their normal habitat are required, not just access to food, water, and nesting facilities. This is why cages in a modern zoo are being replaced by landscaped parks. But a compromise is required because the observer's need to study interaction between animals of a social group is in conflict with the animals' need to roam about for great distances and into inaccessible regions where they are invisible. Primatologists have solved part of the problem by making food available in areas suitable for viewing them. For example, Jane van Lawick-Goodall (1971) used a jungle clearing for offering chimpanzees their favorite bananas, and sweet potatoes were placed on a beach in an open area for the Japanese macaques (see Fig. 3-6) (Jay, 1965). This principle of coaxing an animal to betray his behavior by rewards of food and water is exploited in the operant technique.

Shock avoidance by pressing a lever to de-electrify bars on which the animal stands and the reward of food or water by pressing a lever have been converted by behaviorists Ferster and Skinner (1957) into an extraordinary page in the history of psychology. By using pressure on a lever to elicit a digital electrical signal and running this to a simple printer, an around-the-clock behavioral record of great value could be readily obtained. But this method views the animal in isolation apart from the social group with which his behavior is normally closely integrated.

Direct vision, together with still photographs and motion pictures with videotapes, has been used to study the social interaction of rhesus monkeys at the Yerkes Regional Primate Research Center in Georgia by Bernstein et al. (1974) and at the Oregon Regional Primate Research Center by Eaton (1976). In this case, the compounds under observation were square, about 40 meters per side. The analysis of data and reduction to digital form can be done almost directly by using a series of finger responses to activate a computer program. In the method used by Hinde's laboratory, signs are assigned to the various types of actions disentangled by ethologic observations (White, 1971). When any pattern occurs, such as an infant moving away from its mother, the appropriate keys are punched, giving a digital record of the behavior. Hinde was interested in the social ethologic aspects of behavior, however, he practicably reduced the population to the bare minimum of a single male, several females, and their young; living space was reduced to a cage some four times the body length of the occupant. This is close to the limit, but as long as cage dimensions exceed body length by about one order of magnitude, i.e., 5–10

times, both primates and mice can maintain a fairly well-adapted social group.

Rodents can also be examined from this viewpoint. The boldness with which mice encounter the environment can be observed by determining how many squares of an open field about 10 times larger than his actual body size a single mouse will explore in a given time (Watson, 1972; Watson et al., 1974; Watson and Henry, 1977a), and a few minutes of fighting between a resident and a test animal indicate a measure of individual aggression.

Calhoun (1962) set up colonies of rats in rooms measuring 3 × 4.2 × 2.7 meters (see Fig. 3-2). A 60-centimeter wall partitioned each room into four areas which were interconnected by narrow access routes. Eight centimeters of sawdust covered the floor, and each area contained nesting boxes and food and water. Calhoun's design attempted to follow the natural ecology and to provide an ideal environment for the rats. They were trapped once a month and weighed and checked for pregnancy, lactation, and condition of fur. Records were kept on the quality of nest building and housekeeping, i.e., extent of urine and feces in the nest. The colonies were observed through a 1 × 1.5-meter window on the roof for three to six hours and notes were taken on easily categorized behavior for later analysis.

Mice in our laboratories are studied in population cages or enclosures neither so large as to make it difficult to monitor activity without disturbing them, nor so small as to inhibit adequate development of social behavior in a growing population. One of our techniques followed the approach of Reimer and Petras (1967) with a population cage, based on their design, of standard cages joined by interconnecting runways (Figs. 5-1, 5-4, 5-14) (Henry et al., 1967, 1975a). Each cage, measuring 23 × 11 × 11 centimeters, contained wood shavings and was connected by a 45-centimeter right-angle spur, made of four-centimeter I.D. plastic tubing, either to a one and one-half meter square open-field area or to another standard cage.

The movements of mice during social

interaction were followed by implanting them with small Alnico VIII magnets either in the back, in the belly, or in both. These 9 × 3-millimeter cylindrical implants were tested for biologic and behavioral effects and no significant differences were found between the implanted mice and the normal controls in running on the activity wheel and in exploring the open field; they breed and successfully raise litters (Jarosz, 1977).

Hall Effect devices, which are sensitive to magnetic flux, are placed at the entrance to each cage and generate signals when a mouse passes in or out (Fig. 5-1). These signals are conditioned and encoded by logic circuits with a code that specifies each mouse according to the orientation and posi-

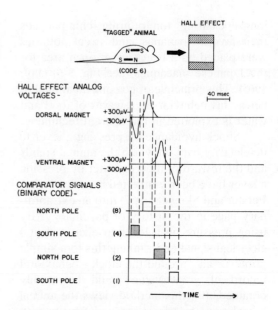

Fig. 5-2. A mouse is implanted with a dorsal or a ventral magnet or both and on going through a portal, the 9.3 × 3 millimeter magnet passes close to Hall Effect detectors that respond with a change of voltage proportional to the direction and amount of magnetic flux. This analog voltage signal is converted into two digital signals corresponding to a positive voltage for the north pole and a negative for the south pole; the duration of these signals can be used to compute velocity. Whether the north or south pole goes first depends on the position of the magnet with respect to the head of a mouse. Each magnetic pole and position is identified by using a binary 8,4,2,1 code as follows: 8 dorsal magnet, south pole; 4 dorsal magnet, north pole; 2 ventral magnet, south pole; 1 ventral magnet, north pole. By identifying the first pole for each magnet, one can determine, for example, that a mouse with a code 6 (dorsal magnet with south pole first and ventral magnet with north pole first) has passed through a portal. Eight mice can thus be uniquely coded.

Fig. 5-1. This eight-unit population cage has Hall Effect detectors at the entrance or portal to each 29 × 18 × 13 centimeter cage. The portal tubes, large enough to permit the passage of a single mouse, connect to a rectangular tube joining all the units. Mice are implanted with magnets so that a record is made each time a single mouse passes through a portal. This system permits an automatic 24-hour observation of mice in their undisturbed home environment *(Ely et al., 1972).*

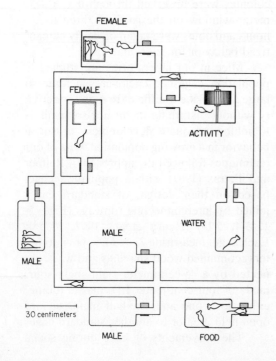

tion of the magnets. The information in the logic circuit is analyzed by a computer and the results are compiled hourly. (Henry J. A. et al. 1974)

Two voltage comparators detect and convert the analog signal generated by the magnet into two digital signals (see Fig. 5-2 legend for code and details). Since mice almost always pass through a portal head first, two mice can be encoded by implanting a magnet with either the north pole or the south pole headward, and eight mice can be identified if two magnets, i.e., in the back and in the belly, are used simultaneously. In the most recent development, rapid scan of a portal as a mouse passes through permits individual poles to be identified. A special program ensures that the poles are in proper sequence and eliminates errors due to hesitancy and other causes. Information from the logic circuits is analyzed by a minicomputer and displayed on a television tube the moment a portal transaction is completed. Data are stored on magnetic tape cassettes for subsequent analysis. As Fig. 5-3 indi-

Fig. 5-3.   One line of this printout is made by the magnetic detection system each time an implanted mouse passes through a portal.

ROBAS-V SYSTEM LOG

TIME	COLONY IDENTITY	MOUSE IDENTITY	BINARY MAGNET CODE	MOUSE DIRECTION	BOX IDENTITY	ELAPSED TIME	HESITANCY	VELOCITY - KM/HR	IDENTITY OF MOUSE CHASED	TIME OF PREVIOUS TRANSACTION
77 158						TUE JUN 06,1977				PAGE: 00017
10.333	SYS2TEST	JIM	0100	UNKN	FOOD	00.019	100	0.06		10.314
10.333	SYS2TEST	TIM	0010	UNKN	NST5	00.067	100	0.81		10.266
05.856	SYS2TEST	KIM	0101	INTO	ACT	05.856	200	4.80	JIM	00.000
10.338	SYS1TEST	TIM	0010	UNKN	NST6	00.101	100	0.11		10.237
10.345	SYS2TEST	DAN	1000	EXIT	H20	00.030	100	0.23		10.314
10.345	SYS2TEST	JIM	0100	UNKN	H20	00.011	100	0.30	JIM	10.333
10.346	SYS2TEST	JIM	0100	EXIT	H20	00.001	100	0.14		10.345
10.346	SYS2TEST	DAN	1000	INTO	H20	00.001	100	1.62		10.345
10.348	SYS2TEST	TOM	0001	INTO	NST5	00.073	100	0.01		10.274
10.349	SYS1TEST	TOM	0001	UNKN	NST5	00.071	100	0.09		10.278
10.353	SYS1TEST	TOM	0001	UNKN	NST6	00.003	100	0.03		10.349
10.364	SYS1TEST	TIM	0010	UNKN	NST1	00.025	100	0.15		10.338
10.364	SYS2TEST	TIM	0010	UNKN	NST1	00.030	100	0.01		10.333
10.377	SYS2TEST	JIM	0100	INTO	H20	00.030	100	0.54		10.346
10.377	SYS2TEST	DAN	1000	EXIT	H20	00.030	100	0.81		10.346
10.377	SYS1TEST	JIM	1000	INTO	H20	00.061	100	0.21		10.316
10.377	SYS2TEST	JIM	0100	EXIT	H20	00.000	100	0.54		10.377
10.377	SYS2TEST	DAN	1000	INTO	H20	00.000	100	1.08		10.377
10.377	SYS2TEST	TIM	0010	UNKN	H20	00.013	100	2.16	JIM	10.364

cates, the immediate information provided includes:

Velocity of passage

Which mouse chased which (chases are transits < 350 milliseconds apart)

Hesitancy at portal (backing up and starting through again)

Elapsed time in each box

Clock time of passage (which mouse passed the portal and the direction)

Time since a particular mouse moved

An evaluation of records from earlier models of this system has permitted detailed quantitative analyses of the behavior of mice in various situations of social significance. In particular it permits differentiation of the dominant mouse from the subordinates (Ely, 1971) and has led to a discrimination between the biochemical patterns that characterize these two types of behavior (Henry and Ely, 1976).

Biologic time is yet another consideration in the field of monitoring. A mouse passes through its entire life-span in two, two and one-half years, which means that a mouse being observed in a colony during the fourth to twelfth month of its life is passing through the equivalent in a man's life from his late teens to the forties (Henry, 1976a). Thus colonies are monitored to determine whether mice are behaving in the same way as man and experiencing the same physiologic changes when exposed to similar psychosocial challenges. If we assume that animals, such as mice and monkeys, can indeed "love" their babes, "hate" members of their own species and those of other species posing a threat to their welfare, and "despair" when cut off from all attachment figures in an environment they are unable to control, then, according to psychosomatic theory, under appropriate conditions we can expect them to suffer from high blood pressure, renal failure, infertility, or peptic ulcers. In other words, because all mammalian nervous systems are built in the same way we should expect to find the same chain of physiologic and biochemical changes in all mammals.

The first step is to observe behavior and to determine whether the behavior of the primate mother and infant resembles that of the human mother and infant; whether the rejected dominant mouse behaves with self-isolation and immobility similar to that found, for example, in the man or woman who has lost both job and spouse.

Techniques for producing behavioral disturbances

An important feature of Calhoun's (1962) work with rats was the observation that their behavior became disturbed as their population gradually increased over the months in a room in which he had attempted to provide them with an ideal environment (see Fig. 3-2). The normal care of the young, the building of nests, and the controlled aggression between males were replaced with failure to reproduce. The few young that were born were neglected and soon died. Finally, aggression between the males became so vicious that it led to severe wounding. This social breakdown appears to be connected with the excessive population growth which eventually made it impossible to care for the young.

The evidence suggests that the early deprivation of opportunity for attachment leads to psychopathy with chronic social disorder. Thus one way to induce behavioral disturbance in a social group is to isolate the young, thus depriving them of both maternal care and of the opportunity to develop attachment between each other (Henry et al., 1967; Harlow et al., 1971).

Another technique is to design the population cage or enclosure so that it is difficult for nesting animals to obtain privacy. Yet another is to force rivals to meet at a single point where they have to tolerate sharing access to the only available food and water supply (Fig. 5-4). Thus the design of an enclosure that makes privacy and territory formation difficult for the individual promotes social disorder and leads to arteriosclerosis, hypertension, and premature aging (Henry et al., 1967, 1975b).

A further method of disturbing behavior is to disrupt the attachment bonds. An infant mammal separated from its mother passes through a sequence that begins with agitation and ends with withdrawal behavior, suggesting depression. An animal formerly established as a member of a group, for example, a female sharing a communal nursery with siblings, or a male dominant in a stable, well-developed hierarchy, is attached to that group. If either is removed from the particular social mileu to which it is adapted and placed in isolation or in another social group as a intruder, it will show a gross behavioral change, such as neglecting the

young and avoiding instead of associating with members of the new group (Henry, 1976b).

As Bernstein and Gordon (1974) have pointed out in their study of the role of aggression in primate social systems, the hierarchy pays the most critical attention to the maintenance of social order. The introduction of a stranger, especially a male, causes violent perturbation in the group which acts in concert to reject it. In fact, although social disorder will eventually develop if there is persistent competition over a diminished supply of food or water, the most consistent stimulus for aggression is the introduction of a strange animal (Southwick, 1967).

Primate experiments

Early development of socialization

No matter how primitive or remote from the human they appear to be, all mammals depend on the right sort of experience during a sensitive learning period in infancy for meeting later social demands. The insect emerges from the chrysalis programmed for effective behavior to preserve the self and species. But not so the mammal. Although the mammal also has an innate program or biogrammar, it must be set in motion by the correct early experiences during a sensitive learning period. Work with rodents shows that even at their stage of evolutionary development, minor changes in early experience can lead to very great changes in their subsequent behavior. Thus monitoring the behavior of rodents has shown that an infant mouse or rat that is handled for a few minutes each day from birth to weaning if challenged later by being placed in an open field, will behave more vigorously than an unhandled rodent that has stayed in the nest all of the time (Denenberg, 1969; Levine, 1969a, 1969b).

Fig. 5-4. This intercommunicating cage system is used to induce social interaction in mice and is usually stocked with 16 males and 16 females. The lucite cages, a standard vivarium (shoebox) size of 29 × 18 × 13 centimeters, are connected into a circle by flexible plastic tubes of 3.8 centimeter I.D. The central hexagon holds food and water and is connected to each cage by short tubes of 3.2 centimeter I.D. *(Henry et al., 1975b).*

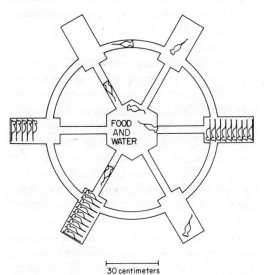

FOOD AND WATER

30 centimeters

Another important factor is how the mother herself was brought up. If she was neglected and had inadequate maternal care when maturing, then when she becomes a mother, she will in turn have deficient maternal behavior. This will reflect on the development of her young (Harlow et al., 1971). Deficient maternal behavior may be the mechanism behind the progressive failure of Calhoun's increasingly crowded rat colonies that developed without population control by emigration or predation in ideal rooms (Calhoun, 1962).

Another factor determining socialization is the number of siblings with whom the infant grows up and the variety of experiences they have available to them as a group. It makes a lot of difference whether there are opportunities to develop motor and social skills by practice during the sensitive learning period. Monkeys, for example, profit by the opportunity to practice chase and escape from each other in a simulated natural habitat where they can both interact with each other and also develop the skill for leaping from one swinging "perch" to another (Sackett, 1968). The critical role of early experience in determining the later adapted and controlled aggressive behavior, which is needed to jockey for position in the social hierarchy, and the attachment behavior, which determines the individual's richness of interaction with others, is presented by Hinde (1974) in his important book *Biological Bases of Human Social Behaviour.* He points to the great complexities resulting from the many early determinants influencing the course of adult behavior. Nevertheless, he presents solid evidence that gross changes in the conditions of early experience have very marked and predictable effects on later behavior. Experiments show the ingredients responsible for attaining skill in maintaining rich and effective attachment to others so that the organism can effectively elicit their cooperation. They also show how to develop the critical but rival capacity to control territory by modulating the aggressive fight and flight responses. Both skills depend on proper learning experiences dur-

ing early development. Effective attachment and territorial behavior as well as the effective behavior pattern characteristic of gender, be it male or female, can be grossly disturbed by experimental manipulation of early mother–infant and peer–peer associations.

Disturbance of attachment behavior

Sackett (1968) has summarized his own work and that of the Harlows at the Wisconsin Regional Primate Center where for years they have made methodical observations of the permanent abnormalities that follow the manipulation of the early experiences of monkeys. For this crucial early work, Harlow used wire cages of a standard design that were small enough to stack in a laboratory room. Females with differing effectiveness in mothering were used. The most maternal were mothers caught in the wild who had already raised at least one infant. The first stage in maternal deficiency used females born in the laboratory and deprived of early maternal experience. When these females had infants, they were called "motherless mothers." The final stage was to raise the young monkeys in a bare cage with only inanimate surrogate mothers made of cloth. In addition, some infants were raised alone with the mother, while others had access to other youngsters of the same age.

Testing included assessment of gross motor activity, vocalization, exploration, and play. Play was tested by having the subject use inanimate objects and by interacting with others. The behavioral categories used were derived from normal rhesus monkeys. Observers scored for nonsocial behavior and interaction on the basis of 150 various responses, such as fear, aggression, play, and grooming. Reliability coefficients were used to establish the competence of the observers. Behavior inappropriate for the test environment was used as the criterion of abnormality; for the situation is so remote from the wild that it is inappropriate to expect caged animals to reproduce it.

In contrast with the normal mother raised in the wild, socially deprived mothers were indifferent and abusive toward their young to the point of causing death. They were deficient in cradling infants and rejected them far earlier than did the mothers raised in the wild. According to the data in Fig. 5-5, this type of behavior is at its worst in deprived mothers, who were not only motherless themselves, but also lacked extensive interaction with peers when growing up (Sackett, 1968). During the first 30 days, deprived mothers withdrew from their infants (A) and were actually aggressive toward them (B)—something which mothers raised in the wild would almost never do. Interestingly, mothers raised in the wild never pushed a newborn away, but, by contrast, they frequently rejected the increasingly explorative four-month-old infant. This is evidence of a biologically valuable inherent programming or biogrammar at work, since, by then, a youngster should be apart some of the time playing with peers. The failure in programming in the deprived mother is seen in her excessive contact with her six-month-old infant. This gives a crossover effect with the experienced mother nurturing the new-

Fig. 5-5. These graphs show the difference in behavior toward their first infant between the motherless mothers and the normal rhesus mothers raised in the wild. During the first month, motherless mothers withdraw more often from infants seeking contact with them (A) and are more often aggressive toward infants (B). Up to six months, they push the infant away more often when it is a helpless newborn, but less often than the feral mothers, months later, when the infant is old enough to fend for itself (C). Finally, they cradle the newborn infant far less frequently just when such behavior is needed (D) *(Sackett, 1968).*

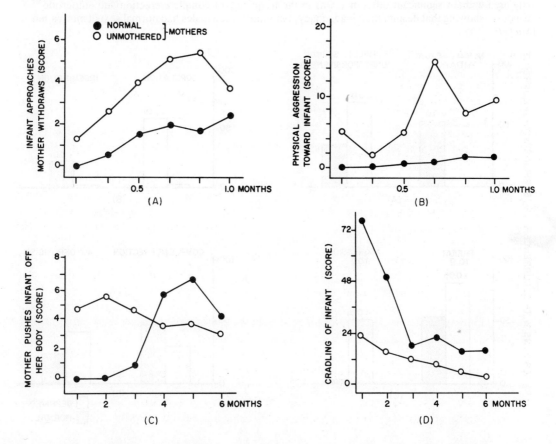

born more and rejecting the older infant more than the psychopathic mother (C). Another feature was that the newborn was cuddled more frequently by the mother raised in the wild (D). In general, these mothers were attracted to all infants, whereas mothers raised in the laboratory preferred association with adults. Sackett (1968) proposes that the lack of early peer association has produced an aversion to physical interaction with others which was incompatible with the behavior demanded by motherhood.

Not only do three and four-year-old infants of such motherless mothers direct more aggression to strangers their own age, but they are also less explorative. Sackett

thinks that mothers from the wild control their infants' behavior by messages delivered by vocalization and facial signals, whereas motherless mothers lacking these skills can control them only by violent physical attacks which are not preceded by such warning signals. The failure of the motherless mother to use more sophisticated threat signals was matched by the reluctance of the mother raised in the wild to proceed from threat to physical aggression.

The results of quantitative studies of sexual behavior of laboratory-reared adult monkeys matched with those of sexually sophisticated males and females reared in the wild are shown in Fig. 5-6. Deprived males are grossly deficient at initiating nor-

Fig. 5-6.   Effects of being reared in the wild as opposed to laboratory rearing on the sexual behavior of adult rhesus males during pairing with sophisticated adult females. There are significant differences in (A) sexual initiation and sexual unresponsiveness; (B) successful intromission and insemination; (C) male threat and aggression against females; and (D) self-clutching and self-biting. The only area without significant difference was in the frequency of complete erection and autoerotic response, showing that despite their inadequacy, laboratory-bred males had normal sexual motivation *(Sackett, 1968).*

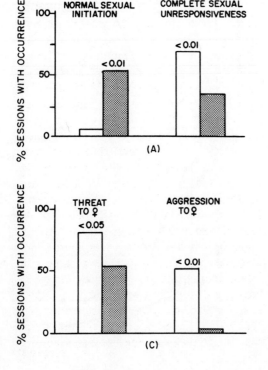

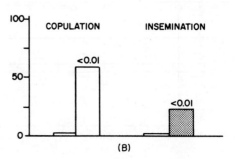

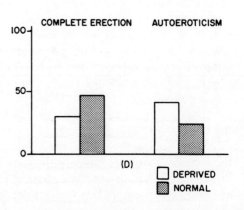

mal sexual behavior and are significantly more often found to be unresponsive (A). They fail at intromission and insemination (B), and, humanlike, try to cover up the deficiency by exhibiting significantly more episodes of threat and actual aggression toward their unfortunate partners (C). Even a modest amount of peer experience at 18–24 months helped the females but not the males. Both males and females raised alone for four years were inadequate. The problem was not a matter of sexual motivation, for erection and autoeroticism were frequent in socially deprived males (D). The problem was with precopulatory and copulatory behavior. There is evidence that fear and anger, i.e., self-clutching, threat, and aggression, with consequent inadequate sexual presentation and activity were responsible for the high rate of failure.

In the sphere of general activity and response to others, Sackett concludes that three months of early isolation produces only transient deficiency of social adequacy; six months led to a definitive reduction of responsiveness; and one year completely devastated social and nonsocial behavior. Thus a normal social response in the rhesus monkey depends on adequate peer contact before the age of six months. The deficiencies include fearfulness, aggressiveness, loss of motor and exploratory behavior, and rejection of complex sensory inputs.

In a striking and important contrast, the classic cognitive or intellectual tests were performed without decrement by isolates once they had overcome a tendency to avoid unfamiliar stimuli. They were as able as the normal controls to solve discrimination problems. Their probability of correct response was also as high as the normal controls in trials in which they had to shift to a new stimulus when the original stimulus was unrewarded.

Sackett concludes that the first year is the critical developmental stage of life for a monkey. Regardless of the inadequacy of the mother, monkeys raised with peers are little impaired except for some hyperaggressiveness. But rearing them without peers or maternal care produces a permanent and gross deficiency in the development of those emotional and motivational systems so essential for responding to complex and novel social situations. However, intellectual deficiencies do not occur as a result of this deprivation.

Mother–infant separation

The work of Harlow, Sackett, and others has demonstrated the devastating effects caused by failure to receive maternal care for prolonged periods (Sackett, 1968). Hinde and Spencer-Booth (1971) have inquired what happens when an infant monkey living in a normal family group is removed and isolated for a week only (Hinde, 1974). Testing occurred in a home pen occupied by a male, two–four females, and their young. Several such groups were studied; each was housed in a five × three-meter exterior cage communicating with a 1.8-meter cube inside a heated building. During observation periods they collected data on check sheets, recording every 30 seconds whether an infant, for example, was asleep, nursing, held by the mother, near the mother, within 60 centimeters of the mother, or farther away. They also used their recording device with a series of coded keys (White, 1971); pressing the appropriate key registered the particular event. The record was fed into a computer and a number of factors were analyzed; they included total time away from the mother, frequency of rejection by the mother, initiation of nursing by the mother, and the infant's role in maintaining proximity. Each time the distance between the mother and infant changed, a record was made of which of the two was approaching or retreating. The proportion of times the infant approached and retreated was calculated, so the extent to which he was responsible for proximity could be determined (see Fig. 2-10). Hinde and Spencer-Booth found that at first it was the mother who was responsible for the increase in time her infant spends away from her and for the distance, for she controls the proximity during the early stages (Hinde, 1974).

Their quantitative technique permitted analysis of the long-term effects of separation, for example, that of removing the mother for six days when the infant was 30–32 weeks old. Following the separation, the usual effect was observed. Infants shifted around aimlessly with their heads sunk on their shoulders and locomotor activity was reduced. Infants spent a longer time than normal being held by their mothers for several days after being reunited (see Fig. 2-10); they developed tantrums more frequently and showed an increase in rough and tumble activity (Hinde, 1974).

Infants who were the most distressed after their mothers' return were also the most disordered after their removal. Thus the behavioral disturbance depended on the preexisting tension between mother and infant. The effects lasted for months, making the monkeys less inclined to join in social activities.

Aggression and its arousal by intrusion

The role of threat gestures in inducing an infant monkey to perform the social behavior demanded by the mother has been outlined. Highly visible displays of aggression are a means of communicating and an effective substitute for inflicting injury on the one threatened (Fig. 5-7). It was found that socially deprived rhesus mothers explode in dangerous physical attacks on their young, whereas, as noted, the normal mothers fuss and threaten but rarely punish physically (Sackett, 1968). This principle extends throughout Mammalia. The hunting cat does not betray his presence until the final aggressive leap. His typical threatening display with raised fur and fluffed tail and low yowling is a communication of irritation directed at the rival male intruding on his territory. Aggressive behavior is very subtly graded and serves the important purpose of prevention, not promotion, of lethal damage

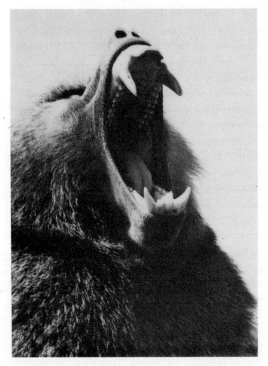

Fig. 5-7. The highly visible canines of this male baboon serve as a means of threat and are used in earnest only in aggression against predators and in bitter fights with rivals. They are not used in routine disciplinary action *(Hall and De Vore, 1965).*

to those of the same species. In the wild state, even a minor injury can have a fatally crippling effect when the individual must compete for his life or use his maximum strength for survival. Hence intraspecies fighting that induces any significant injury may well prove fatal, placing the group at an evolutionary disadvantage.

The work of Rose et al. (1975) with colonies of rhesus monkeys illustrates this grading of aggression very beautifully. They worked partly in the field and partly in the compounds at the Yerkes Regional Primate Research Center in Georgia. Well over 100 animals in various breeding groups consisting of males, females, and young were studied. The question raised was the response of the group to the introduction of new males. They hypothesized that those individuals posing the most significant threat to the existing social order would be the most vigorously resisted and rejected by the group. Among rhesus monkeys with a strongly organized hierarchy, infants and small immature members pose the least threat. Females also constitute little threat to dominant males, but they may be resisted by females, depending on how many of them are in the group and on the male–female ratio. The clue to a newcomer's being accepted is acquiescence to a low rank with a subsequent, gradual working up into the hierarchy. This is in fact the usual mechanism by which unattached males join new social units.

The study involved observation of aggressive interaction with contact, i.e., biting, slapping, pulling, threatening, and charging. Submission was evaluated in terms of grimacing, fleeing, avoiding, squealing, crouching, grooming, and sexual response. Rose and his co-workers confirmed that the maximum response was elicited when a new member was introduced into a healthy group. What impressed them was the dominants' remarkable control of their behavior (Fig. 5-8). When males fought with females, they did so in a stylized fashion; they bit on the neck with their incisors, but never used their heavy canines which could have been lethal. Canines are used for defense against predators and for fighting adult males for dominance. But after the male submits, he is then disciplined with the same nip of the incisors used on females (Rose et al., 1975).

The introduction of strange males or females into a resident group leads to an initial flurry of fighting. But the interaction rapidly shifts from extreme aggression to token gestures of threat. Newly introduced males submit, but with subtle innovation; for they accept the incisor bites at the base of the tail with grimaces and squeals, passively crouching and turning away. Yet they will fight back if the dominant "cheats" and uses his huge lethal canines. The moment the real fighting was over, the dominant moved off, delegating further punishment to the females in his group. When it became their turn, the

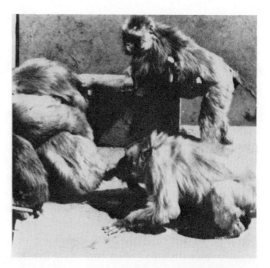

Fig. 5-8. A defeated group is subjected to token attack by members of a victorious group. The male in the foreground bites with his small nipping incisors at the base of the tail instead of biting in a more vulnerable area with his large canines. The female in the rear is participating in punishing physically dangerous larger monkeys despite her ventrally, tightly clinging infant *(Bernstein and Gordon, 1974).*

females rapidly deescalated the affair by replacing body contact with threats and chases. Thus although the dominant males control aggressive competition within the structure of the society, they carefully modulate the severity of the attack, using harmless nips and threats for intruding females or juveniles and reserving their canines for a rival who is close in status. Juveniles, which present no threat to the dominant, were ignored and left to go about their business. The dominant will concentrate on the one male whose size and threat activity indicates that he is able to take over the dominant's position.

As in man, aggression plays an important role in controlling upward social mobility. Serious fighting is at a minimum in a stable group of socially adjusted animals who are free from intruders, since the dominant is challenged only by an animal that has a real chance of taking over. Again, as in man, the most critical factor determining aggression is a perceived violation of the social code, determining the interrelated network of roles and patterns of behavior controlling the various members of the hierarchy (Rose et al., 1975). The formation of alliances between rhesus monkeys was noted by Bernstein et al. (1974) between Japanese macaques by Eaton (1976) and between chimpanzees by Van Lawick-Goodall (1973), underlining the basic significance of who grew up with whom. A male seeking entry into a colony may get assistance from a sibling who is already a member, who recognizes him and is attached to him. The two may even combine to overthrow a resident dominant, and the new dominant may take over without serving time as a low status member.

It is possible for a relationship to extend for two generations because the old female in a dominant position may support a younger female whom she has mothered. The young female's position in such a group is in turn determined by her mother's status and the coalition supporting her; this includes various high or low status males. The female allied with a dominant will have a higher status than rival males because of the help she receives from the dominant. An important part of an infant's socialization is learning the mother's position in relation to all others in the group. Resident females are more likely to attack a female intruder in contrast to males who recognize her as a female even when she is not in estrus. Further, individual male–female preferences do not depend on immediate female receptivity (Bernstein and Gordon, 1974). Rather, the status of a female is conditional on her acceptance by other females, while the male's status depends on his relationship to the dominant male.

Endocrines and changes in social status

Emotional responses to changes in position in a primate social hierarchy are accompanied by changes in the levels of the adrenal medullary and cortical hormones and of the gonadotropins and their dependent hormones. For example, a young animal that loses his parents and is helpless to fend for himself or one that is subordinated and threatened by others will both show an increase in the adrenocorticotropic hormone (ACTH) and in turn in the excretion of adrenal cortical hormones (Sassenrath, 1970) (Fig. 5-9). The depression following the rupture of attachment to a mother who has rejected her growing offspring thus is probably associated with increased levels of ACTH. This hormone, as discussed later, influences the hippocampal cortex, making it easier for the depressed animal to learn new patterns of behavior. (Brain and Poole, 1974). This is advantageous in the struggle for survival.

A further hormonal system that changes sharply with the perception of a change in

Fig. 5-9. With the formation, between three and five weeks, of a consort pair, the new consort's 17-hydroxycorticosterone (17-OHCS) response to the adrenocorticotropic hormone (ACTH) fell, while that of a subordinated rival female rose as her status diminished. The high status dominant male consistently showed a low corticosteroid response *(Sassenrath, 1970).*

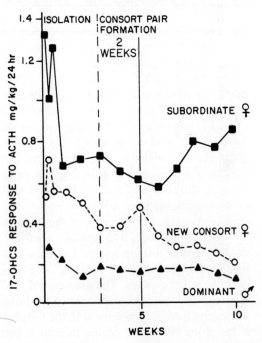

status is the testicular androgen testosterone. In the previously mentioned study of controlled aggression by Bernstein et al., (1974) plasma testosterone levels have been repeatedly measured (Rose et al., 1975). These investigators took advantage of the fact that status in the group determines self-perception and hence behavior and vice versa. By deliberately manipulating status, they determined that an adult male introduced into a group of sexually receptive females and low status males experiences a rise in plasma testosterone as he copulates and achieves a dominant status. By contrast, testosterone level fell sharply when the same male was introduced into a group of aggressive adult males. He was vigorously attacked and had to be removed within two hours (Fig. 5-10). He was then kept isolated in a small cage. In four experiments, different test animals were exposed to attack and then isolated; on each occasion, testosterone level fell by approximately 80 percent.

In later studies, Rose et al. (1975) grouped these four males together and simultaneously exposed them to receptive females. They observed a very high level of testosterone in the male which took over the newly formed group and became dominant (Fig. 5-10).

In further manipulation, the partition between two compounds was opened and the newly established group of four males and 13 females were exposed to interaction with a larger long-established breeding group of two adult males (one of whom was strongly dominant) and 34 youngsters and females. The old breeding group very soon took over and forced the new group into a restricted and subordinated status. The four males still had access to food and water, but they were now subordinate to every member of the larger group, regardless of age, sex, or status. The mob of males, females, and even the young would harass the males whenever they attempted to leave the corner of the compound to which they were confined. The plasma testosterone level of all four now subordinated males was grossly depressed below the original level (Fig. 5-11).

✱ Explain homosexuality

Fig. 5-10.   The testosterone in the plasma of this male rhesus increases when he is placed in a corral without rival males where females in estrus treat him as a dominant. It falls when he is exposed to powerful males who defeat him *(Rose et al., 1975).*

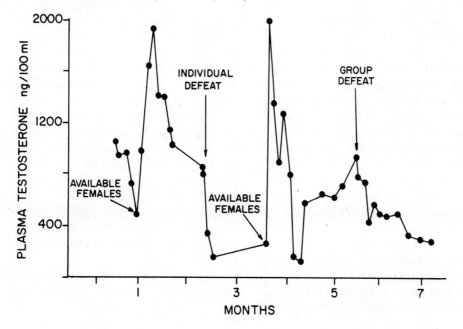

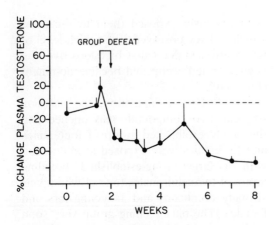

Fig. 5-11. When four members of a group of rhesus monkeys living in a compound in Georgia were defeated by another group (see Fig. 5-10), they showed a progressive and sustained mean loss of testosterone levels which fell to 80 percent of control values *(Rose et al., 1975)*.

Rose et al. (1975) took the results of these studies to indicate that the plasma testosterone level is sensitive to both elevation and suppression by the appropriate social stimuli. Following defeat, there is an associated adaptive fall in testosterone. The word *adaptive* is used because Rose and co-workers suggest that the perception of defeat produces the fall and this lower level of hormone will in turn lead to behavioral changes with a great reduction in the probability of aggressive action.

As discussed in Chapter 7, Sassenrath (1970) has shown a direct relationship between adrenocorticotropic hormone (ACTH) responsive levels, aggressive stimulation, and fear anxiety behavior in groups of rhesus monkeys. The dominant animals had far less adrenal corticosteroid response to an ACTH injection than the subordinates. She concluded that the fear-evoking components of chronic social stress are the predominant stimuli for endogenous ACTH release (Fig. 5-9).

Price (1969) has presented the ethologic argument that yielding behavior and loss of status in the social hierarchy are associated with depression for a good reason. He sug-

gests that the consequent immobilization and "loss of fight" have an evolutionary advantage by suppressing lethal conflict that might otherwise occur if defeated animals kept attempting to regain status. The fall in testosterone and rise in corticosterone are thus associated with a positive feedback—temporarily stabilizing the social hierarchy by preventing attempts to attain dominance.

Rodent experiments

Automatic monitoring of mice in a population cage

Sackett and Harlow's motherless mother rhesus monkeys bear an uncomfortable resemblance to the nonnurturant human mother who goes so far as to desert or to batter her baby or both (Sackett, 1968). Bowlby (1970) has related the effects of social deprivation on the baby primate who develops disturbed emotional response patterns characteristic of human psychopathy. If the mechanisms at fault are subcortical and the critical period for a mother's attachment to her baby occurs early in its development, the question arises as to whether rodents disturbed in infancy might show similar changes. It would be of great value if a tiny animal like the mouse having a total life-span of only two years were to have a similar early learning period during which behavioral cues critical for avoiding social disorder are learned.

The preceding pages described how groups of monkeys respond to the removal of their young or to the introduction of a new member. The automated technique for quantitative studies of colonies of mice, which we have used in our laboratory for the past five years, permits a detailed analysis of their behavior in response to such perturbations (Ely et al., 1976; Henry and Jarosz, 1977; Jarosz, 1977).

Figure 5-3 shows the number of visits made to various cages making up a complex population cage (Fig. 5-1) and the velocity with which each mouse passes through a portal upon entering a cage. Items such as hesitancy at a portal and the number of chases made can be automatically printed out every few hours on a computer. Ely used an earlier version of such a monitoring system to show that some mice are highly active and pursue others. A dominant male described in the preceding chapter made repeated patrols rapidly to a sequence of boxes (Fig. 5-12) to check on the position of various mice in the colony and to identify intruders and other perturbations. He is recognized by a lack of nicks and scars on the rump and tail and has free access to all cages. The contrast is clear between him and the rival who rarely visits the females' nesting boxes and the subordinates whose movements are still more restricted, being confined mostly to the latrine box (Ely, 1971; Ely et al., 1976).

Ely made detailed studies of the effects of marihuana (Ely et al., 1975) and of hippocampectomy (Ely et al., 1976, 1977) on mice. The marihuana study contrasted the low locomotor activity of subordinates with the high activity of dominants; the drug lowered entry–exit rates and patrol patterns of the dominants dramatically. It was possible to demonstrate a significant decrease in a dominant male's aggressive response to an intruder at the dosage of 0.5 milligram/kilogram (Fig. 5-13). In sum, Ely and his associates showed that the behavioral effect of marihuana (Δ 9-THC) on freely interacting rodents of mixed sex living in a population cage depends on the individual's social position in the hierarchy and on the social composition of the group.

The study of social behavior of mice with hippocampus lesions showed that they were less aggressive and failed to develop a normal social hierarchy with dominant–subordinate relationships. A new open-field design was used and movements of mice were monitored by the minicomputer (Fig. 5-14). Figure 5-15 gives a final example from the work of Jarosz; here, as the legend indicates, the loss of dominance due to injection

of an antiandrogen leads to a sharp change in the spatial activity pattern that can be constructed to portray social activity. The size of the sector in a circle (cage) is the percent of time spent in the cage and the width of the interconnecting bands between the circles, the number of visits or transactions. On Day 3 dominant mouse No. 7 shows high activity in all cages and subordinate mouse No. 3 borders on rivalry with his visit to a female box. But on Day 12 after an injection of cyproterone acetate, the now subordinated No. 7 no longer visits females, whereas No. 3, who did not receive the drug, has assumed the dominant role. These examples show that such a system can give a good idea of the social activity in a colony without interfering with the mice and without having to resort to observers (Jarosz, 1977).

Social deprivation and behavior of mice

The question arises as to whether social deprivation would affect the behavior of a group of mice. When the motherless monkeys described by Sackett (1968) become adult, they show a number of ineradicable social defects. They fail to respond to normal social cues because of deficient early experience. One consequence is their unbridled aggression and failure to withhold punishment even when appropriate submissive gestures are made; another is their deficient maternal care with ensuing neglect and destruction of the young.

The work of Watson et al. (1974) with mice that had been raised in isolation from the time they could feed alone, i.e., from about 14 days until adulthood, showed deficiencies similar to those in socially deprived monkeys. All males were equally badly bitten, showing that there was no stable hierarchy and that territory was not respected. As in Calhoun's disturbed rodent colonies, no young were successfully raised by socially disordered female mice (Calhoun, 1962).

In repeated observations, we found that

MALE TERRITORIES

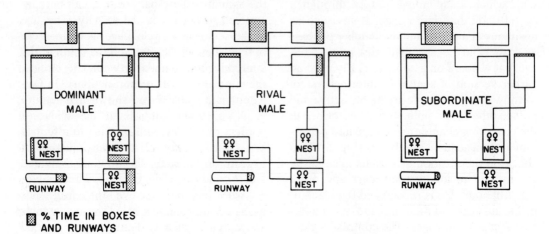

Fig. 5-12. The different territorial distribution of dominants, rivals, and subordinates averaged for a one-week period is illustrated. The dominant mouse has free access to more cages, has the greatest cage entry–exit and patrol activity, is free from scarring on the rump and tail, and has access to females.

Fig. 5-13. Mean of ($n = 6$) dominant male's aggressive responses (entry–exits/hour) to an intruder before, during, and after a single intravenous injection of 0.5 milligram/kilogram marihuana (Δ9-THC). Increase in activity during the control period from 1300 to 1600 hours is due to normal circadian rhythm. Entry–exits for the first intruder period were compared to those of the control period and entry–exits for the second intruder period to those of the first intruder period ($* = p < 0.05$, $** = p < 0.01$, $*** = p < 0.001$; vertical bar = Standard Error of the Mean).

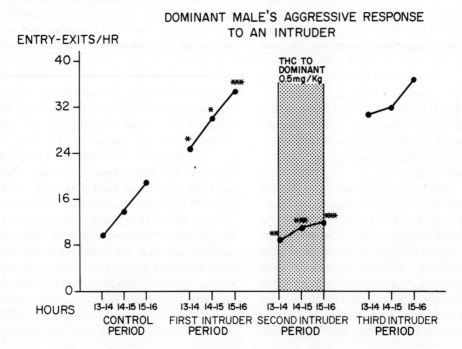

DOMINANT MALE'S AGGRESSIVE RESPONSE TO AN INTRUDER

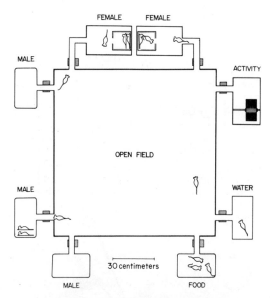

Fig. 5-14. This population cage includes a large open field. Hall Effect detectors are mounted at portals to all eight cages, as also shown in Fig. 5-1. Food and water are placed in single locations instead of in each cage as was the arrangement in Fig. 5-1. The open field permits mice to escape each other, and an activity wheel permits them to run the equivalent of long distances. Nesting boxes in two of the cages encourage females to establish communal nurseries.

colonies of socially deprived mice remain disordered for months on end. As a consequence, they show repeated arousal of the sympathetic nervous system and of the adrenal medulla (Henry et al., 1971a) and cortex (Henry and Stephens, 1977). As this continues for months, the conditions needed to induce chronic disease are fulfilled. These pathophysiologic changes are described in Chapter 8, but it should be pointed out at this stage that the behavior of mice shows the extreme swings of affect, including the arousal of fear and rage, so evident in a socially deprived monkey colony exposed to group living. Thus when socially deprived mice interact with each other or respond to the challenge of an open-field test, they show a greater release of the adrenal cortical hormone than normal mice. Their behavior betrays their emotion because, at that time, they explore less in an open field than normal mice (Watson et al., 1974; Watson and Henry, 1977a).

One may ask what is the emotional state of deprived mice being protected from social stimulation. Plasma renin levels (Fig. 5-16) and the amount of enzymes in the adrenal medulla, which synthesizes adrenaline and noradrenaline, are actually less in these sheltered mice than in normal siblings living with peers with which they have been raised after normal weaning (Fig. 5-17). Their blood pressure is normal and as long as they are in isolation, they have a full life-span without evidence of chronic disease (Henry et al., 1971b). Therefore, we can assume that despite their lack of social skill, as long as no social demands are placed on them, as long as they do not have to make complex adjustments and decisions in the pursuit of food, water, shelter, sex, and the care of young, and as long as they do not have to follow a biogrammar defining their gender identity, and to bond to peers and to young, or to defend territory—they experience little emotional arousal.

The intense aggression of the socially deprived isolated mouse is an expression of failure to adapt to the demands of the social group. All other mice are intruders threatening the narrow autocracy the isolate has enjoyed all of his life. He is without the necessary skills to adjust and hence he overresponds. Such a mouse has a shortened lifespan when placed in a normal colony in much the same way as the socially deprived monkey placed in a wild group dies. If mice isolated for three and one-half months after weaning are exposed to social interaction for several months, then, despite their experience of social disorder culminating in fights, bites, and adrenal arousal, they are even more disturbed when returned to isolation. Like the isolated monkeys (Sackett, 1968), such mice will bite themselves, lose weight, and will show elevated levels of plasma corticosterone and persistent elevation of blood pressure. It appears that they can no longer

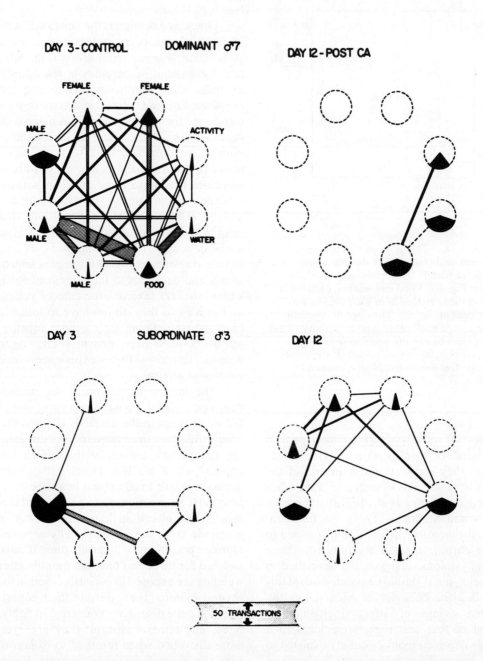

Fig. 5-15. Loss of dominance due to injection of an antiandrogen leads to changes in the spatial activity pattern portraying social activity in a population cage as shown in Fig. 5-14. On Day 3, dominant mouse No. 7 shows high activity in all cages. Subordinate mouse No. 3 borders on rivalry with his visit to a female box. On Day 12, after receiving cyproterone acetate, the thoroughly subordinated No. 7 no longer visits females; No. 3, who did not receive the drug, has assumed the dominant role *(Jarosz, 1977)*.

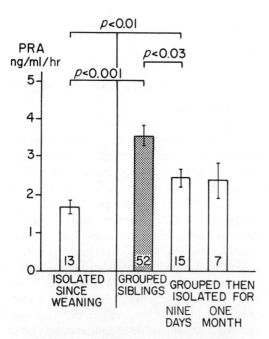

Fig. 5-16. Effects of isolation on plasma renin activity (PRA). The mice isolated since weaning and the normal grouped siblings in cages were six months old. The other grouped siblings were six months old when isolated in the 23 × 11 × 11 centimeter cages for an additional nine days or one month *(Vander et al., 1978).*

adapt to either the low stimulus of isolation or the high stimulus of social disorder (unpublished observations).

Aggression-elicited depression in an intruder

The work of Rose et al. (1975) showed that a monkey intruding on the territory of a social group is immediately set upon. If he is to survive, he must at once communicate his submission to all, including the females and young. He must adopt the posture of a low ranking member waiting for food and accept the less desirable fringes of group territory. His emotional arousal is shown not only by cringing submission but also by the high level of adrenal hormones and the low level of testosterone.

Analogous observations have been made by Ely by placing formerly dominant mice as intruders in colonies with an active, healthy social hierarchy controlled by a strong dominant (Henry et al., 1974, 1975a). The testosterone level of these former dominants fell to near castration levels, i.e., from 1140 ng% to 170 ng%, as they avoided the other mice and tried to find an area of the population cage where they would not be attacked (D. L. Ely, personal communication).

Fig. 5-17. Histograms of mice showing the effects of isolation and chronic psychosocial stimulation on the catecholamine-synthesizing enzymes of the adrenal gland. Left histograms represent standard values as found in normal controls (siblings in groups of six to eight living in 23 × 11 × 11 centimeter cages). With isolation there is a slight reduction of the adrenaline rate-limiting enzyme methyltransferase and of the noradrenaline-synthesizing enzyme tyrosine hydroxylase (middle histograms). Right histograms represent values found in normal siblings exposed to psychosocial stimulation for six months, i.e., from four to 10 months of age) in a population cage of the design shown in Fig. 5-4. Mice develop chronically elevated tyrosine hydroxylase ($p < 0.01$), methyltransferase ($p < 0.001$), and blood pressure ($p < 0.001$). The blood pressure of normal controls does not differ from that of isolated mice. Vertical lines are Standard Deviations.

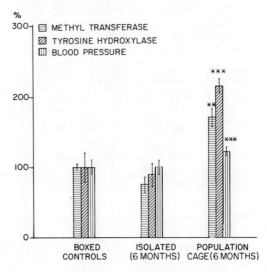

The blood pressure of these former dominants was grossly elevated, attaining 200 mmHg, and their plasma adrenal cortical hormone corticosterone was also significantly increased (Fig. 5-18). Thus the intruding mouse responded to an attack of the social group in the same way as the intruding monkey. We propose, as would be the case in an intruding human, that the mouse was frightened and depressed and indeed betrayed this emotion by withdrawal and high corticosterone levels (Henry et al., 1975a; Henry, 1976b). Their emotional arousal is so great that it is not surprising to frequently find dead mice without gross injuries. As is described in Chapter 9, Barnett et al. (1975) have reported the same findings in wild rats placed in the territory of established dominants, and Von Holst (1972) reports uremia in tree shrews that are forced to intrude unwillingly on a dominant's territory.

Comparison of results for mice and primates

Watson has shown that, unlike motherless monkeys, female mice deprived of early social experience will successfully raise their young if left to do so alone (Watson and Henry, 1977b). The evidence thus far suggests that mice are more fully preprogrammed by a biogrammar than subhuman primates and that social deprivation is not so disastrous for them. The experimental methods already discussed show that mice, however, do need early experience during a sensitive learning period, and if they do not receive it or are unable to follow it, it is fatal for the successful propagation of the species because they cannot form stable demes or breeding groups.

These data for mice show that it is not necessary to use expensive, slow-growing subhuman primates to study the effects of chronic emotional arousal that follows repeated confrontations in a socially disordered group. Mice lacking the necessary attachment and control of territorial behavior can be produced by being raised in isolation, thus depriving them of the maternal and sibling interaction they experience in appropriately designed population cages. Chapter 8 describes chronic blood pressure elevation, high renin levels, eventual early death from myocardial fibrosis, and interstitial nephritis with uremia and suggests that these ailments model the processes by which emotional disorder leads to chronic disease and early death in man.

Fig. 5-18. When a former dominant mouse experienced social rejection because of being placed in a strange social group as a solitary intruder, he was affected by large changes in several biochemical parameters. The level of phenylethanolamine *N*-methyltransferase (PNMT) fell; tyrosine hydroxylase, the rate-limiting enzyme for noradrenaline, did not change, but plasma corticosterone and blood pressure both rose in this study of normal dominants ($n = 7$) after they had spent several days as solitary intruders in a strange colony where they were subordinated. The open columns represent the mean values for seven males while they were still dominants; the hatched columns, the mean values for six males after three to six days of exposure to a strange colony.

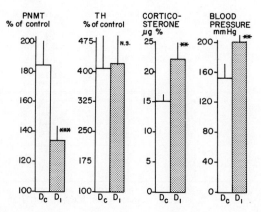

Summary

The skilled observation of primates implemented with a computer backup or the automatic tracking of mice in population

*As we increase in evolutionary scale.

cages can be used to monitor deliberately induced behavioral disturbances. The ensuing behavior can be measured, permitting the effects of various manipulations of the attachment and territorial instincts to be evaluated. Either the habitat or the early experience of the organism may be made deficient. There is now decisive experimental evidence in primates pointing to the crucial role of the first year that the mother–infant dyad spends together. Peer attachment, however, can compensate to some degree for deficient mother–infant bonding. The role of aggression in maintaining the integrity of social structure explains the violent resistance to potentially disruptive intruders and the paradoxic acceptance of active juveniles. Plasma testosterone level in a male increases with positive perception of his recently tested social standing, whereas his plasma corticosterone and ACTH response tend to increase with his perception of loss of control.

By tagging mice with magnets and using Hall Effect detectors at portals to box cages within a complex population cage, a continuous measure of parameters, such as the number and time of box entries and exits, can be made by an appropriately programmed computer. The resulting data can be displayed in diagrams measuring social activity. Social deprivation by isolation from two weeks until maturity at four months produces mice that cannot establish a stable social hierarchy in a colony nor can they raise young. Such social deprivates are aggressive; and if left in the colony, they chronically fight and age prematurely, dying of arteriosclerosis and renal failure. Normal mice that were once dominant but are placed in other colonies as intruders will withdraw. Their blood pressure and corticosterone are elevated; this, together with ruffled fur and avoidance of others, suggest they experience the equivalent of human depression. This evidence suggests that the basic emotions of rage, fear, and depression can be induced in members of both primate and mouse colonies by the proper manipulation.

6

The role of the neocortex and the limbic system in social interaction

Introduction: man's four brain systems

The preceding chapters have dealt with the psychologic aspects of the chain of events leading from the social stimulus past the defenses of social assets to the arousal of the autonomic nervous system and endocrines (see Fig. 1-3). In light of newly discovered principles of the organization of the brain that give insight into the mechanisms of response to stress, this chapter discusses aspects of the neural basis of behavior of importance in controlling neuroendocrine responses to social stimuli.

Altman's basic textbook on the *Organic Foundations of Animal Behavior* discriminates three levels of neural control in mammals (Altman, 1966). The most fundamental and primitive part is the brain stem which is shared in common by all vertebrates and has remained remarkably unchanged throughout evolution. The brain stem carries on the segmental tubular design of the most primitive brains, for it is an extension of the spinal cord and harbors the vital nuclei concerned

with the respiration and heart action as well as the reticular formation controlling alertness and sleeping and waking.

Just beyond the brain stem are the basal ganglia, including the corpus striatum which plays a role in the control of expressive behavior. Together they constitute the most primitive part of a hierarchy of three brain systems. MacLean (1976) has cogently presented the same picture of what he calls the triune brain for many years. Despite the interdependence and interconnection of the brain stem with the limbic system and of both with the cerebral cortex, he argues that they constitute a hierarchy of three brains in one. Each, he maintains, differs in kind from the other. Each has "its own special kind of intelligence, its own special memory, its own sense of time and space, and its own motor functions."

The hypothalamus with the limbic system make up MacLean's intermediate, less primitive brain. The hypothalamus is a group of small nuclei lying at the base of the brain close to the pituitary gland, which controls the endocrines. The hypothalamic nuclei are critically involved in the regulation of the endocrine glands and the basic aspects of eating, sexual behavior, drinking, sleeping, and emotional behavior in general.

This region has strong connections with the rest of the limbic system which is made up of the old regions of the forebrain. It includes the paleocortex, the oldest and most primitive type of cortex, and surrounds the root of the newly evolved cerebral hemispheres which balloon out beyond a limbic noose. This ring of structures is made up of the cingulate gyrus, the hippocampus, the septal area, and the amygdala. They have remained relatively unchanged throughout the evolution of mammals. MacLean has presented evidence that the limbic system operates in relative independence of the brain stem, on the one hand, and of the new cerebral cortex, on the other.

The third system of MacLean, the neocortex, is responsible for cognitive function as opposed to the instinct and affect characteristic of the limbic system. Cognitive function in man involves language and rational, empiric thinking. In the advanced primates the amount of the cortex parallels the great complexity and flexibility of behavior. The most recently evolved projection areas for the analysis of vision, hearing, and sensation are located here in the higher mammals together with the motor cortex. In the cat or rat these areas constitute a major portion of the new cortex, and, even in man, the basic organization of these cortical sensory and motor areas does not differ. However, in man these projection areas are dwarfed by an enormous increase in the association cortex that lies between them.

The fissures covering the human brain increase the area of this two-millimeter-thick cortical mantle still further, so that it contains three-quarters of all the neurons in the brain. These new sheets of complex nervous tissue dominating the human brain are connected by the corpus callosum, a huge band of nerve fibers running from one hemisphere to the other.

Thus MacLean's third system, the neocortex, is found in all mammals, but work on cerebral lateralization, including studies of human patients who have had sectioning of the corpus callosum (commissurotomy), has shown that an extra system has evolved in the form of the so-called dominant hemisphere in man. He has, in fact, four brain systems. Man's two hemispheres are specialized for differing cognitive functions, and by cutting the commissure to disconnect them, the existence of two minds can be detected. Each is specialized in a different way, making them two independent problem-solving organs that can approach the same situation in a different style (Dimond and Beaumont, 1974; Sperry, 1974). Hamburg has lumped these two sets of cerebral association cortices together, calling them a sociocultural brain; he and Washburn point out that this peculiarly human bilateral structure has evolved in the last few million years to deal with the needs of the new toolmaking, talking social mammal (Washburn and Hamburg, 1968). One side is the repository of language and logical skills, and the other, of visual–spatial abilities. Together they permit man to forge and to transmit his extraordinary range of cultures, crafts, and behaviors across the generations; together they form two more systems added to the brain stem and the limbic system; and together they are responsible for the gulf separating civilized man from the animals—a gulf so huge that it distracts from the evidence of his inherited biogrammar (Reynolds, 1976).

This chapter draws attention to these remarkable discoveries about the human brain, not the least important feature of which is that these four relatively independent brain systems permit the metapsychol- *of* ogy of the ego, the id, and the unconscious *loose* to be correlated with neurophysiological thinking. Indeed the differing viewpoints of sociologic and biologic sciences can be seen as deriving from an almost exclusive emphasis on the activity of the two newest and the two oldest brain systems (Galin, 1974, 1976).

The evolutionary origin of lateralization

In their interesting quantitative study Andy and Stephan (1974) have compared the size of the neocortex of higher primates with that of primitive animals, such as the tree shrew. The ratio is about 50:1. This already large figure is three times greater in man. Figure 6-1 shows the enormous area covered by the association cortex in man, as opposed to animals with less flexibility of behavior, such as the cat or rat. The development of the sociocultural brain in the parietal region lying between the projection areas for

Fig. 6-1. The cerebral hemispheres of four mammals, in rough scale, showing the lightly shaded association cortex, differentiating it from the sensory projection areas and the motor region. Scarcely evident in a lateral view of the rodent brain, the association cortex, even in higher primates, is less than one-third that of man. It is the location of this newly evolved sociocultural brain that gives man speech, abstract logic, visuospatial synthesis, insight, and the capacity for making tools with which his societies have been forged (*Harlow et al., 1971*).

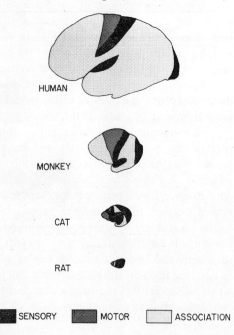

HUMAN

MONKEY

CAT

RAT

■ SENSORY   ■ MOTOR   □ ASSOCIATION

vision, hearing, and sensation and at the frontal poles is the achievement of human evolution. Geschwind (1974) has shown that the left side differs anatomically as well as functionally from the right, i.e., this new brain is subdivided into two spheres: dominant and nondominant. The cells of the speech areas of the dominant, i.e., left parietal association cortex, are responsible for coding language. In the nondominant, i.e., the right hemisphere, the corresponding area is responsible for awareness of spatial relations. Visual discrimination is also involved, so that the regions can be thought of as transmodal, that is, they are involved in forming concepts related to the various adjacent projection areas and are not specifically sensory, auditory, or visual. They may thus be involved in man's capacity for abstract thought and symbol formation.

These association areas are at first equipotential when a young child is learning to speak so that, if as the result of an accident early in life, he loses the speech area in the dominant hemisphere, after recovery he will be found using the speech area of the other hemisphere for communicating. Harlow et al. (1971) comment that the posterior association area in one hemisphere develops the neural substrate of language, while the other side codes spatial relations. The fact that the essential speech area is limited to a particular region of the association cortex in one hemisphere supports the theories of the neural basis of language with coding going on in a strictly delimited area rather than all over the brain. The psycholinguist Chomsky (1972) has presented evidence that a genetically determined neuronal matrix is responsible for syntax, i.e., for the orderly mutual relation of words in a sentence. Instead of being grossly different, all known languages are variations of the same orderly syntactic theme.

Even very young infants have the rudiments of speech perception and discriminate between linguistically relevant sounds like "pah" and "bah." Eimas et al. (1971) point out that they behave as if they were born with "feature detectors" for analyzing the sound patterns of natural languages. Children develop the general rules of language without any training, and psycholinguists of Chomsky's point of view claim that because the child "knows" the rule for forming the past tenses of a word as a result of this predetermined organization of speech, he sticks to "digged" despite correction and stubbornly rejects the irregular verb *dug* proposed by his teacher (Harlow et al., 1971). It appears likely that the evolution of language as a means of communication depended on a capacity for perceiving a common signal which could represent a feature not patterned by individual projection areas for vision, hearing, or sensation: a number, for example, or a word or letter standing for some idea. This capacity would be provided by the combined transmodal interaction of two or more association areas together with the predetermined organization of the speech area of the dominant hemisphere. Furthermore, this region is set up for dealing with long sequences of sounds instead of a rapid simultaneous grasp of overall form characteristic of the nonspecialized associational cortex.

In his discussion of the double brain, Dimond makes the point that both hemispheres of the healthy mammal have separate, important functions and there is no question of one hemisphere being nonfunctional: Indeed, it is now seen as equally important and not even minor or subordinated (Dimond, 1972; Dimond and Beaumont, 1974). Originally, he says, laterality may have developed in the vertebrate to provide control over the different regions of space confronting the animal, i.e., so the stimuli from one side could induce a motor response on that side. Further, by combining the data from two sides, the computation of distance and the perception of three-dimensional space became feasible.

But mechanisms then had to evolve to facilitate integration between the hemispheres to get the two systems to work together. Dimond sees the evolution of cross-connecting fibers as a feature contributing to higher mental processes. In higher vertebrates, the two hemispheres together can accomplish more than the one hemisphere alone because the information being processed is integrated via the callosal commissure. This function is not confined exclusively to one hemisphere; each is an active member in the partnership.

Jerre Levy comes to the same conclusion. She talks of symbiosis in a recent discussion of the psychobiologic implications of bilateral asymmetry (Levy, 1974). Each side of the brain is able to and chooses to perform a certain set of cognitive tasks which the other side finds difficult. Indeed the two sides are logically incompatible. The right side synthesizes space; the left side, time and, hence, can better handle the sequences of speech. People whose lateralization is incomplete have a reduction in either the perceptual or verbal function. If an organization selects its members for verbal–conceptual activity, for example, to work in a scientific technologic environment, both hemispheres of these persons will show the functional development typical of the left hemisphere.

In other words, specialists who actually lack full lateralization and full functional differentiation of the two hemispheres are chosen for the work. Levy postulates that, unlike the right-handed person, these persons have some right-hemispheric as well as the classic left-hemispheric language capability. This bilateral language component intrusion on the right hemisphere interferes with the typically right hemisphere visuospatial mode. This was demonstrated by comparing 10 left-handed graduate science students with 15 who were right-handed. The verbal intelligence of the two groups was the same, i.e., I.Q. 142 and 138, respectively. But there was a large difference in the visuospatial performance scale with the left-handed scoring 117 as against the right-handed group's 130. Thus there was a significant difference between their verbal and visuospatial performances. The left-handed subjects' drive to develop a high level of verbal facility had interfered with their visuospatial performance, presumably by preempting some right hemisphere capability.

Levy asks two questions: Does the typical left-handed person have a superior ability to use language and numbers derived from the transmodal fusion of concepts? Is the survival of the species optimized when a certain number of its members who are neither hunters nor food gatherers are specialized for pure reasoning? In fact it appears that our civilization currently emphasizes left over right hemispheric thinking in the educational process and the rewards for success. The long-term consequences of such specialization have been hinted at by Toynbee (1972) and are discussed in Chapter 11.

Levy speculates that the requirements of a nonliterate food-gatherer society would differ markedly from ours. Yet this was the condition for which our brain was evolved. Those human strains may have survived the best where the majority were generalists, but a minority were already specialists. Assuming that there are different functions to be performed such as hunting, which requires right hemisphere activity, and planning for the hunt, which requires the left hemisphere, then, even at this stage, some specialization is to be expected. For optimum efficiency, she says, there will be a few able planners and many able hunters. If communication by language is feasible, such an arrangement would prove more efficient than one composed of hunters alone.

The presence of a few planners whose advice led to success would soon, by simple conditioning, lead the group to turn to them for guidance. A situation might then develop in which there were a modest number with functionally symmetric hemispheres. Compared with hunters, they would be relatively deficient in depth perception, visual memory, recognition of forms, and directional discrimination of movement. Hence, in the field they would be less able "to make a synthesis of small clues and so spot a lurking lion embedded as a hidden figure in the tall savannah grass." But at the campsite, their better verbalization, logic, and analytic capacity would make them invaluable. Levy concludes that a natural selective advantage went with a differentiation based on some degree of organization for linear, analytic, conceptual thought-processing versus an organization for visuospatial forms. By developing asymmetry, it was possible to utilize the benefits of language without at the same time producing fatal deficiencies in perceptual organization.

Functional differences between the two hemispheres

As Harlow et al. (1971) point out, the classic discipline of psychology has emphasized the directed aspects of thought, the formation of concepts, and the solution of problems with relation to objects in the external environment. There is, however, another thought mode: This is nondirected and involves daydreaming, dreams, and fantasy. One may prove to be just as important as the other for balanced social behavior.

Evidence that this difference is due to physiologic differences between the hemispheres has been discussed by Ornstein (1972, 1973) in two recent texts. It is also argued by Bogen (1969) in his discussion of "the other side of the brain." Bogen contrasts the various types of mental processes, such as digital versus analog and verbal or propositional versus visuospatial and appositional thinking. He comments that each of us appears to have two minds, which differ in content and possibly even in goals and most certainly in respect to mode of organization. The dual system increases the chance of a solution to a novel problem, but it carries the penalty of an increased likelihood of internal conflict. He comments that man, the most innovative of species, is at the same time most at odds with himself (Bogen and Bogen, 1969).

Major implications of the right and left

specializations of the sociocultural brain into separate functioning segments have been discussed recently by Galin (1976) who makes clear that this approach brings certain psychoanalytic concepts into the sphere of objective neurophysiology. He presents the hypothesis that in normal people mental events in the right hemisphere can become disconnected functionally from the left hemisphere by the inhibition of neuronal transmission across the corpus callosum. Galin suggests that they can continue a life of their own in the isolated hemisphere and argues that this implies a neurophysiologic mechanism for repression and an anatomic locus for some unconscious mental contents (Galin, 1976).

Galin's generalizations rest on the massive contributions of Sperry and his associates which have triggered a flood of research on hemispheric function (Dimond and Beaumont, 1974; Sperry, 1974). There is now overwhelming evidence that the sociocultural brain on the left side is organized in a different mode from that on the right. Levy (1974) summarizes the distinction as follows: The left hemisphere dominates when a verbal response is required, for it is specialized for the analytic linear-mode information-processing critical for the peculiarly human capacity for speech. It is also responsible for those nonverbal responses that depend on the recall of auditory images or when linguistic processing is called for, or when abstract conceptualizing based on reason is needed. These are all functions which the right hemisphere performs poorly or not at all.

On the other hand, the right hemisphere is dominant for all visual-matching tasks, regardless of whether the material can or cannot be named, i.e., regardless of whether it can be grasped as a whole or can be analyzed. The right hemisphere is a concrete spatial synthesizer which maps a visuostructural realm. This is nicely illustrated by Fig. 6-2 which shows the superior performance of the left hand of a right-handed man when copying three-dimensional figures. Because his corpus callosum had been cut, the two

hemispheres of this man could not communicate. He could drive his left hand, whose motor skills were poor, by a right hemisphere, whose visuospatial capacities were superior. The other combination put the skillful right hand at the mercy of a visuospatially inept left hemisphere. The outcome was that the left hand-right hemisphere combination did the better job, despite lack of dexterity (Gazzaniga, 1967).

The right hemisphere is specialized for primary process thinking and nonverbal presentations and is more concerned with multiple, simultaneous interactions than with temporal sequencing. The distinction is between the left hemisphere temporal analyzer, which maps input into the details of language structure and is concerned with the abstractions of reason, and the right hemisphere, which is responsible for mental fluency and imagination.

Levy (1974) has illustrated this by arranging that the two sensory images perceived in the right and left brain shall be different and conflicting. Figure 6-3 shows how a visual stimulus such as a portrait can be split down the middle and then recombined and jointed at the midline to make a composite left–right chimera or grotesque monster. The split figure is flashed to the subject whose gaze is centered. The missing half of each image tends to be filled in by each hemisphere as it strives to complete the portrait. Since each hemisphere is cut off from the conscious experience of the other in patients with a split brain, these persons remain unaware of the discrepancy between the left and right halves of these composite stimuli. The left brain verbally describes the face of a man with dark eyebrows and a moustache; the silent right brain ignores the man in a row of faces, and the hands point to the girl who formed the other half of the chimera.

Figure 6-4 indicates that before language develops in the second to third year of life, the child can explore the world with either hand and will establish engrams equally in the two cerebral hemispheres (Fig. 6-

EXAMPLE   LEFT HAND   RIGHT HAND

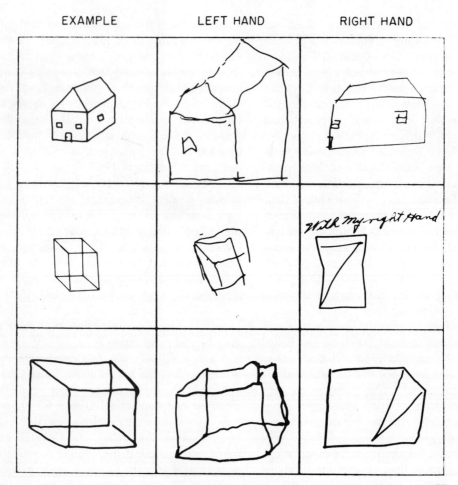

Fig. 6-2. Visual–constructional tasks are handled better by the right hemisphere. A patient whose corpus callosum has been cut, severing connections between the two hemispheres, is left with two possibilities. He can use either his left hand–right hemisphere or his right hand–left hemisphere combination. As the figure shows, the copies he made of three-dimensional drawings with his right hand were inferior, since this task was solely driven by the left hemisphere which lacks visuospatial synthesis. The left hand–right hemisphere combination did a better job, despite lack of dexterity in this right-handed man *(Gazzaniga, 1967).*

4A). Indeed, at this stage there may be little interhemispheric communication. But with maturation, as Fig. 6-4B indicates, the early bilateral verbal processes reorganize, and those on the right shrink in favor of those on the left. Finally at maturity there has been extensive lateralization (Fig. 6-4C). The right hemisphere becomes a visual-spatial processor and calculator; its capacity to analyze words is actually suppressed by transcallosal inhibitory activity, as shown by the arrow. The left hemisphere takes charge,

becoming responsible for syntax, grammar, speech organization, and mathematical manipulations, as well as the activities of a central processing control (Gazzaniga, 1974).

Because it controls language, the left hemisphere system inevitably gains an advantage over the right in a human social context; it powerfully manipulates others and is vital for securing reinforcement from them.

Galin supports Bogen's proposal that

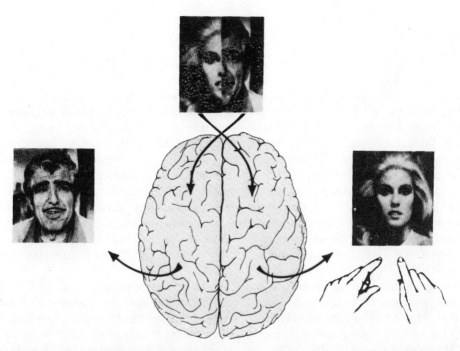

Fig. 6-3. A split figure is flashed on the screen to a patient whose brain has been split by cutting the corpus callosum. If he centers his gaze, the right hemisphere perceives only the left half of the figure, and consequently if asked to respond nonverbally by picking the image he sees out of a group, he must point to and identify the girl. But if asked to say in words what he sees, then he must rely on his left hemisphere; so he describes the man with dark eyebrows and a moustache. *(From Trevarthen, 1974.* © *1974, John Wiley & Sons, Inc. Reprinted by permission.)*

Fig. 6-4. The three parts of this speculative figure indicate stages in the lateralization of cerebral dominance during maturation. In (A) the young child exploring the world uses both hands freely as he establishes patterns in each cerebral hemisphere. At this stage, there is probably little interhemispheric communication. (B) But, as cerebral dominance is established after eight years of age, the original bilateral verbal processes reorganize with those in the right hemisphere, retreating in favor of those in the left. (C) Finally, in the adult a central processor or final decision system in the left hemisphere collects information from throughout the brain. The right hemisphere appears to be inhibited from taking on a similar function. *(From Gazzaniga, 1974.* © *1974, John Wiley & Sons, Inc. Reprinted by permission.)*

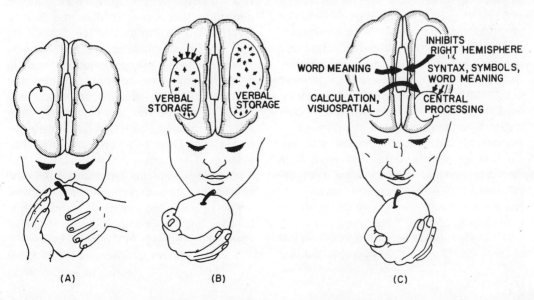

just as there is central control of sensory input for the sensory modalities, there may also be control over the access of right hemisphere activity to the left hemisphere across the corpus callosum (Bogen, 1969; Bogen and Bogen, 1969). It has been said that in the daily life of a technocracy there is little need for the integration of holistic thought of the right hemisphere with the analytic approach of the left, and that the traffic between our two hemispheres may be light compared with the traffic between the frontal and temporal regions within the left or the right hemispheric system. Galin suggests that each hemisphere may treat the weak contralateral input in the same way that men treat observations that do not fit in with their beliefs. First they are ignored; then if insistent, they are actively avoided (Galin, 1976).

Lateralization of emotion

Recent work by Gur et al. (1975) has capitalized on a subtle side effect of the functional asymmetry of the brain. A clue as to the side of maximal cerebral activation is given by the direction of unconscious, minor conjugate, lateral eye movements that are always going on. When reflecting on a question presented by someone facing him, a subject will every now and again briefly avert his eyes by a few degrees. This can be observed, and on the basis of the direction of this eye-flick, he can be classified either as a right or a left eye mover or as bidirectional. Bakan (1969) has hypothesized that this eye directionality is symptomatic of an easier triggering of activity in the hemisphere contralateral to the direction of eye movement. Personality differences between left eye movers and right eye movers have been demonstrated that are consistent with the functional differences between the left verbal–analytical and the right spatial–synthetic or holistic cerebral hemispheres.

Thus in a bold conclusion based on this observation, Gur et al. (1975) predicted that left eye movers would prefer to sit on the right side and vice versa (Fig. 6-5A), and they demonstrated that right-handed subjects are more concerned with sitting on the left side of the classroom for "hard" verbal and analytic topics, such as mathematics and science, than when listening to more synthetic topics like art and the "soft" sciences (Fig. 6-5B). It appears that persons who are moving their eyes to the right because of left-hemispheric stimulation tend to sit on the left side of the room because they prefer not to glance at the wall and vice versa.

Recently Schwartz et al. (1975) also capitalized on this tendency of right-handed subjects to look to the right when their left hemisphere is predominantly involved in processing information. They found that among intact right-handed subjects emotionally charged questions elicit greater right-hemispheric activation than comparable nonemotional questions. Indeed, the affective quality could be distinguished from the more cognitive demands of the questions. Questions requiring both spatial and emotional processing resulted in accentuated right-hemispheric activation; and those demanding both verbal and nonemotional processes, the reverse. An example of a verbal nonemotional question was, "What is meant by the proverb: One today is worth two tomorrows?"; a spatial nonemotional question, "On a quarter does the face of George Washington look to the right or the left?"; a verbal emotional query, "For you is anger or hate a stronger emotion?"; and in a spatial emotional context, "Picture and describe the last situation in which you cried." The data resulting from these carefully constructed and tested lists are shown in Fig. 6-6. There is a significant difference in terms of both left ($p < 0.01$) and right ($p < 0.001$) eye movement frequencies. They concluded that their experiment provides new support for the hypothesis of a special role for the right hemisphere in the regulation of emotional processes in the intact human.

Galin's review enumerates some further

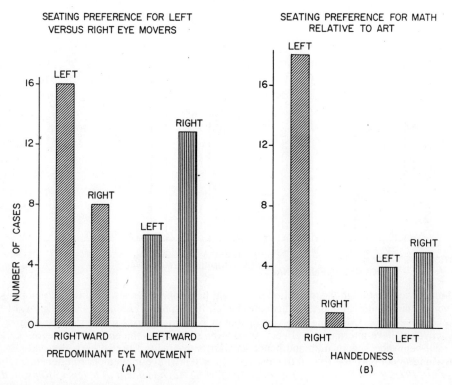

Fig. 6-5.   The directionality of conjugate lateral eye movements can be used as a measure of more easily triggered activity in the hemisphere contralateral to the direction of that movement. The figure (A) shows that when rightward movement of the eyes is being stimulated, persons prefer to sit on the left side of the room and vice versa ($p < 0.05$), and (B) right-handed persons listening to "hard" topics, such as science lectures (left hemisphere activation), prefer to sit on the left. When listening to "soft" topics, such as art (right hemisphere activation), this preference is significantly weaker ($p < 0.05$) *(From Gur et al., 1975.* © *1975, American Psychological Association. Reprinted by permission.)*

evidence of interhemispheric difference in affect (Galin, 1976). He notes that the coping strategy adopted after injury to the left hemisphere differs from that after injury to the right, and there is evidence that the emotional responses differ also. Injury to the less dominant hemisphere is much more often accompanied by denial or by what has been called "la belle indifference" toward the consequent disability. The person with right-hemispheric damage will claim there is nothing wrong with him. By contrast, injury to the dominant hemisphere is more often associated with an acute awareness of the loss and accompanying depression. Similarly, when a small amount of anesthetic is injected into the carotid leading to the left hemi-

sphere, it provokes despair, guilt, and worry about the future far more often than when the same dose is given on the right side. Extensive studies of unilateral electroconvulsive shock treatment suggest a differentiated role of the two hemispheres: the right hemisphere shock being more effective than the left.

Finally, some people are likely to be so influenced by the tilt of a frame around an illuminated rod they are viewing in the dark that they will move it so it is aligned with the frame instead of the sensed vertical; such persons are known as field dependent. Others resist this and perceive the sensed vertical accurately; they are termed field independent. Berent and Silverman showed that

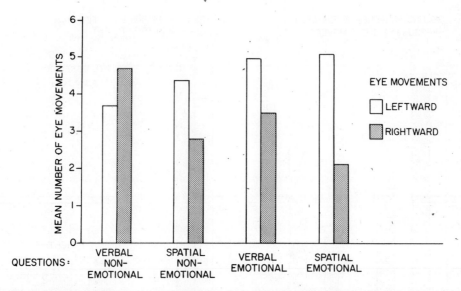

Fig. 6-6. Evidence that in the intact brain, the right hemisphere has a special role in emotions. Abstract, verbal, nonemotional questions activate the left hemisphere, producing more rightward conjugate eye movements. Questions involving spatial or verbal responses with accompanying emotional activation have intermediate effects. Finally the spatial plus the emotional categories maximize right-hemispheric activation and hence leftward movement. The two extremes differ significantly in terms of both left ($p < 0.01$) and right ($p < 0.001$) eye-movement frequencies. *(From Schwartz et al., 1975. © 1975, American Association for the Advancement of Science. Reprinted by permission.)*

highly field-dependent mental patients discriminated pairs of forms better than pairs of words (Cohen et al., 1973). To them this suggested a relative left-hemispheric deficiency. They argued that electroshock therapy (ECT) to the left hemisphere should make their rod and frame error-score higher, i.e., make them still more field dependent. The result confirmed this. All 12 patients with ECT on the left side showed more field dependence after treatment. But to the surprise of Cohen and his co-workers, all of their control cases with right-side ECT actually improved, showing more field independence. Thus, field dependence seems to be associated with a relative right-hemispheric dominance rather than a dysfunction of the left hemisphere. For had field dependence been due solely to left-hemispheric deficiency, the right-sided ECT of the controls would not have affected the results (Cohen et al., 1973).

Galin notes that the characteristics of

persons with high field dependence have been regarded by our social system as inferior and primitive. Reviewing the evidence on culture and life style, he points out, for example, that the unitary world view of some Pacific Islanders can be contrasted with our linear analytic style and viewed as an emphasis on the right as opposed to the left hemispheric skills. Field-dependent subjects may then relate better to a global integrative mode, which, in turn, relates better to the biogrammer of the limbic system than to the linear analytic mode of the field independent (Galin, 1976).

Flor-Henry (1976) has considered the previously mentioned studies and has added further observations of his own, suggesting that affective responses may be a function of the nondominant hemisphere. He speculates that the connections from the new association cortex in the right parietal and frontal regions to the limbic system determine affective responses. Paradoxically they appear to do so under the monitoring and control of frontal mechanisms in the left dominant hemisphere.

Cerebral lateralization and sexual differentiation in man

In man, important aspects of his recently evolved sexual differentiation of behavior depend on the neocortex and on lateral specialization (Hamburg, 1975). In female but not male newborn, the left superior temporal region in which the speech facility is to develop is already larger than the right. This specialization and earlier maturation in the left hemisphere is compatible with female attentiveness to and preference for verbal interaction in contrast with the male interest in rough and tumble motor skills. The greater verbal skills of preadolescent girls as opposed to boys of the same age is well documented. By simultaneously presenting different stimuli to the right and left eyes or ears, functional differentiation along a verbal–nonverbal dimension has been demonstrated. These tests show that young males are more proficient at processing nonverbal stimuli. An additional factor favoring girls is that in mother–infant interaction they often receive more verbal stimulation than boys, thus further enhancing the verbal skills that are so important in the practice of attachment behavior or social bonding (Hamburg, 1974, 1975).

A long learning period with an intense mother–infant attachment and a developed language permit the transfer of information from the sociocultural brain of one generation to that of the next one. Detailed information of the flora and fauna of diverse areas, the knowledge of animal cycles, and the recall of rare events are vital to group survival. The male with his greater proficiency in spatial tasks has been shown to be dependent on nondominant hemisphere activity. As noted previously, in persons with split brains whose corpus callosum has been severed, this hemisphere has been shown to be superior in the recognition of geometric figures and spatial representation in special tests using nonverbal expression. Similarly, though behind on verbal tests in the evaluation of spatial disorientation, boys more than eight years old did better than girls.

Male–female specialization of function regarding the hemispheres gives the species an evolutionary advantage. The superiority of women in verbal skills may reflect the need to communicate with the young which encouraged the use of language for teaching. These skills become supremely important as language contributes to the increasingly complex social organization of the hunter–gatherers. On the other hand, man's superiority in spatial skills as contrasted with those of other primates is connected to hunting with weapons over a huge territorial range. The adaptive advantages for hunting, warfare, and gathering food, of having excellent topographic localization and a good sense of geography and terrain are evident. Spatial skills are also related to the aimed throwing of objects at animals of prey. As man evolved, his accurate use of weapons at a distance offset the effectiveness of the specialized predators (Hamburg, 1974, 1975).

The limbic system: affect and programmed behavior

The concept that certain subcortical regions are involved with emotion was convincingly advanced by Papez (1937). Starting with MacLean (1958), the combined efforts of many workers have demonstrated that the phylogenetically old cingulate, the hippocampal cortex, and, related structures have a profound importance in emotional behavior (Fig. 6-7).

MacLean points out that a clue to the function of the paleocortex and of the nuclei of the limbic system is given by the fact that intense emotions and drives accompany the

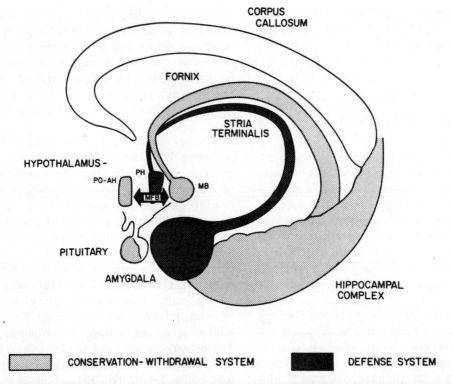

Fig. 6-7. This highly schematic diagram shows the relation of two important temporal lobe structures to the hypothalamus. It depicts the connections of the hippocampus and contrasts them with those of the amygdala. The fornix is shown as it leads from the hippocampus to the mammillary body, thence via the medial forebrain bundle (MFB) to the preoptic anterior hypothalamic region (PO-AH). (The pituitary actually lies medial to the temporal lobes and has been enlarged and placed in a slightly anterior position.) The stria terminalis connects portions of the amygdalar nuclear complex with the defense system in the posterior hypothalamus (PH), which in turn activates the sympathetic system.

march of an epileptic attack that has its origin in this region and passes through the various parts of the circuit. The electroencephalographic and neuroanatomic evidence shows the close connection of the limbic cortex with the hypothalamus. MacLean (1975) sees the septal–hippocampal region as working with the striatal complex in establishing the ancestrally learned territorial and attachment behaviors connected with the preservation of the species. He enumerates on selecting homesites, establishing and defending territory, hunting, mating, rearing young, and forming social hierarchies. He suggests that the corpus striatum and the globus pallidus are repositories for a biogrammer of inherited motor acts which can be integrated with well-learned behavior patterns. They are under the influence of the limbic paleocortex, and the question arises as to how these patterns become integrated into the activities of the new brain cortical systems.

Insight into the general aspects of limbic function comes from the final chapter of Isaacson's (1974) recent text on the limbic system. The extrahypothalamic parts of the system clearly exert a regulatory influence on the hypothalamus and the midbrain. In effect, the limbic or emotional brain regulates the programmed instinctively determined drive systems. A close relationship with the primary process of the nondominant or right hemisphere is not surprising. For Flor-Henry (1976) and Schwartz et al. (1975) have both presented evidence that the nondominant hemisphere is the most closely related to the emotional response system and hence to the limbic structures. Thus the pathway from the logical analyzer of the left hemisphere to the value-attaching mechanisms of the subcortical regions appears to be across the corpus callosum and via the nondominant right hemisphere. This region, which recent observations would connect with fantasy, dreaming, and gestalt thinking, i.e., the primary process, proves to be a critical link between the language-processing, analyzing, left sociocultural brain and the neuroendocrine response systems of the more primitive limbic structures and the hypothalamus.

The hippocampus and territory: the amygdala and reward

The ancient hippocampal complex is paleocortex. It is a part of the forebrain's layered sheets of neurons that form a more readily programmed computer. It contributes flexibility to the limbic system which itself represents a new higher control superimposed on the ancient, rigid system of the reptiles and the more primitive vertebrates. The suppression of one behavior and the substitution of a more appropriate one, a hallmark of the mammal with his new cortex, are attributed to the intervention of the limbic system. Apparently the more the forebrain tissue increases during the phylogeny of mammals, the greater their ease in forming temporary associations. According to Isaacson (1974), the hippocampal paleocortex comes into action during times of uncertainty, thus permitting the organism to suppress the accustomed way of responding by initiating behavioral changes based on new information. With the vastly greater forebrain development in primates, much of this new data will come from the still more adaptable neocortical association areas via the frontal lobes.

As the previous chapters have indicated, one of the most important factors controlling the behavior of mammals is an awareness of their exact position in the often rapidly shifting social hierarchy. This is crucial for primates, but even so simple a social mammal as a mouse must know its place in the social structure. In our own laboratories, Ely et al. (1976) have made a detailed analysis of the 24-hour/day behavior of male mice interacting socially in a complex population cage equipped with a sensor at the portal of each of the eight chambers. They noticed a dramatic change in behavior which included a loss of difference between the behavioral patterns of the dominant and the subordinates in a group of mice with hippocampal lesions (Fig. 6-8).

The normal behavioral constraint which forces the subordinate to restrain his movements in the urgent search for food and water and to avoid the places marked by the dominant as his territory was missing in those with hippocampal lesions. They are not concerned with each other's behavior, and males eat freely in each other's presence. Their normal aggressive male defense of territory is replaced by flight, but it is suspected they do not use the strategy of freezing and the gestures of submission. Ely et al. (1976, 1977) suggest that the hippocampal lesions lead to a modification of emotional control in a colony. Their data indicate that mice were confused as to the position of the colony chambers and that this was responsible for their continued high rate of exploratory activity. Having faulty spatial mapping, they failed to identify details of territory and consequently could not initiate aggression and establish a hierarchy despite intact amygdalar fight–flight mechanisms.

The proposal of O'Keefe and Nadel (O'Keefe and Dostrovsky, 1971) suggesting that the hippocampus functions as a cognitive mapping system has recently been confirmed by others. They see the structure as providing information for place-learning (O'Keefe et al., 1975) by which the organism knows how to approach or how to avoid a particular location in the environment by any available route. The hippocampus appears to have a modifiable neural map

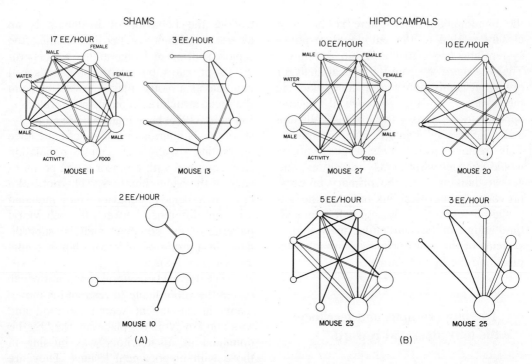

SHAMS   HIPPOCAMPALS

17 EE/HOUR   3 EE/HOUR   10 EE/HOUR   10 EE/HOUR

MOUSE 11   MOUSE 13   MOUSE 27   MOUSE 20

2 EE/HOUR   5 EE/HOUR   3 EE/HOUR

MOUSE 10   MOUSE 23   MOUSE 25

(A)   (B)

Fig. 6-8. Contrasting the behavior of a control group of mice with one having hippocampal lesions. In the sham-operated group a dominant (Mouse 11) emerges whose behavior differs from those of the subordinates, i.e., greater box entry and exit rate (EE) and use of all available boxes. Note how little the subordinated Mouse 10 moves. The lesioned mice do not show this restraint. They act freely in each other's presence, and a dominant mouse cannot be identified *(Ely et al., 1976).*

containing cells which represent the spatial arrangements among the features of an environment; these cells locate the animal's position within that environment. There is also evidence of a system of cells which signals a mismatch between the stored representation of the environment and the animal's present perception of it. When a mismatch is perceived, exploratory activity is generated; the animal then ceases to practice old patterns and rapidly learns new information with which to update the cognitive map into a pattern more suitable for the new facts of the situation. Whereas, O'Keefe and co-workers discuss this primarily in terms of location in the physical space, the ethologist's concept of territory includes that of social dominance and of subtle positioning within a hierarchy, and we would point to a role for the hippocampus in this crucial aspect of social behavior.

O'Keefe et al. (1975) have recently demonstrated that rats with lesions in the fornix (a major afferent–efferent pathway of the hippocampus) failed on a water-finding task when place learning was required but succeeded in the same task when simple cue learning of associating a light with the water was the only requirement. This evidence that the hippocampus functions as a cognitive mapping system is supported by Pisa's related studies of impaired incidental place-learning in fornicotomized rats using an *H* maze. Lesioned rats had significant impairment of information about place location (Pisa, 1976). Branch and co-workers have also followed up on the proposal by O'Keefe and Dostrovsky. By using an eight-arm radial maze designed to maximize the spatial aspects of behavioral organization in animals, they found that single cell activity in the dorsal hippocampus was determined by spatial characteristics encountered during a discrimination task in the maze. The spatial characteristics of all cells were stable and persisted for repeated samplings of the same maze space. They viewed their data as supporting the O'Keefe and Nadel hypothesis that the hippocampus is intimately involved in spatially organized behavior (Branch et al. 1976).

The role of the more primitive amygdalar nuclear complex was seen by Isaacson to be an accentuation of arousal and activation of the hypothalamic system when conditions are appropriate. In their analysis of the brain's reward system, Rolls (1975) and Isaacson (1974) follow up on Olds's (1976) discovery in the 1950's that electrical stimulation of the appropriate pathways in the brain will provide reward, and that animals will learn a task and work to obtain stimulation. Motivational behavior, such as eating and drinking, is rewarded by sensory stimuli that can be shown to have the same effect on the hypothalamic cells as the psychic stimulus. This only occurs as long as these animals are in a susceptible state due to hunger or thirst. But, whereas the hypothalamus is the effector for responses to brain stimulation, the amygdala is higher up the line, receiving sensory inputs, and by attaching "value" to them, connects them to the reward or punishment mode. Animals with bilateral damage to the amygdala have difficulty in discriminating between the various naturally rewarding and aversive stimuli. They cannot choose between food and poison, nor do they avoid punishing situations. This region appears to give positive and negative value to stimuli, and, in turn allows a sensory stimulus to influence the hypothalamic reward level (Rolls, 1975).

Evidence is presented in Chapter 7 that the hippocampus and the orbitofrontal part of the sociocultural brain system may be involved in generating the depressive behavior that develops after a defeat, when the organism loses control of his position in social space and his access to desiderata. On the other hand, the amygdalar complex of the limbic system appears critical for making reward or avoidance judgments that are crucial for maintaining the organism's value

system and hence for the vigorous pursuit of desiderata (Rolls, 1975).

Patterns of thinking and susceptibility to psychosomatic disease

The question arises as to whether these great subdivisions between the cerebral systems, i.e., between the right and left hemispheres, and between their analytic and synthetic cognitive functions, on the one hand, and the affects of the related limbic system on the other, can be related to subjective patterns of emotion and experience. Galin's suggestion that inhibition of neuronal transmission across the cerebral commissures can lead to a functional disconnection between the hemispheres gives a neuropsychologic mechanism for some aspects of repression and an anatomic locus in the right hemisphere for the primary process with its access to "unconscious" mental contents through fantasy and dreams. As Galin (1976), Gazzaniga (1974), and Bogen and Bogen (1969) have all proposed, activation and deactivation of the psychoanalyst's unconscious may be a matter of suppression and release of interhemispheric traffic by the neurons of the corpus callosum.

The presence of frontal–limbic pathways connecting the cognitive with the affective sphere raises the further question whether there may not also be a psychologic consequence of a similar inhibition of communication between the limbic and the cognitive systems. Figure 6-9 attempts to illustrate the possible relation of well-known psychologic concepts to the major functional subdivisions of the central nervous system described previously. Following the thesis of Altman (1966) and MacLean (1976), the brain is divided into the three systems which have been superimposed on one another in the course of evolution. There is the medulla which, together with the mesencephalon and the hypothalamus, takes care of the basic

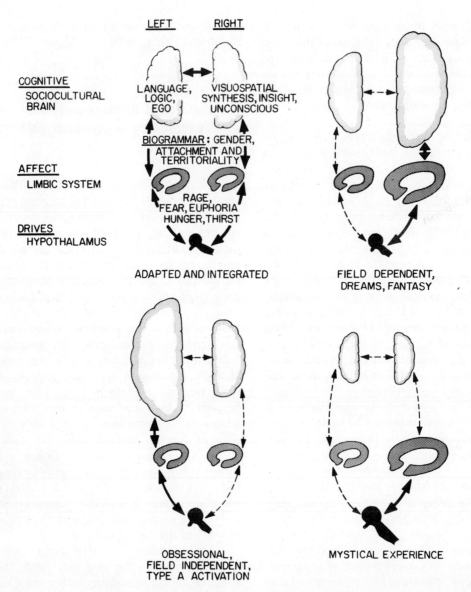

Fig. 6-9. A schematic of the relation between the three systems of the human brain: the cognitive, using the association cortex; the limbic, dealing with affects; and the hypothalamic, the locus of basic drive mechanisms. New theories of the role of interhemispheric communication and of the connections between the three basic systems have led to this schema, depicting the relation of familiar psychologic concepts to these major functional subdivisions of the brain. Different states of consciousness and possible mechanisms of their production are presented. See text for details.

needs of the organism, such as to maintain metabolism and to reproduce. The next level is that of modifiable capacities which meet what MacLean calls self- and species-preservative needs. These are identified by Altman with paleocephalic control of recurrent catering activities which are intimately associated with feelings and emotions. Finally,

for Altman, there is the neencephalon found only in mammals which is responsible for novel, variable, highly adaptive cognitive activities displayed in response to new challenges. This he calls the cognitive integrative level. In man, this development is so overwhelming that it may be considered as a new sociocultural brain. The left and right subdivisions of the hemispheres constitute two more systems corresponding to the ego and the personal unconscious. The corpus callosum connects the two hemispheres and can inhibit the transmission of stimuli between them to a varying degree by repression (Galin, 1976).

The limbic system is credited, among other things, with gender identity and the instincts of attachment and territoriality. Tiger and Fox (1972) might consider it the locus of biogrammer activities. The diagram (Fig. 6-9) is replicated with modifications to cover four states of significance in relation to the theory of psychosomatic disease.

In the first portion, integration and adaptation are depicted as a state in which there is free access of information between the right and the left hemispheres and between the affective and the cognitive systems. Equal size is therefore given to each form.

In the second portion of the diagram, which represents neuroticism with its related fantasy, field dependence, and dream states, the size of the right hemisphere and the right limbic system to which it is connected by the right frontal–limbic pathway is drawn larger than that of the left to emphasize that the right side is the functionally dominant region in this mode. The transcallosal arrows are reduced to indicate poor communication with the left hemisphere, i.e., the ego. This would be on a fluctuating basis of the type already demonstrated for the classic sensory pathways (Livingston, 1976). A similar failure of transcallosal communication is suggested in the field-independent obsessional: the person with the so-called Type A personality—this is the alexithymia of Sifneos et al. (1978) and may be related to an impaired emotional expression associated with an increased susceptibility to disease, such as lung cancer.

The domination by the left hemisphere and the downgrading of right-hemispheric activities, including communication with the limbic system and its biogrammar, are indicated by the increased size given to the left side.

Finally, the last section of the diagram suggests that in meditational states there is a shift of emphasis from the cognitive to the affective mechanisms and even to the basic drives of the brain stem itself.*

The evidence that susceptibility to chronic diseases can be increased by a defect in the mechanism for the expression of emotion is detailed in Chapter 10, where Kissen's (1967) painstakingly acquired evidence on approximately 1000 inpatients in hospital chest departments awaiting medical diagnosis is discussed. In nearly 50 percent, the final diagnosis was lung cancer. Kissen observed a disturbance of emotions before anyone had identified the condition as cancer. Greer and Morris (1975) have recently developed evidence of a similar mechanism in breast cancer. Friedman and Rosenman (1974) have indicated that one of the deficiencies of the Type A person in our society is in emotional expression. Such a person is especially prone to think in objective terms and is numbers oriented. In their earlier work, Nemiah and Sifneos (1970) regarded "operational thinking," (first described by Marty and de M'Uzan (1963)) as characteristic of patients with psychosomatic disease, observing that these persons have impoverished fantasy lives and very poor dream recall. But in further work, Sifneos used the word alexithymia (of Greek derivation: "a" for lack, "lexis" for work, and "thymos" for emotion) to describe these characteristics and has published a number of papers on the subject which are referenced in his latest work (Sifneos et al., 1978).

Sifneos sees the condition as one in which feelings exist but are denied. He draws a distinction between feelings and emotions. Others can tell we are experiencing emotion because of our behavior and its confirming neuroendocrine changes. Emo-

---

*An alternative Jungian treatment of this problem is presented by J. P. Henry as "Comment" to Dr. Ernest Rossi's paper, "The Cerebral Hemispheres in Analytical Psychology," in the *Journal of Analytical Psychology* 22(1):52–57 (January), 1977.

tions are based in the limbic system. Feelings, by contrast, involve subjective fantasies and thoughts. According to Sifneos, emotions do not necessarily require neocortical activity but feelings do. Alexithymia as a disorder of feeling may thus apply to the deficiency in interhemispheric communication postulated by Galin.

Twenty-five patients suffering from diseases, such as asthma, hypertension, and ulcerative colitis, were compared with 15 controls from a psychiatric hospital staff by Sifneos who used a special questionnaire. He repeatedly demonstrated alexithymic traits in more than half of the psychosomatic group but the number of traits in the

Table 6-1. *Contrast between the Characteristics of Alexithymic and Neurotic Patients*[a]

	Alexithymic	Neurotic
Presenting complaints	Endless description of physical symptoms, at times unrelated to underlying medical illness	Less emphasis on physical complaints; elaborate description of psychologic difficulties (symptoms or interpersonal problems or both)
Other complaints	Tension, irritability, frustration, pain, boredom, void, restlessness, agitation, nervousness	Anxiety described as fantasies and thoughts rather than physical sensations; depression described as feelings of worthlessness, guilt during sleepless nights, etc.
Thought content	Striking absence of fantasies and elaborate description of trivial environmental details (*pensée opératoire*)	Rich fantasy life; marked ability to eloquently describe feelings
Language	Marked difficulty in finding appropriate words to describe feelings	Appropriate words to describe feelings
Crying	Rare; at times copious but seems unrelated to appropriate feeling, such as sadness or anger	Appropriate to specific feeling
Dreaming	Rare	Often
Affect	Inappropriate	Appropriate
Activity	Tendency to act impulsively; action seems to be a predominant way of life	Action appropriate to situation
Interpersonal relations	Usually poor, with tendency toward dependency or preference for being alone, avoiding people	Specific conflicts with people but generally good interpersonal relations
Personality makeup	Narcissistic, withdrawn, passive–aggressive or passive–dependent, psychopathic	Flexible
Posture	Rigid	Flexible
Countertransference	Interviewer or therapist is usually bored by patient who they find frightfully ''dull''	Easy communication with patient who the interviewer or therapist finds ''interesting''
Relationship to social, educational, economic, or cultural background	None	Considerable

[a]Sifneos et al. (1978) have contrasted the characteristics of the alexithymic who is suspected of faulty interhemispheric communication with consequently impaired perception of emotions with the neurotic whose emotions are obtrusive.

control group was significantly smaller. Sifneos contrasts the neurotic with the alexithymic patient, painting a vivid picture of the two (Table 6-1). An important clue may be that following commissurotomy, as reported by Hoppe (1975), dreams, fantasy, and symbols are deficient. Such studies question the function of the one to two hours of dreaming-sleep the average human being experiences every day. Could there be some sort of deficiency of interhemispheric communication in social groups and individuals who have an abnormal lack of activities demanding fantasy, who do not pray or meditate, who do not dream with recall, who devalue poetry and art?

Galin's (1976) observations suggesting a disturbance in interhemispheric transfer of information is at the basis of a split between the ego and the unconscious has been equated with alexithymia as suggested by Sifneos. A similar concept may be applied to the limbic system which is the locus of the programs of self- and species-preservative behavior; here, a deficiency may be termed neurotic or dyssymbolic. The hypothesis may be formulated that it is as important to have continued communication between the limbic system and the cortex as between the hemispheres. This transfer of information may occur especially during dreaming sleep. It has been held that dreams represent information coming from the various "depths" of the unconscious. If Galin (1976) is correct, dreams might represent information coming from the limbic system by way of the right hemisphere during the special state of rapid-eye-movement (REM) sleep.

Experimental sleep disturbance and failure of communication between the limbic system and the neocortex

In a detailed neurophysiologic analysis of the function of dreaming, Jouvet (1975) attached great importance to the high level of REM sleep *in utero* and immediately after

birth. In reviewing the phylogenetic evolution of dreaming, he also noted that there were no signs of the REM phase of sleep in amphibians or reptiles. Jouvet hypothesized that REM sleep is needed for the increasingly complex nervous system of mammals. Perhaps mammals, especially the young, have special problems in adapting and matching their old brain of reptilian inheritance to the learned behavioral patterns worked out by the superimposed neocortex. Jouvet postulated that, since cellular growth and differentiation continue in the brain while the young mammal is developing its final patterns of behavior, dreaming or the REM phase may be important in the organization of the biogrammar of complicated behavioral sequences that involve the defense of territory, hunting, and mating. He suggests that the function of dreaming may be to stimulate neurons that command a network responsible for programming patterns of behavior characteristic of the species' response. These patterns would be related to incoming stimuli derived from the experiences of the individual. Such programming, he said, would not likely occur during wakefulness when the command neurons were responding to external stimuli, but the alteration of synapses through learning in response to the needs of genetic programming might occur during REM sleep when the command neurons were less engaged by the environment.

Recent work is compatible with this theory. Lucero (1970) observed that the duration of REM sleep increases after a learning experience. This observation was confirmed and extended in several other studies by various groups (Fishbein et al., 1974; Hennevin et al., 1974; Smith et al., 1974). If REM sleep is prevented for two to three hours immediately after the experience, a deficit in learning occurs. Kitahama et al. (1975) showed that the REM-suppressing substance α-DOPA slows maze learning, and Pearlman and Becker (1973) found a similar effect when imipramine or chlordiazepoxide was used during bar pressing. Of special interest, from the point of view of social situations, Pearlman and Becker also reported that REM deprivation prevented a rat from assimilating the significance of a companion's skilled bar-pressing behavior. The question arises as to whether the learning involved in the acquisition of territorial and maternal behavior needed by a hierarchially organized colony also falls into the REM-dependent category of a biogrammar.

Earlier chapters indicate that the peer interaction of animals is essential to the development of normal social behavior, and that responses to social cues are poorly established in socially deprived monkeys. We have cited the experiments of Watson et al. (1974) showing that when socially deprived mice were exposed to each other for 30 minutes of social interaction, they had a much higher plasma corticosterone response than group-reared mice. They were also less active in the open field. Furthermore, when these formerly isolated mice were put into a complex population cage, they failed to adapt socially to chronic psychosocial stimulation, with resulting high levels of aggression and hypertension. Thus, repeated social interaction after weaning enables the mice to acquire certain behavior patterns of value during adulthood. These patterns increase the tolerance of external stimuli and modify adult activities so as to decrease the intensity of social stimulation arising within the group.

As Jouvet (1975) and Greenberg and Pearlman (1974) suggest, dreaming or REM sleep may be important to the developing central nervous system as it integrates and reprograms emotionally arousing experiences into fresh social behavioral patterns. If REM sleep does indeed provide opportunity for the adaptation of inherited species-specific repertoires, i.e., biogrammar, to appropriate external cues, then animals repeatedly deprived of all sleep (including REM sleep) following socialization might not exhibit the full effects of early socialization as adults. Watson and Henry (1977a) have recently completed a study to determine whether the socialization of CBA mice

could be inhibited during maturation by systematically depriving them of a few hours of sleep by walking a treadmill following each period of interaction. Figure 6-10 shows the experimental design, which may be viewed as a 2 × 2 factorial, for testing the effects of socialization and treadmill experiences on mice in five different categories. All experiments began and ended with isolation and socialization and treadmill were varied as follows:

Isolation	I
Isolation/socialization	I-SOC
Isolation/treadmill	I-TM
Isolation/treadmill/ socialization	I-TM-SOC
Isolation/socialization/ treadmill	I-SOC-TM

The sequence, treadmill first, then, socialization (I-TM-SOC) would permit mice to sleep immediately after socialization and so to integrate their experiences. The reverse sequence, deferring the treadmill might defer sleep—REM sleep—sufficiently long to impair the memory of socialization in young mice. Thus isolated mice (I) and mice with treadmill (I-TM) or with socialization-

Fig. 6-10. A 2 × 2 factorial design for testing the effects of socialization and treadmill experiences on mice in five different categories (see text). I-SOC includes two and one-half hours of socialization. Each complete horizontal bar represents 24 hours. Shading is proportional to time spent on treadmill and in socialization, and their relative positions represent the sequence of events *(Watson and Henry, 1977a)*.

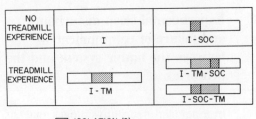

treadmill (I-SOC-TM) were lacking either in social interaction or in the opportunity to sleep immediately after social interaction. Our hypothesis suggests that these mice would develop high blood pressure when exposed to social interaction in a population cage. They would also be aroused by exposure to an open field, which they would explore very little, and would react with elevated corticosterone.

On the other hand, mice with socialization only (I-SOC) and those with treadmill-socialization (I-TM-SOC) might be expected to show good social integration either because of socialization and uninterrupted sleep (no treadmill) or because treadmill preceded daily socialization which permitted them to consolidate their memories and to sleep immediately afterwards. Thus the hypothesis suggests that these two groups (with the SOC at the end of the acronym) will be socialized and the other three will be disordered and hypertensive.

The procedure was as follows: Twenty pregnant CBA females were placed in pairs in 28 × 17 × 12 centimeter nest boxes and were allowed to deliver. Litters were reduced to eight pups at birth and were not disturbed further until weaning at 21 days of age. The males were then individually placed in one-half liter jars containing wood shavings; twelve were assigned at random to each of the five experimental categories as shown in Fig. 6-10. Mice assigned to socialization were removed from their jars and placed for two and one-half hours in an intercommunicating six-box population cage where they could explore and engage in social activity (see Fig. 5-4). The experiments were initiated one week after weaning and continued until the mice were four months old.

The treadmill experience consisted of placing mice on a drum (7 centimeters in diameter) rotating at 2 rpm so that they remained isolated while walking (Fig. 6-11).

Fig. 6-11.   A treadmill with a rotating 7-centimeter diameter central shaft (2 rpm) forces mice to keep moving slowly. The partitions ensure isolation and ice on the floor prevents them from sheltering there. Exposure for three–five hours daily was started at the age of one month and continued until maturity at four months *(Watson and Henry, 1977a)*.

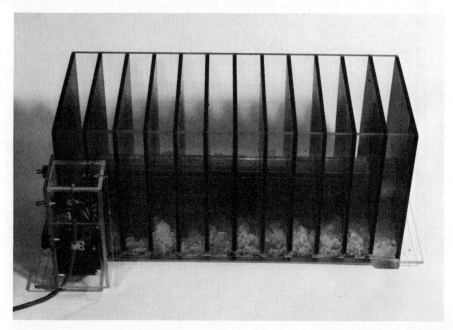

They were returned to isolation each day after the experiment, and treadmill and socialization procedures were continued five days a week until the mice were four months old. Each mouse was then tested in an open field and the number of squares traversed during a two-minute interval was recorded (Watson et al., 1974). A retro-orbital puncture to collect blood was made 15 minutes after each mouse's initial exposure to the open field; the plasma was removed and frozen for corticosterone assay.

The final phase of the experiment was then commenced. Six males from each of the five experimental categories were assigned to separate six-box intercommuni-

cating population cages for two months to interact socially among themselves as well as with 12 females that were assigned to each group (see Fig. 5-4). During this socialization, systolic blood pressure was measured (four times) once every two weeks by tail plethysmography. Data for each mouse were then pooled and averaged; statistical analyses were based on an analysis of variance by the Neuman-Keuls procedure.

The principal findings are summarized in Figs. 6-12 and 6-13. Socialized mice traversed significantly more squares during open-field tests than isolated mice ($p < 0.01$). There was significant interaction between treadmill and socialization experi-

Fig. 6-12.   Depicting the number of squares traversed in two minutes of open field activity and the various corticosterone responses to the experience of the five treatment combinations. There is a significant difference between the performance of groups permitted to sleep after the daily socialization period and of those for which it is deferred because a three–five-hour treadmill episode follows ($p < 0.01$) *(Watson and Henry, 1977).* See p. 112 for explanation of abbreviations.

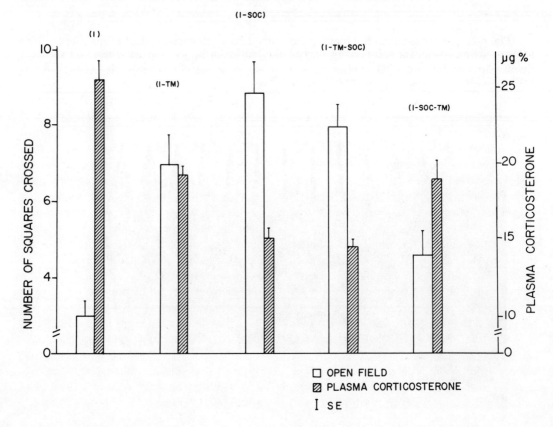

□ OPEN FIELD
▨ PLASMA CORTICOSTERONE

⊥ SE

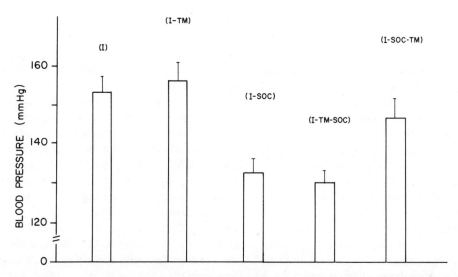

Fig. 6-13.   A contrast of the blood pressures of the five groups of mice, as outlined in Fig. 6-11, after they had been living in a population cage for two months (see Fig. 5-2 for design of the intercommunicating box system). Mice that remained isolated in their bottles and those removed only for daily solitary treadmill exercise lack social experience. They fight and develop high blood pressure; so do those that are socialized daily, but exposed to the treadmill immediately afterward. On the other hand, isolated mice that experienced daily socialization followed by the opportunity to sleep fought less and had lower blood pressure ($p < 0.01$) *(Watson and Henry, 1977).* See p. 112 for explanation of abbreviations.

ences; treadmill increased the activity ($p < 0.001$) of isolated mice (I-TM) and decreased their corticoid response to open-field tests ($p < 0.01$). Moreover, both mice with treadmill-socialization (I-TM-SOC) and with socialization only (I-SOC) traversed significantly more squares ($p < 0.01$) than mice with socialization-treadmill (I-SOC-TM). The socialized mice also had significantly lower plasma corticosterone response after open-field tests ($p < 0.01$) than isolated mice.

Isolated mice (I) had significantly higher blood pressure ($p < 0.001$) than socialized mice, while living in the population cage. In addition, mice with socialization-treadmill (I-SOC-TM) had significantly higher blood pressure than mice with socialization only (I-SOC) that had had the regular two and one-half hour periods of socialization ($p < 0.01$) or than mice with treadmill-socialization (I-TM-SOC) ($p < 0.01$) (Fig. 6-13). Presumably isolated mice (I) and mice with

treadmill only (I-TM) could not control their aggression and submit to an ordered dominance–submission hierarchy characterizing socialization. Intensive fighting among males and general social disorder persisted throughout the two months in the population cage. Minimal fighting was observed in socialized (I-SOC) and treadmill-socialized (I-TM-SOC) groups, and a distinct subdominant emerged within three weeks. Thus when the daily period of socialization was immediately followed by sleep it proved sufficient for mice to develop normal adult social reactivity and social behavior.

Mice have critical periods in their development when they must be exposed to members of their own species to acquire the necessary social aggressive–defensive behavior. During their daily socialization, young male weanlings of the socialized group (I-SOC) roamed about a complex six-box intercommunicating population cage specifically designed to impose maximum control of aggressive interaction. As they matured during the weeks, they participated in various play activities, learning the appropriate gestures with their associated external sensory cues. From the many repetitive experiences throughout their sensitive learning period, it is assumed they gradually acquired social aggressive–defensive behavior. The experiences of mice with treadmill-socialization (I-TM-SOC) were also successfully integrated each day during the sleep period immediately following their return to isolation in jars.

Standing in contrast to these two groups, socialization-followed-by-sleep, were the two that lacked the socialization-followed-by-sleep experience: isolated mice (I) and those with treadmill experience (I-TM). There was no question about the social failure of these mice. When they were placed in the population cage for two months, they could not achieve a stable hierarchy and their sustained fighting led to sympathoadrenal arousal and high blood pressure.

The fifth group of mice with socialization-treadmill (I-SOC-TM) was the most critical to our hypothesis. Their repeated socialization was futile because each time they were forced to wait four–five hours on the treadmill before they could relax, sleep, and consolidate their social experiences. Mice eat every two hours; and since their life expectancy is one-thirtieth that of ours, we can assume that each of their daily treadmill experiences may have lasted the equivalent of at least 48 hours of a man's life. These mice whose treadmill experience came last presumably forgot and failed to profit from their daily opportunity to socialize. Hence they remained as aggressive as the isolated mice and they fought vigorously in the population cage. Their blood pressure of 145 ± 5 mmHg supports our original hypothesis.

Mice that were allowed to sleep after socialization would have had opportunity to integrate their recently acquired social experience during the regular period of REM sleep, thus developing the appropriate defensive–aggressive hierarchy. Certainly these mice adjusted to a complex social environment during adulthood more readily than mice that had not been socialized or had been deprived of sleep after socialization. Thus the observed phenomena are compatible with the hypothesis that deprivation of REM sleep prevents socialization and delays integration of the limbic system's programs for attachment and territorial behavior with the higher cognitive processes in the cerebral hemisphere. It is to be assumed that for man, in particular, REM sleep may also permit the interchange of information between the right and the left hemispheres.

Observations of humans by psychologist Bakan (1976) support this conclusion. He points to recent demonstrations of a shift toward greater electroencephalographic activity in the right hemisphere during both REM (dreaming sleep) and active sexual fantasy just before orgasm. He cites Penfield's findings with conscious patients undergoing brain surgery that dreams and visual illusions were induced by stimulating the right but not the left hemisphere. During REM sleep, he says, the brain stem blocks motor activity, making dreaming possible without acting out the dreams. Although the vivid imagery of everyday details carried by the dream should be attributed to the right hemisphere, its content of basic biogrammatic symbols, such as parent and child, male and female, dominant and subordinate, presumably derives from the limbic system.

Summary

In addition to the huge frontal poles, the associational neocortex that evolved in man became specialized in the left parietal region into a verbal–analytic processor subserving communication, and into a visuospatial brain on the right. The right-hemispheric complex is closely linked with emotions, dreams, and fantasy. Its performance is critical for the sense of form and structure, not only with relation to perception of the environment, but also perception of the more abstract aspects of social and cultural organizational activities. This double system gives extra brain space, permitting the emergence of language whose grammatical foundations are inherited, and whose detailed syntax and vocabulary are a cultural tradition passed on from mother to child. Evolution has added this peculiarly human, logical, analytic brain to the holistic mute hemisphere which is the apparent locus of primary process thinking. This latter nondominant hemisphere may have a more direct neuronal involvement with the biogrammar of attachment and the territorial programs of our common mammalian heritage whose locus appears to be in the paleocortex and the subcortical regions.

Together these two newly evolved cognitive brain systems are responsible for man's progressive upbuilding of society. The imagination and fantasy of the right hemisphere, contributing to the stimuli influencing subcortical systems, are counterbalanced by the left hemisphere's logic and by the social assets of a cultural inheritance embracing all brain systems. Work with the lower animals that lack the traditions generated by the new sociocultural brain permits experimental discrimination between the contributions of culture that occupy the attention of anthropologists and sociologists, and those of the paleocortex and the brain stem which involve ethologists and neuroscientists. The subcortical limbic structures of the amygdala appear to control the value put on the source of the stimulus and hence to determine the motivation: to become attached or to reject. The hippocampus, which appears to be critical for spatially organized behavior, including territoriality, determines the turning off of the drive and the development of inhibitory depression when there is a failure to maintain social position. There is evidence to support the theory that the dream state is an activity linking the learned experiences of the hemispheric cognitive systems with an innate, genetically programmed, behavioral biogrammar with limbic roots.

7

Neuroendocrine responses to social interaction

Our objective is to trace the way in which the psychosocial stimulus results in disease. The first five chapters recount the work of anthropologists, ethologists, and psychologists who describe the motivation of organisms in terms of attachment and territoriality, of dominance and subordination, and of maternal care. Chapter 6 discusses the work of neurophysiologists who have made remarkable discoveries concerning the cognitive and affective roles of the hemispheres and the limbic system.

The topic now shifts to endocrine responses involved in emotional arousal. The hypothalamus is the effector for these changes (see Fig. 6-9). Not only do its paraventricular and supraoptic nuclei release the antidiuretic hormone (ADH) vasopressin passing down the nerves to the posterior pituitary gland, but the various regions of this tiny, cell-packed area produce the releasing factors for the corticotropin, thyrotropin, gonadotropin, prolactin, and growth hormone inhibitor being transported by portal blood vessels to the anterior pituitary.

Together, the hypothalamus and the pituitary form the crucial outflow for the control of the neuroendocrine apparatus by converting nerve impulses into hormonal responses, thus linking the brain to the regulatory mechanisms, whose disturbance in turn leads to disease (Haymaker et al., 1969).

The hippocampal paleocortex transmits responses to the pituitary adrenal-cortical mechanism acting as a regulator during conditions of uncertainty (Isaacson, 1974). Its mapping function is probably important in determining the workings of the instinct of territoriality (O'Keefe et al., 1975). When the unexpected happens and expectations are not met, i.e., during failure to control territory and to achieve the desired goals, the hippocampus, sensing the mismatch, may initiate the social withdrawal and neuroendocrine changes of depression; it stimulates the adrenal cortex by way of the hormonal chain involving the releasing factors for adrenocorticotropin (ACTH) of the anterior pituitary. Another major pathway, which involves the orbital frontal cortex, the amygdalar complex, and the sympathetic adrenal–medullary defense response, is associated with the fight–flight response and is activated by a challenge to attachments. Figures 7-1 and 7-2 together with Figs. 6-7 and 6-9 summarize this picture of a dual stress pathway.

As the perceived stimulus takes effect in the higher centers, it results in the activation of lower limbic system structures, unless the pathways are blocked by the individual's patterns of coping and social assets. The organism that has always achieved goals of food, water, parental care; that is gifted

Fig. 7-1. A conceptual model summarizing the theme of this book. If the psychosocial stimulus perceived by a mammal is not inhibited at higher levels by interaction with coping patterns and social assets, then a response of the limbic system will ensue. The amygdala and the sympathetic adrenal-medullary system are activated when the organism is challenged in its control of the environment. By contrast, when there is loss of territorial control and failure to meet expectations, the hippocampal pituitary–adrenal–cortical system becomes more involved as the conservation–withdrawal response is aroused. The physiologic consequences of these two response patterns differ as shown; the horizontal arrow indicates no change (see also Figs. 6-7, 6-9, and 7-2) *(Henry, 1976a,b).*

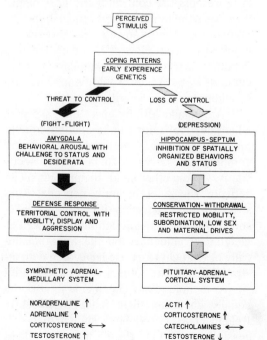

physically; that is fortunate enough to live in a society with adequate resources will react—as the dominant does—with active coping efforts to a challenge to its accustomed control. As a result, its responses contrast with those of the depressed subordinate who has lost or has never held a position of control. This chapter presents evidence that the contrasting behavioral response patterns ensuing from a perception of self as dominant, as opposed to subordinate, result in differing patterns of neuroendocrine activation mentioned elsewhere (Ely et al, 1974; Henry and Ely, 1976).

The frontal lobes and amygdalar and hippocampal function

The preceding chapter referred to frontal–limbic connections, suggesting that the frontal association areas are interposed between the social analyzer of the parietal neocortex and the affect-determined and motivational regions of the limbic system. This chapter is concerned with the mechanisms by which different neuroendocrine responses are triggered by emotional states, such as rage or depression. Man's frontal poles, whose associational cortex matches his huge transmodal parietal association area in size, are believed to have a considerable role in these responses. There is a question as to whether other mammals really have a frontal cortex in the sense that it exists in primates and especially in man.

Extensive research in man and animals indicates that the frontal association areas give an extraordinary stability to man's behavior by keeping the action programs going, but they give flexibility too, so that when the approach being used is perceived as failing, appropriate affective responses are activated. For example, the organism may have a choice of triggering a response that seeks to overcome the difficulty by perseverance and aggressive action. At a lower level this corresponds to the affect of rage with fighting. An alternative mode may be recognizing the problem and attempting to escape with the intention of reopening the issue at a more favorable time. The affect is fear leading to flight. A third possibility can be conservation–withdrawal in which the approach is abandoned; failure is recognized and after a period of lying low, fresh actions aimed in a new direction are initiated. The affect is depression leading to submission, relearning, and reorganizing the behavior patterns. A choice is made between these possibilities, depending on the circumstances.

According to Nauta (1971), the frontal cortex is not only critical in making decisions but the ensuing neural associations explain its unique and subtle role in planning behavior. It is the end point for long neuronal chains coming from the parietal association areas relating somatic sensory, visual, and auditory inputs. Information from the olfactory and limbic systems is also received. The frontal cortex is like the parietal cortex in being a cross-modal area. Both the external environment and the neural codes, which relate to motivational states and their visceral concomitants from the limbic system and the hypothalamus, are represented. Thus the frontal cortex receives data from the internal and the external environments. Nauta suggests that it both receives and modulates affect as represented by the limbic mechanisms with which it stands in reciprocal relationship.

As the major mediator of information exchanged between the cortex and the limbic system, the frontal cortex may be responsible for the strategic making of choices, such as turning off an unrewarding response pattern, as previously mentioned. The efferent connections of the frontal lobe going to the hippocampal gyrus are rich and originate dorsally. Associations with the amygdalar nuclei are also present; however, they are made by way of the temporal cortex and arise ventrally, as opposed to dorsally. Thus there is functional differentiation in the frontal region and the depressive and the

fight–flight responses not only have separate neuroendocrine bases, but they may derive from separate responses of this highest decision-making area (Nauta, 1971).

The amygdala and Cannon's sympathetic adrenal–medullary defense pattern

The amygdalar nuclei in the anterior portion of the temporal lobes consist of a corticomedial and a basolateral group. Although this division suggests separate functions, they have not been fully defined and analyzed. The stria terminalis is one of the two main efferent bundles (Fig. 6-7) giving the complex close ties to the hypothalamus (Isaacson, 1974).

The controlling influence of the amygdala on the activity of the lower centers, including the sympathetic system, has been demonstrated recently (Lang, 1975; Lang et al., 1975). The medulla and the ventral brain stem structures are concerned with maintaining resting blood pressure. The amygdala represents the control at the next higher level, i.e., the limbic system. In a laboratory preparation, they showed that the rise in blood pressure typical of lower center activation, which follows the stimulation of the cut ends of the vagus, could be inhibited by simultaneously stimulating the amygdala.

Amygdalar lesions upset the ease with which new behavior can be elicited, attachment is disturbed, and lack of induced competitiveness results in a loss of social status. On the other hand, the amygdala can activate the hypothalamic neuronal substrate for the expression of emotions (Isaacson, 1974). Amygdaloid inhibitory as well as facilitatory influences on the hypothalamically based fight response have been demonstrated in the cat. Others who have used a similar technique have been able to alter the equally important flight reaction. Recently Roldán et al. (1974) have shown that successfully eliciting these fight or flight responses depends on electrically stimulating this region only and doing so with very limited shocks. If the stimulus is not carefully controlled, it will induce paroxysmal discharges interfering with the amygdalohypothalamic substrate of the defense response.

In his study of *The Brain and Reward*, Rolls (1975) associates the amygdala with the formation of reinforcement associations. He sees it to be crucial for normal behavior. For example, when the organism perceives that access to a source of valued responses is being challenged, this region will trigger the fight response with the aim of securing continued access to the desired object, be it food or young.

In keeping with Rolls's conclusion and after scanning a large and varied body of evidence, Isaacson (1974) considers that the role of the amygdala is to arouse and activate the hypothalamus when external conditions are appropriate.

Peripheral effects of the sympathetic adrenal–medullary response

The peripheral effects of activating the fight–flight response were studied in the 1900's by Cannon who, with his associate de La Paz, showed an increased output of adrenaline in the venous blood coming from the adrenal of a cat exposed to a barking dog (Cannon and de La Paz, 1911). Cannon formulated an emergency function or stress theory of adrenal–medullary activity; he suggested that fear and rage responses helped the cat to cope with a threatening situation (Cannon, 1929). This was supported by the later demonstration that stimulation of the reticular formation in the posterior hypothalamus (Fig. 7-2) elicits responses behaviorally and physiologically identical with Cannon's concept of a defense reaction. This, as Folkow and Neil (1971) point out, is a state highly suited for either attack or flight which is activated by induc-

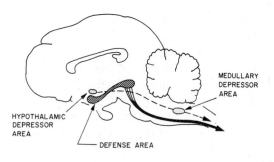

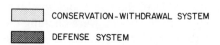

Fig. 7-2. A schematic of the general region occupied by the hypothalamic depressor and the defense areas. The former, an aspect of conservation–withdrawal, is inhibitory and connects with the medullary depressor area, which in turn determines the fainting response. The defense area is critical in the organization of the fight or flight response with its control over the sympathetic adrenal-medullary system (see also Figs. 6-7, 6-9, and 7-1) *(Folkow and Neil, 1971).*

ing tenseness and alertness in anticipation of challenging events, such as a confrontation with a rival of comparable achievements and potential. The behavior is typical of all mammals, primates included, with modifications for the different species. In the cat, whose display is particularly dramatic, it includes hissing, spitting, arching the back, and raising the hair on the back and tail. At the same time, sympathetic cholinergic vasodilator fibers to the arterioles of the skeletal muscles are activated. There is a violent excitation of the adrenergic fibers to all other parts of the vascular bed and the heart, and the release of catecholamines from the adrenal medulla is greatly enhanced.

In primates, including man, this sympathetic adrenal-medullary arousal results in an increase in arterial pressure, cardiac output, and heart rate. The increase in cardiac output is taken up in skeletal muscle blood flow, while the flow through the kidney is redistributed and reduced. Such changes have been induced in rodents by direct stimulation of the lateral hypothalamus (Folkow and Rubinstein, 1966). By using chronically implanted electrodes, they were also able to induce a chronic moderate elevation of systolic pressure in otherwise normal unanesthetized rats by exposing them to several months of mildly alerting, daily stimulation of the hypothalamic defense area (Fig. 7-3). Typical blood flow changes in the kidneys and muscles could be induced by stimulating anesthetized rats in the same location, suggesting that the electrodes were eliciting the same cardiovascular response as mental stimuli. Folkow and Neil (1971) describe this response as a central anticipatory adjustment of the cardiovascular system. Cocking the trigger, it alerts the muscles by preparing them for explosion into an all-out fight or flight response, should it be needed.

The biochemical accompaniments of these complex neurophysiologic and cardiovascular changes were shown to involve two hormones, one of which, the versatile nor-

adrenaline, differs from adrenaline by only one methyl group. Noradrenaline as the adrenergic transmitter has a major physiologic role. An impressive mass of related psychophysiologic work during the past two decades was reviewed (1975) by Marianne Frankenhaeuser: Any threatening or rewarding event perceived by the organism as emotionally arousing will be accompanied by an increased adrenaline output. Noradrenaline was seen as differing from adrenaline in being associated with circumstances in which an effort is made to achieve a goal.

In their multidisciplinary pilot study of hard-pressed workers in northern Sweden, Frankenhaeuser and Gardell (1976) go still further. Essentially they confirm the early and much challenged generalization of Funkenstein (1956) that adrenaline is associated with fear, and noradrenaline, with irritation. They studied sawmill workers who were relentlessly paced by their machines and had a short work cycle of a few seconds. They

Fig. 7-3. Solid line: Gradual change in resting mean blood pressure of six rats exposed to three months of intermittent, weak stimulation of the hypothalamic defense area. The stimulus was not strong enough to induce any observable behavioral changes. Broken line: Resting mean blood pressure of six controls with identical electrode implants, but without stimulation. There is a return toward normal when stimulation was withheld and a rise with resumption *(Folkow and Rubinstein, 1966).*

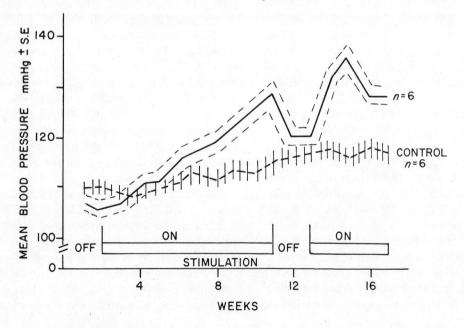

contrasted the neuroendocrine responses of such workers with those of maintenance men who paced their own work. Frankenhaeuser and Gardell found an increased adrenaline release was typically induced by brief work cycles which are measured in seconds [Fig. 7-4(A)] and by extremely repetitious work [Fig. 7-4(B)]. Sawmill edgers and graders were involved in such tasks, having a low degree of control and much physical strain. They also suffered from a restriction of social interaction. As can be seen from the two figures, the higher their adrenaline level, the less their sense of well-being. By contrast, noradrenaline, which

Frankenhaeuser and Gardell saw as related to factors affecting blood pressure homeostasis, increased when the workers expressed irritation. This anger could have been caused by cramped work posture [Fig. 7-5(A)], or by not being able to self-pace the work [Fig. 7-5(B)], or by being so hurried that the job could not be given its due measure of skill and experience.

Although these preliminary data were derived from groups of 5–14 subjects too small for statistical analysis, the authors are impressed by the consistency of the trends and the meaningful patterns that emerged.

Other studies now support Funken-

Fig. 7-4.   (A) Per cent of increase in excretion over resting levels of adrenaline in the urine of men exposed to differing lengths of work cycles is compared with their assessed feeling of well-being. Although not susceptible to statistical analysis, the data show a strong consistency of pattern and trend. The longer cycles are perceived as more desirable; note, they are accompanied by less adrenaline excretion. (B) The extent to which the work was repetitious also shows a good correlation with the biochemical measure *(Frankenhaeuser and Gardell, 1976).*

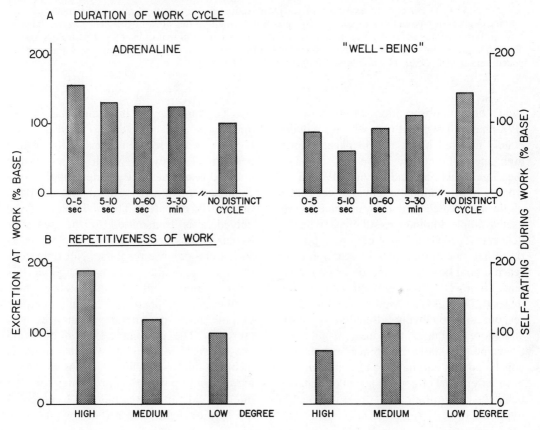

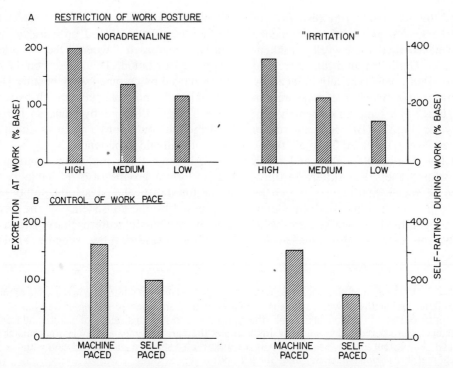

Fig. 7-5. (A) Per cent of excretion of resting noradrenaline in urine of men who experience varying degrees of having to maintain the same posture throughout the working day. The excretion for three different degrees of restraint is matched against self-estimates of irritation at these restraints. (B) The procedure is the same, but the independent variable is the extent to which the work was machine-paced versus self-paced *(Frankenhaeuser and Gardell, 1976).*

stein's original observation. Friedman et al. (1975) have shown that men who were deliberately irritated had a rise in plasma noradrenaline, but that their adrenaline remained the same. Lawrence and Haynes (1970) have worked out the animal behavioral correlates of the two catecholamines in mice. They used a simple dominance–submission test to determine which member of a pair pushed the other out of the way in attempting to reach a goal box at the end of a one-meter-length tube. Their young five to 15-week-old males (C57 blacks) showed more submissive responses on receiving adrenaline (p<0.01) and more dominant responses from noradrenaline (p<0.001). Lawrence and Haynes concluded that adrenaline and noradrenaline have differential effects on social dominance behavior appropriate for the Funkenstein hypothesis.

To summarize: If circumstances are appropriate, the amygdala is aroused, perhaps, from the orbital regions of the frontal neocortical analyzer which activates the defense response. An example of this is a challenge to status by a rival who has been previously defeated. The activation of the amygdala is transmitted to the posterior hypothalamus, inducing a rise in blood pressure and a defense response. Not only does the cardiovascular system engage in this defense mode, but adrenal catecholamine synthesis is stepped up. Initially, cardiac output and peripheral resistance will increase. The ensuing elevation of blood pressure is accompanied by increased levels of blood lipids and glucose as the organism assumes a posture appropriate for the intense and rapid expenditure of energy of the fight or flight pattern (Folkow and Neil,

1971). Thus a chain of events that starts with a certain type of psychosocial perception leads to bodily changes of potential significance in producing disease.

The hippocampus and adrenocortical secretion

O'Keefe and Nadel's proposal that the hippocampal formation functions as a cognitive mapping system (O'Keefe et al., 1975) has recently been confirmed by others (see Chapter 6). Not only may this mapping function apply to location in physical space, but also to the concept of territory and home range in their broadest sense. Social organizations require their members to have an acute sense of location; they must "know their place" not only in the physical, but in the hierarchic space. This premise holds true for all mammalian societies, but for civilized man the need to recognize relations between various features of a milieu becomes enormously complex and refined.

The basic concept of hippocampal function as a cognitive mapping system fits in with Isaacson's previously mentioned perception of its role as regulating other regions of the brain during mismatches between stored representation and present perception of the environment, i.e., when old patterns of responding fail to pay off with anticipated rewards. In Isaacson's context, it is a mechanism by which the more well-established response patterns are turned off when the unexpected happens and control is lost (Isaacson, 1974).

Certainly, blocking hippocampal outflow by lesioning the fornix eliminates the diurnal variation of corticosterone, and Moberg et al. (1971) present evidence that there may be both inhibitory and excitatory fibers in the fornix, permitting the hippocampus to play a part in control of the adrenocorticotropic hormone (ACTH)—corticosterone mechanism. Kawakami et al. (1968) have shown that, depending on the circumstances, opposite effects can be produced by hippocampal stimulation. Under the stress of

forced immobilization, hippocampal stimulation will inhibit the increase in corticosteroid biosynthesis that would otherwise occur. When not under stress, the same stimulus increases biosynthesis. These results are compatible with Endröczi and Lissák's (1963) observation that by changing the frequency with which the hippocampus is stimulated, ACTH release can be increased or inhibited.

At the hypothalamic level, Goldfien and Ganong (1962) have shown that endogenous adrenaline secretion plays no part in the activation of pituitary adrenocortical function. Indeed, Van Loon et al. (1971) found a negative correlation between plasma corticosterone and the catecholamines in the central adrenergic system. Their demonstration that intracerebral α-methyltyrosine increases corticosterone by decreasing catecholamine synthesis supports their hypothesis. Bohus et al. (1968) have shown that implanting the ventral hippocampus with corticosterone leads to increased pituitary adrenal-cortical function, and that amygdalar implants produced an inhibitory effect. The stimulus following the placement of a subject in a new environment was necessary to produce this effect. Russo et al. (1976) have shown that despite the difficulty an animal has in learning passive avoidance after destruction of the amygdala, the pituitary adrenal response of rising plasma corticosterone to the stress of active avoidance of a shock to the foot remains unimpaired. They saw this reaction as compatible with the thesis that the pituitary–adrenal mechanism is independent of the amygdalar fight–flight complex. Thus the evidence indicates that the hippocampus has control over the pituitary–adrenocortical system, especially during periods of failure to overcome challenges. Furthermore, it appears to be acting in a direction opposite to and independent of the amygdala and the sympathetic adrenal–medullary system. The latter may also influence the ACTH response, but this may not be by means of a normal physiologic pathway. For example, McHugh and Smith (1967) showed that plasma 17-hydroxycorticosterone (17-OHCS) is increased in conscious monkeys by electrical stimuli to the amygdala, but only by those strong enough to evoke after-discharges. They explain that the amygdala itself may not be involved but the discharges have probably recruited related areas, such as the hypothalamus.

The idea that the hippocampal formation has primary involvement in control of the pituitary ACTH adrenocortical mechanism is in keeping with Mason's (1968a) convincing detailing of the evidence that psychologic influences are potent releasers of cortical hormones (Mason et al., 1976). This includes the alarm response first described by Selye (1950) who frequently elicited responses from conscious animals during his studies.

In a crucial demonstration Bronson and Eleftheriou (1965) showed that mice previously exposed to a fighter will develop increased plasma corticosterone merely when they see their opponent and feel threatened by it. This is in keeping with the pioneer studies of Davis and Christian (1957), who showed that the higher the social rank of an individual rodent, the less its adrenal corticoidogenesis was affected when placed with other rodents. Partially domesticated male mice descended from a wild strain were isolated at weaning until two months old. They were then placed in groups of six for four hours a day in an open space and returned to isolation for the remaining 20 hours. This procedure was repeated for 10 days. Social rank was determined by observing the fighting going on in the open space; and, on the last day, by round-robin contests—each mouse was pitted in turn against another. Adrenal weight measured in mg/100 gm body weight was significantly greater (p < 0.01) in the low- than in the high-ranking animals. Body weight was greater in the dominant animal.

Louch and Higginbotham (1967) followed up on this experiment by placing mice that had been isolated since weaning in groups of four either for six or for 24 hours

and watched for the development of aggressive behavior and hierarchies. Control mice were maintained in separate cages; their corticosterone level was 9.3 ± 0.6 micrograms/100 milliliters. That of the dominants did not differ significantly, being 11.9 ± 1.0 micrograms, while that of the subordinates was 19.9 ± 1.0 micrograms. These results support Christian's (1971) conclusion that defeat is an important stimulus acting on mice to produce an adrenal response after fighting. Dominant mice who initiate and win their fights show no increase in plasma corticosterone, but subordinate mice consistently show a significant increase. Wounding was not a factor, since the winners were often injured as badly as the losers.

Ethel Sassenrath (1970) in working with subordinate rhesus monkeys compared them with dominants and got similar results. She found a statistically significant association between ACTH response levels, aggressive stimulation received, and fear–anxiety behavior, i.e., the dominant animal had far less adrenal corticosteroid response to injection of ACTH than the subordinates (see Fig. 5-9). She concludes that the fear-evoking component of chronic social stress is the predominant stimulus for endogenous ACTH release.

Depression and the pituitary–adrenocortical mode

In a recent survey of neuroendocrine abnormalities in depressive illness, Sachar (1976) has presented evidence that the mean hourly cortisol concentration of depressed patients is significantly higher in the afternoon, evening, and early morning hours (Fig. 7-6). They secrete extra cortisol during the time secretion normally ceases rather than during the interval from 5 A.M. to 11 A.M. when the bulk of the day's cortisol is normally excreted. He concludes that there is an excessive driving or removal of inhibi-

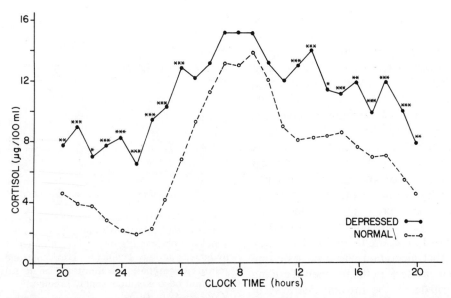

Fig. 7-6.   Mean hourly plasma cortisol concentration over a 24-hour period for seven depressed patients compared with the mean for 54 normal subjects. Each point represents the mean cortisol concentration during the preceding hour: * $p < 0.05$, ** $p < 0.01$, *** $p < 0.001$ *(Sachar, 1976).*

tion of the hypothalamic cells secreting the corticotropin releasing factor (CRF) as an intrinsic part of severe depressive illness.

Recently Carroll (1976) has established that a dysfunction occurs in a depressed man's limbic system which affects the pituitary control of the adrenal cortex and leads to an elevated plasma cortisol. This condition occurs in primary depression found after bereavement, but not when the individual behaves similarly but suffers from a schizophrenic disturbance of the cognitive (reasoning) process. He also showed there was an impaired response to dexamethasone that normally suppresses the release of cortisone by competing, and so eliminates the feedback to the ACTH mechanism. In primary depression the limbic drive overrides the normal feedback.

The subjective behavioral stimulus for this, as both Weiss et al. (1976) and Seligman (1975) have demonstrated, is a failure of the organism to see that its efforts are bringing results. If the self is perceived as achieving control over the environment, the success provides the needed information and behavior is reinforced. This effect has been demonstrated in the rhesus monkey by the studies of Hanson et al. (1976). When given control over an unpleasantly intense noise that would otherwise induce an elevation of plasma cortisol, their cortisol stayed at control values. But monkeys without any possibility or expectation of being able to turn off the noise developed a behavioral disturbance with a significant diminution of social contact. At the same time, they had a marked cortisol response. Monkeys deprived of control after successfully learning to use it were even more disturbed, responding with aggressive behavior and an intense elevation of cortisol. Thus a conservation–withdrawal pattern of behavior involving social avoidance developed in subjects without expectations. This contrasted with the aggressive, i.e., amygdalar fight–flight, arousals of subjects whose expectations were denied with sufficient ambiguity for them to think there was a possibility of regaining control (Hanson et al., 1976).

Weiss and his associates made related experiments evaluating the physiologic consequences of exposure to inescapable stressors. They contrasted the incidence of gastric ulceration in yoked rats, one of which could avoid electric shocks by touching its nose to a panel, while the other received the same shocks, but had no control. They found that the passive rat had more lesions and higher levels of plasma corticosterone (Weiss, 1972b). These researchers have also shown a depression in brain noradrenaline levels when rats were exposed to inescapable shock. This depression was less marked with repeated exposure to shock. Thus they conclude that ulceration and corticosterone response increase with the number of coping attempts made by the rat and decrease in proportion to the volume of feedback indicating success, while noradrenaline in the brain moves in the opposite direction (Weiss et al., 1975).

In a related study of the effects of expectance on the pituitary–adrenal system, Coover et al. (1973) showed that during shuttlebox avoidance learning, the plasma corticosterone levels of rats rise sharply during the acquisition phase. But after learning was stabilized, the increase was significantly less intense (Fig. 7-7). They concluded that during the later stages of avoidance, fear and arousal are decreased as rats learn to predict and to control the situation, thus permitting a set of expectancies to develop about the stimulus contingencies.

Observations by Conner showed that a single rat exposed to repeated shocks has higher plasma ACTH levels than paired rats receiving the same intensity. Paired rats fight when shocked, and it might have been expected that this combination of shock with fighting would have elicited a greater pituitary–adrenal response than either stimulus alone. The reverse, in fact, was the case and ACTH levels were lower in the fighting pairs (Fig. 7-8). Since the overall level of physical activity was the same in both cases, Conner and co-workers concluded that the difference in ACTH response was related to a

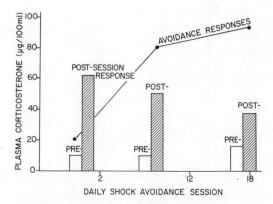

Fig. 7-7. Plasma corticosterone responses of rats to daily shock-avoidance sessions of 10 shocks at one-minute intervals. Although avoidance activity levels out, corticosterone returns toward base line after the session as the situation becomes increasingly predictable *(Coover et al., 1973).*

change in behavior. The paired rats directed attacks at each other instead of attempting to escape as did the single rat. It would appear that pairing changes the animals' perceptions. The single animal probably experiences helplessness and depression due to uncontrollable shock; the fighting pair experience an arousal of the classic Cannon sympathetic adrenal-medullary response, as perhaps each suspects the other of having

Fig. 7-8. The ACTH level in plasma of solitary rats exposed to several minutes of repeated electric shock rises higher than in paired rats. Paired animals direct attacks at each other and presumably perceive the situation as offering more possibility for control *(Conner et al., 1971).*

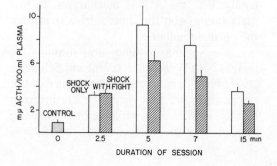

something to do with the problem (vertical bars, S.E.: $p < 0.05$) (Conner et al., 1971).

Weiss et al. (1976) have followed up on these studies with a demonstration that if paired rats can fight, their exposure to foot shocks will not induce as severe a gastric ulceration as if they receive equal shocks in isolation. Weiss suggests that the act of aggression serves as a "relevant feedback" and, in effect, the organism perceives itself as achieving expectations. It has been known for some time that administering inescapable stimuli for a number of days, such as repeatedly dropping a bound rat in a rotating drum (Mikulaj and Kvetňanský, 1966); daily subcutaneous injections of two percent of formalin, producing inflammation and therefore eliciting pain; or daily repeat-ed immobilizations for two–three hours by holding the paws apart (Mikulaj and Mitro, 1973); eventually leads to a decreased response of the adrenocortical mechanism [Fig. 7-9(A)]. Yet the hypophyseal–adrenocortical system is not exhausted, for it will respond vigorously to fresh stimuli.

This falling off of response can be contrasted with observations of increased adrenal and urinary adrenaline [Fig. 7-9(B)] and the noradrenaline-synthesizing enzyme tyrosine hydroxylase [Fig. 7-9(C)] during an identical series of immobilizations made by Kvetňanský and Mikulaj (1970) and Kvetňanský et al. (1970). Here there is a progressively enhanced ability to replace catecholamines. It would seem that with repetition the rat changes its response to the experi-

Fig. 7-9. Composite diagram of data from three experiments; in each rats were exposed to upwards of 40 daily episodes of immobilization stress, each lasting two hours. (A) mean plasma corticosterone level after the fortieth episode was half of that following the initial immobilization *(Mikulaj and Mitro, 1973).* (B) By contrast, excretion of adrenaline in the urine was doubled at the fortieth episode ($p < 0.001$) *(Kvetňanský and Mikulaj, 1970).* (C) Concentration of tyrosine hydroxylase, the noradrenaline-synthesizing enzyme, in the adrenals was even more elevated ($p < 0.001$) *(Kvetňanský et al., 1970).* These changes indicate a shift from stimulation of the adrenal–cortical to the adrenal–medullary system as the stimulus becomes more predictable.

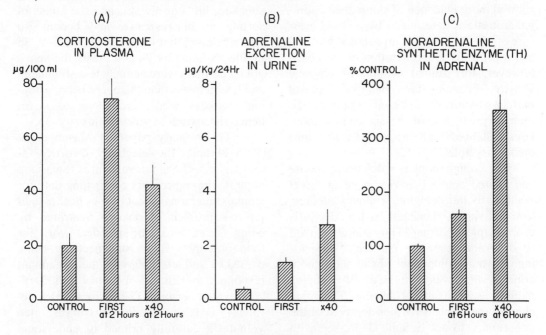

DAILY EPISODES OF IMMOBILIZATION STRESS

ence. Early events, it could be argued, are seen as a threat which cannot be escaped and against which the rat is helpless, having no coping defenses. Later, although just as noxious, the event is perceived as having a predictable outsome. Once more, a change from a Selyean conservation–withdrawal response, with a pronounced pituitary–adrenocortical arousal, toward a Cannon pattern, involving the fight–flight reflex, can account for the observed decrease of pituitary adrenocortical involvement and the progressive increase of sympathetic adrenal-medullary involvement.

A final example of the dichotomy of response patterns comes from the work of Corley et al. (1975) with excitable squirrel monkeys. They confined pairs of monkeys to pillory chairs for eight hours a day. The average test was one month, but, in the six groups tested, they ranged from four days to three months (K. C. Corley, personal communication, 1977).

The coping monkey of the pair had to turn off a light once a minute, but since both were wired in series, both received identical shocks to the tail. The coping monkey showed more evidence of sympathetic adrenal arousal, as determined by a blood pressure of 150–110 mmHg, myocardial fibrosis, and myofibrillary degeneration of the heart; however, this animal maintained physical activity, outlasting the "helpless" control partner which could not control or cope. To their surprise, five of the six control monkeys collapsed with bradycardia and four died in asystole.

The coping monkey's defense response and related active behavior were in direct contrast to the debilitating clinical depression and vagally mediated fatal bradycardia of the helpless partner. Thus stimulation led to different response patterns, depending on which component of the neuroendocrine system was activated. The coping monkey saw itself as having a fighting chance; the helpless partner deprived of the opportunity to act became depressed with characteristic arousal of the conservation–

withdrawal response and vagal stimulation. Had they been human their response might well have been termed despair.

When Corley repeated the study by exposing previously naive monkeys to a single 24-hour session of shock avoidance, the situation was reversed, and myocardial damage and cardiac arrest were more readily induced in the coping monkeys. The shift in vulnerability from the helpless partners to the coping monkeys could be attributed to the added stress of an avoidance situation to which they were now exposed without having previously experienced shock avoidance (Corley et al., 1977). In the earlier study, monkeys had been repeatedly trained to avoid shock in one-hour sessions. But the new approach speeded up the process, forcing the coping monkeys to react to being shocked while at the same time trying to learn how to respond to avoid it. It is true that the naive coping monkey receives sufficient feedback to tell him that his behavior is or is not leading him to avoid shock. But the full realization of how to avoid shock consistently has not yet been achieved. He sometimes responds in a way to avoid being shocked, but not always, and the stress of sorting out his responses may become so overwhelming that he gives up and dies. So in this continuous 24-hour test, the naive yoked partners were actually less stimulated and less helpless than the overwhelmed coping monkeys who were trying to learn, hence the switch in vulnerability.

The summary paper by Mason et al. (1976) outlining the selectivity of corticosteroid and catecholamine responses to various natural stimuli presents contrasting data for animals and humans that throws further light on this problem. Monkeys frustrated by being forced into hard physical work for food or depressed by unexpectedly being passed by and left hungry by their attendant responded to their loss of control with sharply elevated urinary 17-hydroxycorticosterone (17-OHCS) excretion. By contrast, men volunteers carefully primed to understand and cooperate in an experiment showed no change in 17-OHCS excretion during three hours of exhausting exercise; this occurred despite a near doubling of urinary catecholamine excretion. The sense of control these men retained protected them from helplessness. It did not, however, prevent them from experiencing unpleasantness when forcing themselves to those same limits that Frankenhaeuser et al. (1969) have associated with an increase in adrenal-medullary secretion.

Endocrine characteristics of dominant and subordinate status in animals

An animal that perceives the possibility of maintaining control responds to a challenge with increased activity and aggression. His neuroendocrine system is activated in the amygdalar and sympathetic adrenal-medullary response pattern. By contrast, the defeated and immobilized subordinate animal withdraws from associations and experiences activation of the adrenocortical hormones. This is not to deny that states of acute arousal or mixed emotions will not activate both systems (Mason, 1968a,b). Furthermore, this is but one of many neuroendocrine changes. Plasma testosterone in a previously successful animal falls in response to a decrease in gonadotropins during a defeat (see Figs. 5-10, 5-11). This is accompanied by a feedback affecting the hippocampus (Rose et al., 1975).

Indeed, aggressiveness is not only a function of the effect on the brain of the gonadotropic axis and testosterone levels, but also of the adrenocortical hormones. This was difficult to analyze because the chronic behavioral effects of corticosterone are opposite to those of the adrenocorticotropic hormone (ACTH), which, nevertheless, induces corticosterone. However, by using dexamethasone to suppress ACTH and adrenalectomy to keep corticosterone levels constant, the following conclusions

have emerged from the work of Brain and Poole (1974). Chronic administration of ACTH decreases isolation-induced intermale aggressiveness in mice by controlling levels of corticosterone or testosterone or both, while dexamethasone, which suppresses ACTH, increases aggression. Apparently ACTH enhances the rate at which hypophysectomized rats acquire both active and passive conditioned-avoidance responses. Hence, subordinated animals with elevated ACTH can more rapidly change their behavior and avoid attacks by dominants either by escaping or by displaying a subordination response (Brain and Poole, 1974). In a social group that is acquiring a new hierarchy due to a change in membership, the feedback effect of ACTH on the hippocampus reduces the amount of overt fighting by inducing a conservation–withdrawal mode in those experiencing subordination. Subordinate behavior is an aspect of depression, and evidence that it is the same as the human primary depression described by Carroll (1976) comes from the similarity of behavioral and hormonal responses. Both man and animals undergo withdrawal and immobility and develop elevated plasma cortisone (corticosterone in rodents). Psychologist Seligman (1975) reviews this parallelism between the behavior of animals and the behavior in humans in his excellent text on *Helplessness*.

Sassenrath's (1977) recent observations on the behavioral sequelae of weaning strategies in colony-born rhesus monkeys are relevant. She showed that infants with no previous social experience who develop high levels of pituitary adrenocortical activation as a result of postweaning stress will develop submissive responses. By contrast, animals with low cortisol response assume the highest dominance ranks and display less submissive and clinging behavior. Other observations from her laboratory indicate that such initial endocrine influences can have long-term effects since young rhesus monkeys are consistent in maintaining either dominant or subordinate roles as they mature. She perceives the association of high cortisol with submissive behavior as a primate psychosocial counterpart to the ACTH enhancement of learning and the retention of avoidance behavior.

Candland and Leshner (1974) have measured urinary 17-hydroxycorticosterone (17-OHCS) and total catecholamine levels in previously isolated squirrel monkeys immediately after they had formed an order of dominance. The subordinates had higher 17-OHCS levels than the dominants, whereas urinary catecholamines increased in the mid-ranking monkeys who successfully fought to maintain status, but decreased in those who were unsuccessful and became further subordinated.

Recent biochemical observations of mice by Ely et al. (1974) support the preceding studies. Groups of five normal sibling males and 12 females were placed in population cages where the males were left to work out their social hierarchies during the ensuing three months. Several such colonies were studied, i.e., four at two weeks, seven at six weeks, and five at 15 weeks. During intense social interaction early in the study, plasma corticosterone levels of 10 future subordinates were significantly higher than those of four future dominants. Later, after a month or so when a relatively stable hierarchy had developed, the emerging dominant was no longer challenged, expectations were formed and met, and corticosterone levels of subordinates returned to normal (Fig. 7-10).

In a subsequent experiment, Ely added a restraint stress technique by placing both dominants and subordinates in wire mesh tubes two hours a day for about three weeks. When their corticosterone was measured at 16 and at 25 days, subordinates had significantly higher levels than dominants ($p < 0.05$) (Fig. 7-11). After a suitable recovery period for the mice, Ely then applied Sassenrath's technique of giving ACTH to both dominants and subordinates (see Fig. 5-9). Again the plasma corticosterone in subordinates rose significantly higher than in dominants whose level did not change signif-

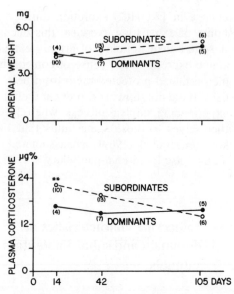

Fig. 7-10. A contrast of adrenocortical responses of sibling males in a mouse colony as they form a hierarchy of dominants and subordinates. This is normal socialization accelerated by the presence of females in the cages. *Abscissa* is the time in days. Measurements were made at termination of different colonies at 14, 42, and 105 days. Top: Adrenal weight shows no change, indicating that the social stimulus was not intense. Bottom: Plasma corticosterone is significantly higher ($p < 0.01$) in the still-competing subordinates at 14 days. After colony dynamics had stabilized, this difference vanished as the now thoroughly subordinated mice accept the dominant *(Henry and Ely, 1976).*

icantly from those of controls. These experiments support earlier observations and indicate that the adrenal–cortical mechanism of a mouse that has lost territorial control will respond more to a threat than that of a dominant mouse.

In the population cage study (see Fig. 7-12), the adrenal–medullary content of the enzymes tyrosine hydroxylase (TH) and phenylethanolamine *N*-methyltransferase (PNMT) was also measured. The TH, under sympathetic control, is the rate-limiting enzyme in the chain of synthesis of noradrenaline and adds a hydroxyl group to tyrosine, and PNMT is the enzyme which con-

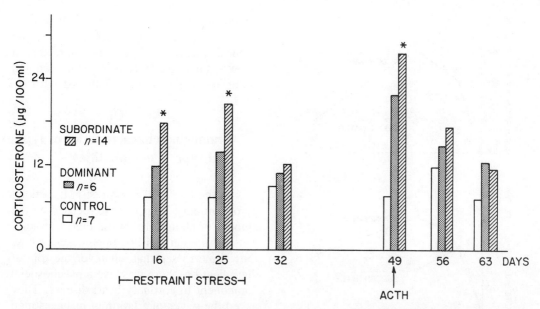

Fig. 7-11. Groups of dominant and subordinate mice were submitted to restraint stress for two hours on days 16 and 25 of their mutual 63-day exposure to a population cage. Plasma corticosterone in subordinates measured significantly higher ($p < 0.05$) than in dominants. Values for the controls (unstressed boxed-siblings) are shown in the open columns. On day 32, when plasma corticosterone was measured for all groups now lacking restraint stress (dominants, subordinates, controls), no significant difference was indicated. But on day 49, when ACTH was given to dominants and subordinates, the subordinates again showed a significantly higher rise ($p < 0.05$). On days 56 and 63, during a final control period, when neither restraint stress nor ACTH was used, there was again no significant difference between the three groups. Thus adrenal-cortical hormones in the plasma of subordinated mice rose more with restraint stress and ACTH than in dominants *(Ely, unpublished data, 1976).*

verts noradrenaline to adrenaline by adding the methyl group; the two form a measure of catecholamine synthetic activity. After an initial rise in both dominants and subordinates, TH continued to significantly higher levels in the dominants; PNMT not only increased in dominants but continued to rise and was falling in subordinates as they adapted to their loss of status (Ely et al., 1974; Henry and Ely, 1976).

The adrenal weights of all the males remained normal throughout, emphasizing the subtlety of their social interactions, for adrenal weight is a sensitive index of the intensity of social stimulation in males (Davis and Christian, 1957 p. 126). All values return to normal in colonies that have been interacting socially for three months, an indi-

cation that these neuroendocrine disturbances are to be found only when the hierarchy is unstable and when expectations are not being met and social disorder exists. The blood pressure of the dominant male mouse actually rose after social order was established, which suggested that he experiences a continuing stimulus, possibly because he cannot expel subordinated males from the close quarters imposed by the population cage (Fig. 7-13). Preliminary evidence indicates that when this responsibility is relieved, the blood pressure elevation subsides (Ely, 1971). Further, if food and water are available in only one box, the dominant's systolic blood pressure does not rise, but the subordinates may weaken and die within 35 to 42 days. This difference may exist because the

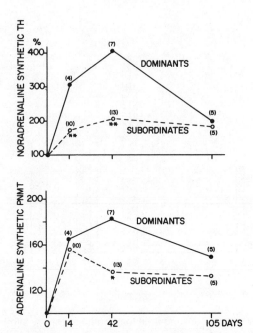

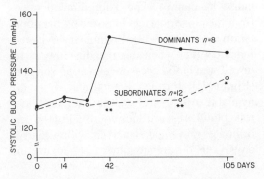

Fig. 7-12. A further aspect of the study described in Fig. 7-10 contrasts the adrenal–medullary content of tyrosine hydroxylase (TH), the noradrenaline-synthesizing enzyme, and of phenylethanolamine *N*-methyltransferase (PNMT), the adrenaline-synthesizing enzyme, in the adrenals of the same dominant and subordinate mice. The TH is significantly higher ($p < 0.01$) in the dominants at 14 and 42 days, but PNMT shows a significant difference only at 42 days. The data point to increased sympathetic activity in the dominants *(Henry and Ely, 1976).*

Fig. 7-13. The experimental design is that referred to in Figs. 7-10 and 7-12. This time the measure is blood pressure which is significantly elevated ($p < 0.01$) in the dominant at 42 and 105 days, but not during the first 14 days. Since all eight boxes in the population cage have food and water, this design may unduly stimulate the dominant because he cannot control all boxes simultaneously *(Henry and Ely, 1976).*

dominant can deny access to a single box, but not access to eight boxes; hence, the subordinates can escape him more readily in an experiment designed to provide food and water in every box (Figs. 7-10 and 7-12).

Endocrine characteristics of type A and type B personalities

In the late 1950's, interest in the etiology of coronary heart disease focused on the amount of cholesterol in the diet. Cardiologists Rosenman and Friedman describe how they came to see that whatever the role of diet might be, there was also a psychosocial component to coronary heart disease. They asked the wives of a group of business men that they regarded as vulnerable to coronary heart disease to detail their diets and were frustrated to find no difference between the diets of husbands and wives, despite a six-fold difference in incidence of the disease. At this point, one of the wives, the President of the Women's Auxiliary of the Junior Chamber of Commerce, pointed out that Rosenman and Friedman were barking up the wrong tree. Since the wives ate the same diet as their husbands, perhaps a psychologic stress factor was at work. She pointed out that their husbands as members of the Junior Chamber of Commerce had quite a different set of social interactions, and, consequently, different social pressures than their own.

Friedman and Rosenman (1974) evolved the idea of splitting up the men and women they interviewed into Type A and Type B behavior patterns. For Type A they lumped all those persons whose behavior evidenced the urgency of time pressure, excessive competitive drive, or undue hostility when thwarted. Type B was used to cover about an equal number interviewed who did not fit into the Type A category. Rosenman, Friedman, and their associates have recently published the impressive results of an eight-year follow-up of 3000 men. Those with Type A behavior patterns were shown to carry an approximately two-fold risk of coronary heart disease (Rosenman et al., 1976).

From the viewpoint of this chapter's concern with neuroendocrine responses to psychosocial stimulation, the question arises as to whether there are physiologic and biochemical differences between someone with the Type A behavior pattern and the rest of the population. If an appropriate social stimulus were used, it might be possible to tell from individual responses whether the two groups differ in the set of their neuroendocrine systems.

The observations of Jones et al. (1970) on the differences in urinary noradrenaline excretion and changes of plasma 11-hydroxy-corticosteroids when different types of persons are stimulated suggest that this distinction may be feasible. They studied male medical students during a critical oral examination in anatomy, measuring their biochemical changes while they were under the influence of this challenging psychosocial stimulus. Jones and his co-workers typed them into two groups: one had the highest muscularity and the lowest component of fat; the other, a long thin body and limbs and lower muscularity. Those with high muscularity had the most marked noradrenaline response to stress. On the other hand, they showed a significantly lower response ($p < 0.005$) of the adrenal-cortical hormone plasma cortisol than the linear men. Jones suggested that in the muscular individual the challenging social stimulus may have primarily evoked anger, activating adrenal-medullary activity with the release of noradrenaline, which has been associated with active aggressive behavior (Frankenhaeuser and Gardell, 1976). Whereas, the pituitary adrenocortical mechanism may have been more readily activated in the predominantly linear type whose personality exposed them to a withdrawal response (Jones et al., 1970).

The biochemical studies of Friedman et al. (1969) certainly suggest a difference between the responses of the hypothalamic pituitary–adrenal system in the two contrasting types of subjects whose behavior

they have been observing since the late 1950's. They found that the average levels of cortisol were the same in both Type A and Type B. However, when persons showing the fully developed Type A response pattern were challenged with large doses of the adrenocorticotropin hormone (ACTH), they excreted significantly less cortisol than Type B subjects ($p < 0.01$) [Fig. 7-14(A)].

The group then used a mental contest to contrast the plasma catecholamine response of Type A coronary-prone subjects to a specific challenge with that of Type B subjects. They invited subjects of opposite types to sit at either end of a table in a small room where they were given 15 minutes to solve identical puzzles. The first to finish would receive a bottle of good French wine that was placed on the table between them. The subjects were simultaneously exposed to background music from two rock and roll radio stations.

Type B subjects appeared relaxed at the idea of competing in this manner, but Type A subjects were tense, hyperalert, and impatient; and when told at the end of the test that no solution was possible, they became angry, whereas, Type B subjects remained unperturbed. The mean plasma noradrenaline value for Type A subjects (0.54 ng/ml) during the contest was significantly ($p < 0.05$) different from the resting value (0.41 ng/ml). There was no significant difference between the corresponding values of Type B subjects (0.41 versus 0.44 ng/ml) [see Fig. 7-14(B)] (Friedman et al, 1975).

Thus the Friedman group found contrasting responses: The pituitary adrenocortical system of Type B individuals responded more to the ACTH stimulus, and the sympathetic catecholamine system of Type A responded more to the stimulus of competition.

In another study they contrasted the urinary excretion of noradrenaline in the two groups. Both noradrenaline and its metabolic end product 3 methoxy-4 hydroxy mandelic acid increased significantly more in Type A persons during a tense working day than in the Type B [Fig. 7-14(C)]. Yet during bed rest at night, neither Type had an increase (Byers et al., 1962).

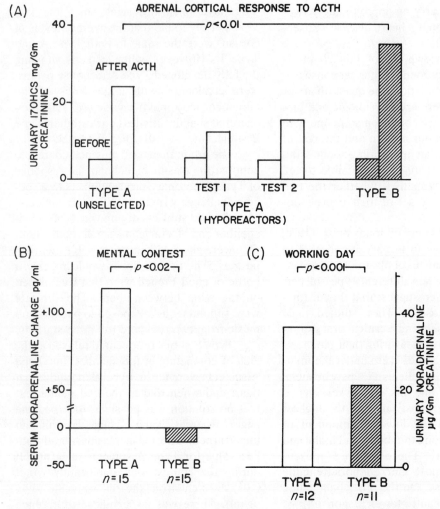

Fig. 7-14.   A composite of three experiments contrasting the neuroendocrine responses of subjects with personalities defined as Type A with those defined as Type B. (A) A fixed dose of ACTH induced significantly more excretion of 17-OHCS in urine of the Type B than the Type A persons ($p < 0.01$). Of the total of 18 Type A persons, six were hyporeactors who hardly responded at all. Similar differences are found in dominant monkeys (Fig. 5-9) and mice (Fig. 7-11) *(Friedman et al., 1969)*. (B) When Type A persons were pitted against Type B persons in a mental contest, their serum noradrenaline level rose, while that of Type B did not change *(Friedman et al., 1975)*. (C) When the excretion of noradrenaline in urine of Type A persons was contrasted with that of Type B during the working day, it was significantly higher *(Byers et al., 1962)*. Taken together, these studies suggest that the Type A and the Type B persons differ in the responsivity of their sympathetic adrenal–medullary and pituitary–adrenocortical systems in the same way that dominants differ from subordinates. *(Reprinted by permission of the publishers.)*

A Type A employee might be an advertising executive supervising an exacting job under the pressure of deadline. A contrasting Type B counterpart might be a municipal employee performing routine accounting duties without time pressure. The difference between the two groups was approximately two to one and highly significant, i.e., ($p < 0.05$) for the mandelic acid and ($p < 0.001$) for noradrenaline [Fig. 7-14(C)] (Byers et al., 1962).

The behavior of Type A persons

appears related to that of a dominant animal being challenged, whereas, that of the Type B has more of the relaxed noncompetitive aspects of subordinates who have accepted their position. The excessive production of noradrenaline by the Type A person being stimulated is compatible with the higher level of tyrosine hydroxylase found in dominant mice by Henry and Ely (1976). The noradrenaline produced by the enzyme tyrosine hydroxylase in the adrenal medulla is increased in dominant mice being challenged to maintain territory, but, as shown in Fig. 7-12, this does not occur in subordinated mice. The behavior of the two groups fit: The dominants are aggressive and free from bites, whereas the subordinates avoid conflict and are repeatedly nipped in the rear.

As already noted, Sassenrath (1970) found a lower level of adrenal-cortical response to ACTH in dominant monkeys (see Fig. 5-9), and Ely reports the same findings in mice (Fig. 7-12). The biochemical work of Friedman et al. (1969) mentioned earlier showing that the adrenal response to excess ACTH is less in Type A individuals supports the results of these animal studies and suggests that dominant versus subordinate role differentiation is at the basis of A and B typology, at least to the extent that Type A is competitive and readily slips into a sympathetic adrenal-medullary mode, whereas Type B is more inclined toward an adrenal–cortical mode (Fig. 7-14). Plasma cortisol levels of Type A and Type B subjects were the same, but the diurnal urinary noradrenaline levels of Type A were significantly higher (Friedman et al., 1960).

In his review of stress behavior patterns and coronary heart disease, Glass (1977) sees Type A college students as more ambitious; they earn more honors and more go on to graduate school. Treadmill tests showed that Type A men push themselves harder and suppress feelings of fatigue. They work closer to the limits of endurance, and when they are defeated in spite of their efforts, according to Glass's data, they experience the loss of control as more threatening. If the loss was obvious, they were more vulnerable to a helpless response than Type B's. Glass sums up his data by speculating that when Type A perceives a threat to his control of the environment, he struggles to reestablish control. During this period, he says, the active coping efforts will be associated with increased plasma noradrenaline but adrenaline is unchanged. Upon perceiving that control has been lost, Type A will become passive and give up, and his noradrenaline levels are likely to decline. The more frequent and the more intense the cycling between the sympathetic nervous system arousal of the effort to control and the onset of helplessness with parasympathetic activity, the more vulnerable the individual may be to the acceleration of pathophysiologic precursors of coronary heart disease (Glass, 1977).

In a related study of psychoneuroendocrine sex differences in adaptation to the psychosocial environment, Frankenhaeuser (1978) repeatedly demonstrates that boys and girls and adult men and women differ in their adrenaline response to challenge. Active periods like mental tests, examinations, or other tasks led to a significantly greater elevation of adrenaline in men. She concludes that men are more dependent on their hypothalamic adrenal-medullary system to overcome a challenge. According to their own accounts, Frankenhaeuser found that feelings of success, confidence, and mastery were common among challenged men, whereas feelings of discomfort and failure were predominant in women working at the same task at the same level of performance. High discomfort was correlated with poor performance in men, but with a good one in women. At first sight, a man's response falls into the Type A category, but a woman's would appear to be closer to Type B and would fall into the Selyean distress or conservation–withdrawal mode more readily. However, subjective reports may be deceptive and more work is needed.

Finally, there are now two comprehensive series of anatomic studies showing that the adrenal cortex is richly innervated, especially in the inner zones (Mikhail and Amin,

1969; Unsicker, 1971), plus three recent independent reports showing that adrenal denervation disturbs biochemical processes, such as cortical steroidogenesis and the synthesis of cyclic adenosine-3', 5'-monophosphate (cyclic AMP) (Paul et al., 1971; Ciaranello et al., 1976; Henry et al., 1976; Henry and Stephens, 1977). It is therefore proper to consider the possibility that nervous stimuli as well as the hormones ACTH and aldosterone influence adrenalcortical function.

The inverse relation between the gonadotropic hormones and the defense and alarm reactions

The classic studies of Christian (1971), which he has recently reviewed, demonstrate that the various endocrine responses developing in crowded animal societies result in decreased natality and point to increased ACTH and decreased gonadotropin levels. Christian has presented an interesting control systems analysis of the various behavioral–endocrine feedback systems that may be involved in increased mortality and decreased natality. Recently Bronson (1973) has successfully demonstrated that the gonadotropic hormones of subordinated male mice decrease during fights to establish social order. At the same time, as shown in the studies by Henry and Ely in Fig. 7-10, the adrenocortical hormones remain slightly more elevated in subordinates than in dominants (Fig. 7-15). Concurrent effects on androgens were indicated by a decrease in the size of the androgen-linked sexual accessory preputial gland of the subordinates (Fig. 7-16). Dominant animals show the reverse trend with a conspicuous enlargement of this gland, which is located close to the urinary bladder; its secretions mingle with urine to produce an identifying odor for marking territory. It is thus a most valuable index of social status.

Fig. 7-15.   One hour after male mice had been placed together in a small cage and were fighting to establish rank, an intense rise in their plasma corticosterone was noted. By day 3 when the hierarchy had been established, the corticosterone level in subordinates was higher than in dominants, but the difference vanished by day 6 as the hierarchy stabilized. Each point represents four–five corticosterone samples for dominants and the mean of 10–14 for subordinates. These results are more intense and rapid but compare, nonetheless, with a slower course of events during the formation of hierarchy in a complex population cage. Vertical lines represent Standard Error of the Mean (see Fig. 7-10) *(Bronson, 1973).*

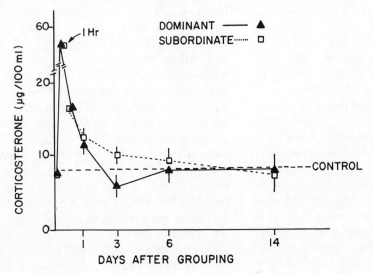

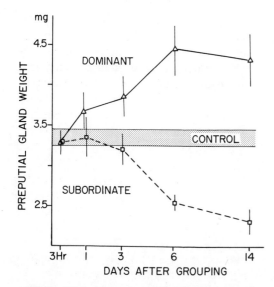

Fig. 7-16.   In an extension of the study with mice described in Fig. 7-15, Bronson demonstrated that by day 3 the weight of the preputial gland of dominants had become significantly larger than that of subordinates, increasing steadily thereafter until twofold at day 14. Each point represents five–seven weight measurements for dominants and 10–17 for subordinates. Vertical lines represent Standard Error of the Mean. The size of the preputial gland is a measure of self-perception of position in the social hierarchy *(Bronson, 1973).*

The work of Sachar et al. (1965) with human subjects hypnotized under friendly relaxing circumstances, that of Bourne (1971) in Vietnam with combat personnel exposed to danger but perceiving high self-worth in their performance of emotionally rewarding duty, and that of Katz et al. (1970) with psychiatric scoring of defenses of women awaiting biopsy reports of a lump in the breast—all show that the feelings of social acceptance and of high personal value, which commonly accompany effective psychiatric defenses, are associated with decreased activation of the pituitary adrenal-cortical mechanism (Fig. 7-17). The work of Carroll (1976), cited earlier, is also compatible with this conclusion—for primary depression accompanied by a lack of self-worth is associated with elevated plasma

cortisol. On the other hand, a variety of observations, including the dramatically increased incidence of complications of pregnancy observed by Nuckolls et al. (1972) in women evaluated as having weak defenses in situations characterized by a high occurrence of social change suggest that the human reproductive system is adversely affected by depressing social perceptions (Fig. 11-1).

Indeed, Abernethy (1974) has recently reviewed considerable evidence from primatology and psychiatry suggesting that male dominance facilitates male–female copulatory behavior and that female dominance inhibits it. Along this line, Jonas and Jonas (1975) in their study of sex and status maintain that a high-ranking social position with a feeling of inner worth is as critical for the human's ability to form bonds and to breed as it is for other mammals. Continuing this theme, Akiskal and McKinney (1975), who recently completed an overview of depression research, recognize the role of early object loss and of failure to control the envi-

Fig. 7-17.   For hospitalized women awaiting biopsy of a lump in the breast, a regression line ($p < 0.01$) can be drawn relating their excretion of urinary hydrocortisone to the extent to which a team of psychiatrists assessed them as demonstrating failure of defense responses and loss of social acceptance and personal worth *(Katz et al., 1969).*

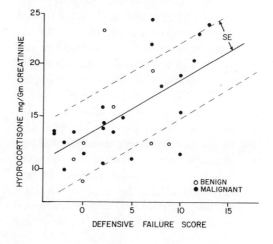

ronment in precipitating disturbance of critical homeostatic feedback loops in the mammal. They speculate that it may result from a shift in balance between the noradrenergic and the cholinergic toward the cholinergic side. The reverse pattern of success and increased status has been shown to be associated in the male with more dominant behavior, an increase in plasma testosterone level, and lower 17-OHCS levels (see Figs. 5-9, 5-10, and 5-11).

Summary

The response of animals or men striving to maintain status contrasts with those who are not competing. The amygdala with inputs from the frontal cortex is associated with the formation of reinforcement associations giving value responses, indicating which goal continues to be worth pursuing. Lacking this reinforcement, the fight–flight reaction will not be triggered by frustration. Amygdalar control leads to a chain of responses, activating sympathetic efferents to the peripheral vascular bed and elevating adrenaline during a general arousal and plasma noradrenaline during an irritated fight response as in a would-be dominant or Type A personality. By contrast, the hippocampus, with inputs from other areas of the frontal cortex, appears to regulate the activities of the corticotropin-producing hypothalamic cells when control of the territory has been lost during conditions of uncertainty. When old patterns of responding fail to pay off with anticipated rewards and when control of the surrounding space vitally important to life is lost, the depressive response is precipitated along with the release of ACTH and activation of the pituitary–adrenal system. Behavioral evidence indicates that this occurs when coping attempts are thwarted and a potentially disastrous threat is perceived which cannot be escaped or controlled. The physiologic and biochemical consequences of these responses are described with examples of dominance–submission conflicts in rodents, subhuman primates, and man. Finally, the inverse relation between the activity of the gonadotropic hormones and these responses is described.

8

Functional and structural changes in response to psychosocial stimulation

Distinction between Cannon and Selyean stress

The preceding chapters outline the mechanisms by which a psychosocial stimulus can lead to a change in autonomic and endocrine activity, whereas this chapter is concerned with the eventual consequences of the regulatory disturbances resulting from these functional and reversible changes of neuroendocrine activity. We are considering a delicate no-man's land between a purely physiologic shift in equilibrium, which may last for only minutes or hours, and irreversible pathology, such as cardiac hypertrophy with gross arteriosclerosis; pathophysiologic changes in the adrenal cortex; kidney damage by interstitial nephritis; or even formation of malignant tumors. It is precisely at this point, that to many the chain of evidence linking the higher centers of the brain with pathophysiology is the weakest and the arguments are the most strained. This chapter outlines the progress made in this area.

The question may arise as to the num-
ber of stress response patterns. Figure 7-1 has indicated that at the very least a dichotomy must be considered. We discriminate between Cannon's fight–flight or rage response, which leads to an increase in sympathetic and adrenal–medullary activity and eventually to cardiovascular deterioration due to arteriosclerosis, and the Selyean response that primarily involves activation of the adrenal-cortical mechanism. The latter is associated with withdrawal behavior, indicative of depression, and with increased vagal activity. The diseases associated with chronic activation of the Selyean stress response do not appear uniformly the same as those elicited by chronic arousal of the Cannon fighting response. As seen in later chapters, while high-renin high blood pressure characterizes the Cannon response, increased corticosterone characterizes the Selyean and may contribute to a failure of immune response mechanisms. This may pave the way to the formation of tumors as well as bacterial and viral infections.

Another feature may be heightened vagal activity (see Fig. 7-1) that may contribute to cardiovascular collapse and to peptic ulceration, as well as add to problems induced by the Cannon response. If both are present at the same time, the failure of the gonadotropins opens the way to disease of the reproductive system, especially when arteriosclerosis and undue responses of the vascular bed are at work, together with activation of the adrenal medulla, or the cortex, or both. Indeed the disentanglement of the Selyean from the Cannon neuroendocrine chain has only now become feasible; and during intense or intermediate states of arousal, both response patterns are activated simultaneously.

Changes primarily related to the sympathetic adrenal–medullary response

Radius changes in resistance vessels

There is no better example of initially reversible and quite normal responses to physiologic stimulation than that of vascular changes in hypertension. Starting as physiologic adjustments, they can conclude in a series of positive feedback loops creating an unstable condition. The vascular bed becomes increasingly responsive to a given autonomic stimulus, and finally the organism is dragged down to pathophysiologic disaster. For more than 20 years, Folkow has studied the structural adaptive changes in the vascular bed determining resistance in essential hypertension, and his evidence for the critical effects of simple physical changes is now overwhelming (Folkow et al., 1958; Folkow et al, 1973; Folkow, 1975).

Resistance vessels in precapillary regions are the key to primary hypertension. The overall resistance (R) to flow through the combined vessels of a region is a measure of the average internal radius of those vessels. But this radius is also a measure of the average length of the vascular smooth muscle strips that encircle the lumen. The resistance R is the ratio between pressure drop (PA-PV) and flow (Q). Any change in internal radius becomes greatly amplified when expressed in terms of this resistance because it is inversely proportional to the fourth power of the radius. Thus a decrease in internal radius of five percent which cannot be measured by histologic methods still implies a 20–25 percent increase of resistance. This is enough to be of great functional significance. Flow resistance can be determined when the vascular smooth muscle is completely relaxed and is at a given low transmural pressure to allow for variations in distensibility. If this is done, then the minimum flow resistance (R min) provides a measure of the resting length of muscle elements that make up the internal radius of the vessel. If the vessel complex is now exposed to various procedures changing its radius, minimum flow resistance will provide the needed base line against which the respective levels of smooth muscle activity in the two states can be compared (Folkow and Neil, 1971; Folkow, 1975) (Fig. 8-1).

Folkow has used this concept of determining the ratio between the resting and the active flow resistance to study the possibility of the structural design of precapillary vessels changing in hypertension.

Structural autoregulation in man

Looking for evidence of this proposed change in structural design, Folkow, Grimby, and Thulesius tackled the problem of human hypertension in the 1950's. They studied the response of the forearm by contrasting normal with hypertensive subjects and induced maximal dilatation by combining ischemia, intense muscle exercise, and external heating. Estimating R min for both groups by plethysmography, they found it significantly elevated in essential hypertension. Resistance to flow in the steady resting state also increased in approximate proportion to the increase of arterial pressure. This

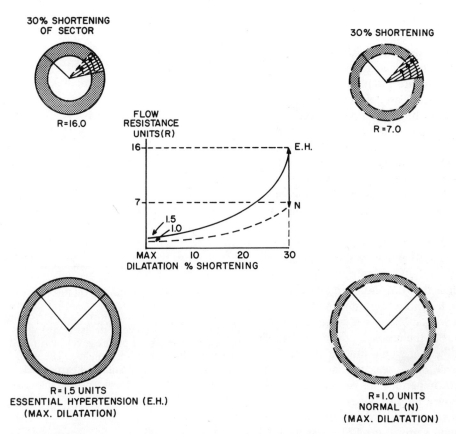

Fig. 8-1.   The changed relationship, in arbitrary figures, between the degree of vascular smooth muscle shortening and the increase in flow resistance, once a structural adaptive change in wall/lumen ratio has occurred in essential hypertension (EH) (left side of diagram). At maximum dilatation, the normal vessel (N) (right side of diagram) has a resistance of 1.0 unit against the 1.5 unit of the wall-thickened hypertensive vessel. This is shown in the central diagram by the contrasting points at which the hypertensive and normal curves cut the ordinate. At 30 percent shortening, the resistance (R) of the normal vessel (bottom right) increases to 7.0 units (top right). *R* for the hypertensive vessel increases for the same 30 percent shortening from 1.5 (bottom left) to 16.0 units (top left). Thus shortening alone, without the thickening of the wall structure, will not account for the greatly increased resistance in essential hypertension *(Folkow and Neil, 1971).*

meant that the ratio of resting resistance (*R*r) to minimal resistance (*R*m) of flow was approximately the same in both groups. Thus, despite the increase in resistance, there was no evidence of increased smooth muscle activity in the forearm muscle beds of resting subjects (Folkow et al., 1958).

These intitial studies with humans suggested that resistance vessels in the forearms of essential hypertensives had structurally narrowed lumina and that the base line for resistance control in the sys-

temic circulation had been set to a higher level. In addition, as Fig. 8-1 indicates, the logic of physics demands that this decrease in internal radius due to wall hypertrophy results in an exaggerated increase of resistance for any given degree of smooth muscle shortening. In Fig. 8-1 the curve *N* for resistance vessels of normotensives, with a normal ratio of wall thickness to radius, can be compared with the curve *EH* for resistance vessels of essential hypertensives, with thicker walls and hence a reduced radius.

These two curves relate the degree of smooth muscle shortening to the resulting resistance increase. Curve *EH* has a steeper slope because there is a greater mass of wall to be pushed toward the lumen in the thick-walled resistance vessel of the hypertensive. This increases the rate at which radius is reduced, and hence the vascular resistance increases rapidly as the smooth muscle shortens. The result is an increase in the reactivity of the blood vessel without any change in that of the smooth muscle composing it (Folkow and Neil, 1971; Folkow, 1975).

In 1970 Sivertsson used the vascular bed of the hand to explore the human hypertensive's sensitivity to noradrenaline. He showed that the threshold resistance responses in hypertensive subjects were not associated with an increased smooth muscle sensitivity. For the minimal concentration of noradrenaline that would initiate any particular response curve was the same in both normal and hypertensive vessels. But, as Fig. 8-2 shows, the responses were exaggerated, once suprathreshold concentrations of noradrenaline were used. The data demonstrate that in man the so-called hyperactivity of resistance vessels is, in fact, a mere physical expression of an increase in the ratio of wall thickness to internal radius (Sivertsson, 1970).

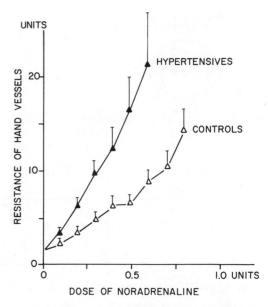

Fig. 8-2. Dose response curves showing the change in resistance of the hand vessels as the muscle in the vessel is progressively shortened by increasing doses of noradrenaline. The solid triangles are Mean and Standard Error of Mean (SEM) for 16 hypertensive patients; the open triangles, for 16 matched controls. The curves may be related to those in Fig. 8-1 *(Folkow, 1975)*.

Distribution of vascular changes

Folkow concluded that if such changes were generalized, they would be sufficiently severe to explain the increased blood pressure and resting resistance to flow without changing resting smooth muscle activity. But if, in addition, there was also functional excitation of the nervous system, then further increases in the resistance of these thickened vessels could occur due to the damaging effects of positive feedback.

Recently other investigators have used the hemodynamic approach in confirming a structurally determined reduction in the radius of precapillary resistance vessels (Furuyama, 1962; Folkow and Neil, 1971; Folkow et al., 1973; Folkow, 1975).

Members of Folkow's group have made extensive studies of the isolated hindquarters and renal vascular beds of spontaneously hypertensive rats. Their ingenious technique was to study all resistance vessels of the hind limbs at one time by applying the principles of biophysical and pharmacologic analysis of isolated muscle strips (Fig. 8-3). These experiments incorporated constant flow perfusion with artificial plasma substitutes and simultaneously compared matched pairs of hypertensive and normotensive vascular circuits. Curves showing the resistance for various doses were obtained by giving noradrenaline in equal progressive steps. This resulted in increasing perfusion pressures up to the point of peak contractile strength of the vascular bed (Fig. 8-4) (Folkow, 1975; Hallbäck, 1975).

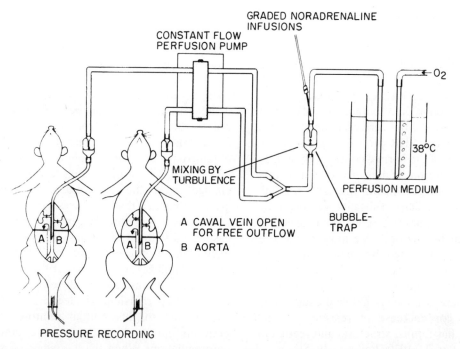

GRADED NORADRENALINE INFUSIONS

CONSTANT FLOW PERFUSION PUMP

O₂

38°C

PERFUSION MEDIUM

MIXING BY TURBULENCE

BUBBLE-TRAP

A CAVAL VEIN OPEN FOR FREE OUTFLOW

B AORTA

A B A B

PRESSURE RECORDING

Fig. 8-3. Schematic of the hindquarter perfusion of paired rats. This technique permits warm perfusate to first pass through a common tube into which graded doses of noradrenaline are infused. Emerging from the mixing chamber, the tube bifurcates and the same fluid is pumped through the aortic cannalae into a spontaneously hypertensive rat and a normal control. The ensuing curves relating resistance to smooth muscle shortening are seen in Figs. 8-1 and 8-4. The perfusate freely exits by way of the cut vena cava, and perfusion pressure is measured in the artery of the tail *(Weiss, 1974).*

Fig. 8-4. In the left diagram, experimental data have yielded average "resistance curves" of the type shown in Figs. 8-1 and 8-2; Fig. 8-3 shows the perfusion setup for spontaneously hypertensive rats (SHR) and normal controls. The right diagram shows mathematically deduced resistance curves for two hypothetical vessels whose characteristics are changed as shown; the hypertensive differs from the normal only in 30 percent increase in medial thickness (see Fig. 8-1). The result is some encroachment on the lumen even at maximum dilation. Note the threshold at which resistance starts to increase sharply is at the same point in both rats, indicating that the hypertensive has the same vascular smooth muscle sensitivity to noradrenaline as the normal control *(Folkow, 1975).*

EXPERIMENTAL RESULTS (A) CONTRASTED WITH HYPOTHETICAL RESISTANCE VESSELS (B)

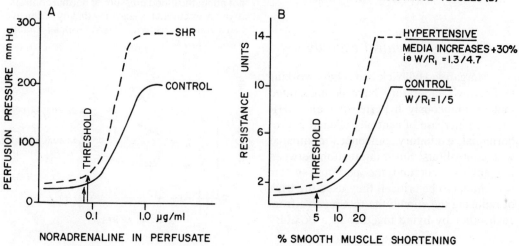

Neither a decrease in the number of available arterioles nor a changed sensitivity to constrictor influences would account for hypertension in the spontaneously hypertensive rats (SHR). In every case the resistance vessels of the SHR proved less distensible than those of the normal controls; they had a reduced internal radius associated with a thicker, stronger medial muscle. Not only are the precapillary resistance vessels of the SHR hyperreactive to constrictor agents in that their lumina decrease more because of their changed design, but they are also more responsive to all types of dilator influence. Thus, merely because of vessel wall thickness, there is a locally induced exaggerated increase or decrease of resistance which Folkow has termed structural autoregulation (Folkow et al., 1970; Folkow, 1975).

Exposure of the vessel to an increasing load would appear to be responsible for this medial hypertrophy. For if arterial pressure is reduced in the hind limbs by aortic occlusion, the design of the vascular bed changes and the walls become thinner, thereby reducing the ratio of wall thickness to internal radius. The same effect is obtained by keeping the pressure low from the time of birth by using an immunologic technique to destroy the peripheral sympathetic nerves. The fact that local transmural pressure is critical raises the question of what affects this pressure. What triggers the pressure increase that gradually induces structural changes (Weiss, 1974)?

The role of central excitability

Margareta Hallbäck and others working in Folkow's laboratory have demonstrated that spontaneously hypertensive rats SHR show an increase of centrally elicited neurohormonal excitatory influences compared with control rats. Since interaction between the environment and the nervous system was shown to be critical, they used the trick of reducing the stimuli the rats receive from each other by living together in a box. By housing the SHR separately for seven months, their blood pressure and structural changes in heart and vessels could be decreased, the mechanism being the elimination of stimuli resulting from social confrontations (Fig. 8-5). The opposite effect was obtained by creating excitation with light, noise, and vibration (Hallbäck, 1975), for changes were then accelerated. Folkow's group concluded that there was a close interaction between the neurogenic changes associated with arousal following controlled excitation and the blood vessels' structural factors (Hallbäck and Folkow, 1974); together, they determine the development of chronic hypertension. A feedback effect occurs due to this mutual reinforcement between functional excitation and structural autoregulation. When the average transmural pressure rises, the structural changes become intensified; these, in turn, lead to a further increase of pressure. As a matter of fact, experimental psychologists working with monkeys have induced changes along these lines.

Fig. 8-5. The two sets of curves contrast the blood pressure of spontaneously hypertensive rats (SHR) living in isolation with that of normal controls living in groups. Isolation significantly reduces the rate at which the blood pressure of hypertensives rises with age (two upper curves), resulting in a difference between 15–20 mmHg. But isolation from normal group stimulation did not affect the blood pressure of normal controls (two lower curves), suggesting that hypertensives had a greater sensitivity to psychosocial stimuli *(Hallbäck, 1975).*

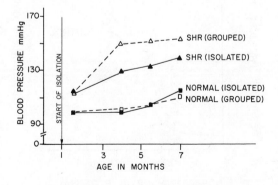

High blood pressure following operant conditioning schedules

In recent years a number of researchers have used operant conditioning schedules to induce high blood pressure. Forsyth has shown that high blood pressure will accompany long-term avoidance schedules in restrained rhesus monkeys whose arterial pressure was measured continuously by implanted arterial catheters. The monkeys were exposed to shock avoidance schedules which forced them to press a lever within a few seconds after a light flashed on; their systolic pressure rose to 150–160 mmHg in response to this chronic stimulus (Fig. 8-6). No consistent relation was found between bar-pressing behavior, number of shocks received, and blood pressure. However, as Forsyth (1969) noted anecdotally, experimental monkeys became more excited and

Fig. 8-6. Up to six months, rhesus monkeys were exposed to predictable, daily shock-avoidance schedules, while sitting in restraint chairs. After three months had elapsed, both systolic and diastolic pressures increased significantly ($p < 0.001$); during the last two months, a diminution in pulse rate was observed *(Forsyth, 1969)*.

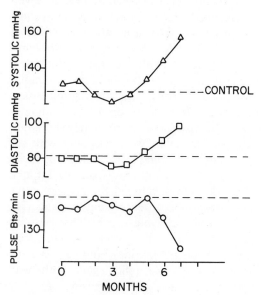

hyperactive during transferring and handling. This change in behavior suggested they were responding to operant conditioning stimuli with emotional arousal.

Very similar results have been obtained in experiments with squirrel monkeys. They were restrained in a pillory chair and trained to press a key a fixed number of times to turn off a light associated with shock; meanwhile their mean arterial blood pressure was chronically measured by implanted aortic catheters. Herd and his co-workers reported that an operant conditioning schedule forcing a monkey to behave in this manner induced a persistent elevation of mean arterial pressure. But further experimentation showed it was not even necessary for the animal to press the key: A schedule was arranged to provide biofeedback so that the increase of blood pressure in itself would turn off the light and so prevent the noxious stimuli from occurring. Thus these monkeys could sustain a depressed mean arterial blood pressure by training them with a schedule so arranged that a decrease in their mean arterial pressure terminated the light (Herd et al., 1969).

Harris and co-workers have shown that baboons can be conditioned to accept food and exposure to shock as "contingent consequences," i.e., rewards or punishments for appropriate self-induced changes, of diastolic blood pressure. After 40 or more 12-hour daily conditioning periods, they were able to induce a 30 mmHg or more sustained elevation of both systolic and diastolic pressure. When the stimulus was turned off at the end of the 12-hour training session, the elevated heart rate and blood pressure both returned to near basal values. These pressure elevations were associated with increased peripheral resistance (Harris et al., 1973).

Recently Friedman and Dahl (1975) made studies of rats having a genetic susceptibility to high blood pressure. The rats were subjected daily to a conflict situation in which they inevitably received a shock, despite responding correctly by repeatedly pressing the lever for a pellet of food. The shock was given during a programmed interval after they had received a pellet, occurring randomly about once every eight presses of the lever. The blood pressures of subjects exposed to this conflict were considerably elevated, measuring up to 170 mmHg (Fig. 8-7). After 13 weeks of such stress, the rats were allowed to recover for an equal length of time; blood pressures of most rats slowly dropped to normal with an expected lag, in view of Lundgren's (1974a) evidence that structural changes reverse slowly (Friedman and Dahl, 1975).

Diminished baroreceptor gain

In 1956 McCubbin and his colleagues Green and Page showed that in renal hyper-

Fig. 8-7. The increased systolic mean blood pressure of rats who were exposed to an electric shock of the tail as an unavoidable consequence of eating. Pellets of food were given in response to pressing a lever at a certain time after a light appeared, but the unpredictable time interval made it impossible to achieve a sense of control. Furthermore, after an unpredictable number of presses, they received a shock, creating a conflict because their already random response to obtaining food was also punished, but in an unpredictable manner. Control rats had *ad lib* access to food and were not exposed to pressing the lever or shock ($p < 0.01$ for 11 of 13 weeks) *(Friedman and Dahl, 1975).*

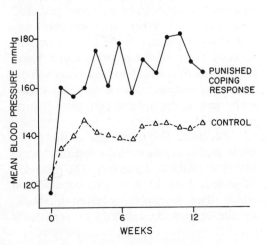

tension, discharges in the nerve from carotid sinus baroreceptors of a dog are "reset," so that it takes a greater elevation of pressure to produce the same rate of discharge (McCubbin et al., 1956). Sleight (1975) has recently confirmed this important work, and Aars (1968) made similar studies of the sensitivity and threshold of aortic receptors in rabbits.

The work was concerned with the fact that if the baroreflex gain is lowered either by damage to the arterial receptors or by splinting them (i.e., surrounding them with a nondistensible material), there will be an increase in peripheral sympathetic nervous activity as the discharge decreases. This leads to tachycardia, increased peripheral resistance, and smooth muscle tone, all of which will increase blood pressure. An increased sympathetic tonus will also increase renin release from the kidney, and the ensuing rise in the pressor agent angiotensin is a strong stimulus to further sympathetic discharge (Zanchetti and Stella, 1975).

Such an upward resetting of the baroreceptors will occur in hypertensive dogs due to changes in the vessel walls following a sustained pressure elevation. Sleight, who used single-fiber preparations, showed that the carotid sinus receptors of hypertensive dogs do not begin to fire until pressure levels are reached which would produce a continuous discharge from a normal receptor (Fig. 8-8). Although the receptor discharge appears qualitatively normal in hypertension, not only is the threshold raised, but it is also not as sensitive to further increments of pressure. Thus the receptors are failing to buffer the rises in pressure as they should.

The preceding work was done with animal subjects. But in a follow up with humans, Sleight's group used a discriminating technique developed for a quantitative assessment of baroreflex gain; they incorporated cardiac slowing which follows a transient rise in pressure produced by the pressor agent phenylephrine. Finding a striking diminution of baroreflex gain both with hypertension and with increasing age, they suspected an increasing stiffness of the

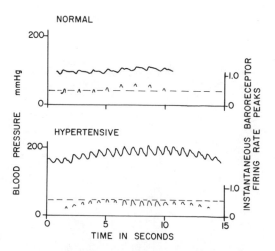

Fig. 8-8. The activity of single carotid baroreceptors from a normal dog and a dog that has had renal hypertension for five weeks is contrasted. In both records, a curve represents tracings of systemic arterial pressure (above) and a computer-derived curve of instantaneous firing frequency (below). The latter was obtained from a study of action potentials of single baroreceptor units. Note that the firing rate resembles the arterial pressure contour, and that although the pressure of a hypertensive dog is approximately double that of a normal dog, the peak instantaneous baroreceptor firing rate is actually not as high as for the normal dog. This demonstrates the upward resetting of the threshold in disease *(Sleight, 1975).*

arterial wall as well as a possible primary change in receptors. They cited studies of human hypertension as a probable result of baroreceptor damage and of the opposite effect of a fall in blood pressure in patients who had atheromatous deposits removed from the interior of carotid vessels, causing an increased carotid sinus discharge in the now more flexible vessels. Thus these changes are not confined to animals. A very gradual stiffening and hence splinting due to decreased distensibility of the carotid vessels and of the aortic baroreceptors can also occur in humans. This can be secondary to the frequent development of degenerative lesions in vessel walls (Sleight, 1975). Although attributing a disturbance of the central reflex arc in hypertension partly to this change, they agree however that central

modulation of the arc by repeated "defense" reactions to the daily environment also plays an important role.

Rate of development and regression of vascular changes

The rate at which these cardiovascular changes develop has been studied by Lundgren and others of Folkow's group. They have shown that cardiac hypertrophy and an increase in the ratio of precapillary wall thickness to internal radius in the spontaneously hypertensive rat (SHR) (Fig. 8-9) are completed in several weeks after the onset of experimental hypertension induced by constricting the renal artery with an adjustable clamp devised by Goldblatt. Folkow speculated that this type of structural adaptation is probably far slower in man, taking months. They further demonstrated that if a Goldblatt hypertension is reversed by removing the constricting clip from the renal artery, changes will gradually regress over a period of three weeks. Preventive treatment for the SHR by appropriate drug therapy in early life prevents structural cardiovascular changes. In fact, from all indications, it is fairly easy to hinder or to reverse structural changes during early stages of hypertension when hypertrophy is still uncomplicated (Lundgren, 1974).

However, Folkow's group confirmed that after prolonged periods of hypertension, it becomes very difficult to reverse these changes. Wolinsky's (1970) work on the rat aorta throws light on this; as an increased stretching pressure persists, vascular muscle cells begin to produce collagen filaments and other fibrous proteins. Vascular walls become infiltrated by increasing amounts of these fibrillar supportive tissues. Such reorganized smooth muscle elements fail to regress when the load is removed. Thus hyperplasia and muscular hypertrophy are now infiltrated by a large amount of fibrillary protein elements which stay in the vessel walls despite a reduction of blood pressure (Wolinsky, 1970, 1971, 1972).

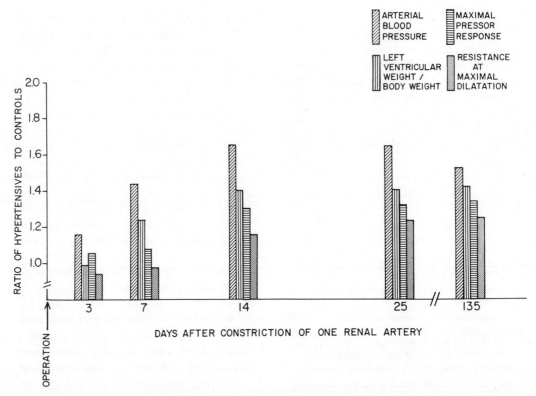

Fig. 8-9. The time course and extent of adaptive cardiovascular changes in normal Wistar rats made hypertensive by a constriction of renal arteries. *Abscissa,* days after artery constriction. Data were obtained from constant flow perfusion of paired, hindquarter vascular beds (see Fig. 8-3 for technique). *Ordinate,* ratio between arterial blood pressure of renal hypertensive rats and normal controls (diagonal shading); ratio of left ventricular weight to body weight (vertical shading); maximal pressor response to noradrenaline (horizontal shading); resistance at maximal dilatation (see Fig. 8-1 also) (stippled shading). Structural adaptive changes of the left heart ventricle and the resistance vessels are almost completed; thus they start with the pressure rise and not as a sequel to it *(Lundgren, 1974b).*

Studies in our laboratory indicate that these changes signaling the advent of true irreversible pathophysiology develop during the second half of an animal's life span. In man they commonly appear at the corresponding decade of the forties and represent the beginning phase of clinically fixed hypertension.

Social stimulation and plasma lipid levels

Folkow's demonstration of the subtle consequences of change in the ratio of wall thickness to internal radius of small arteries, occurring with an increase in the central activation of the defense response, has been described in detail because it represents a uniquely cogent chain of evidence that connects long periods of psychosocial overstimulation with the gradual onset of pathophysiologic deterioration. The next change to be considered, also a response to stimulation of the sympathetic system, concerns evidence that a disturbance of lipid metabolism follows acute emotional arousal in man.

Lipids are continuously mobilized from adipose tissues for release into the blood plasma as free fatty acids. They are bound to the albumin and transported to and utilized in the different organs, such as the skeletal and heart muscle, kidneys, and liver. Lipid oxidation accounts for more than 50 percent of the total oxygen consumption in the body during fasting. Our understanding of the mechanisms underlying the turnover of free fatty acids and triglycerides is limited and represents a complete biochemical problem still undergoing analysis and elaboration. It is, however, agreed that the catecholamines are of major importance in stimulating the release of glycerol and free fatty acids from adipose tissue (Havel, 1968). Vasoconstriction which follows excitation of the receptor sites on the sympathetic effector cells—the classic response to noradrenaline—is not the only factor at work here. Indeed, Ballard and Rosell (1971) have shown that with respect to lipolysis the response of subcutaneous adipose tissue to both circulating catecholamines and sympathetic innervation is specially adapted, and with continued stimulation or sustained infusion of noradrenaline an initial mild constriction will often revert to vasodilatation.

The sympathetic nervous system is physiologically important for regulating vascular reactions and releasing lipids from such adipose tissues as the omental fat pad of the abdominal cavity (Ballard et al., 1971, 1974). Kathryn Ballard and her colleagues also showed that there is an extensive capillary network and perivascular plexus of nerve in adipose tissue. There are interesting questions concerning the possible cell-to-cell transmission of information, and details of the innervation of various types of adipose tissues are still being studied. In recent work Ballard (1973) has shown that, in addition to nervous action, increased levels of circulating noradrenaline can also produce beta receptor-mediated vasodilation in adipose tissues.

Levi extended these observations made on animals by working with human volunteers. He and his co-workers studied the effect of a two-hour period of rest followed by two hours of sorting small, shiny steel balls of four different sizes while being exposed to loud industrial noise (100 decibels), a flickering light, and unfair criticism for working too slowly and inaccurately. Mobilization of free fatty acids increased during this stimulus. Since both systolic and diastolic pressures and urinary excretion of catecholamines were also increased, the lipolytic effect on adipose tissue appears to have been due to increased nervous system activity. The free fatty acid increase was approximately 30 percent and was significant to the $p < 0.001$ level (Levi, 1967).

In related observations, Taggart and Carruthers (1971) took plasma samples from experienced automobile racing drivers at various times for three hours following an international contest. It was chosen instead of an athletic contest, such as ice hockey, so as to represent extreme emotion and aggression combined with minimal physical exertion in terms of oxygen consumption. Noradrenaline and adrenaline were both moderately but significantly increased, i.e., total catecholamines rose from 0.8 to 4.0 units. At the same time, the level of free fatty acids in the plasma tripled. Triglycerides also rose, but took one hour. There was some evidence of interconversion between free fatty acids and triglycerides. The work thus demonstrated that emotions, which arouse submaximal plasma catecholamine responses, will trigger maximal lipid responses (Fig. 8-10).

A further study showed that an oral dose of the sympathetic nervous system beta receptor blocker, oxyprenolol, abolished the plasma free fatty acid response when it was given orally one hour before a professional racing car contest (Taggart and Carruthers, 1972). This result with its suppression of tachycardia, despite the excitement of the contest, is similar to that reported earlier by Eliasch et al. (1967) who demonstrated that the beta blocking agent, propanolol, will prevent an increased cardiac output observed during an exacting experience of testing in a Link trainer.

These studies of the plasma lipid increment accompanying psychosocial stimula-

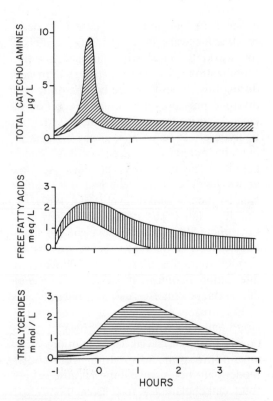

Fig. 8-10. Plasma total catecholamines, free fatty acids, and triglycerides during the fight-flight response arousal elicited in 16 men by a brief episode of driving a racing car. The shaded area represents the range of the response. The catecholamines, chiefly noradrenaline (a fight response), are grossly elevated immediately before and during the event but rapidly subside. Free fatty acids, also elevated before the event, take 60 minutes to subside, whereas triglycerides rise gradually, peaking only a full hour after the event *(Taggart, 1971)*.

tion indicate that it occurs in response to sympathetic adrenal-medullary stimulation. In certain cases, this arousal may be repeated day after day, with the possibility of leading to prolonged functional disturbance. In his hypothesis on aggression and atheroma, Carruthers (1969) has suggested that an excess of free fatty acids could be converted to endogenous triglyceride in the liver and under the action of raised cortisol levels could be deposited in the arterial walls,

causing atheroma. They may also initiate thrombosis by increasing platelet adhesiveness.

Social stimulation and adrenal-catecholamine biosynthetic enzymes

The preceding observations raise the question as to what will happen to animals living in constant turmoil. What happens to colonies of socially disturbed mice unable to find relaxation becase a stable hierarchy fails to develop due to their lack of social experience and the confrontation–stimulation design of their population cage? We first measured the content of the catecholamine-synthesizing enzymes in the adrenals and later used plasma corticosterone as a measure of adrenal cortex activity.

In Fig. 5-17 the measurements of blood pressure, tyrosine hydroxylase and methyl transferase in normal socialized mice living in boxes are given an arbitrary value of 100 percent (left column). The second column shows that mice isolated for the first 10 months of life have normal blood pressure and their tryosine hydroxylase and methyl transferase are actually lower due to the lack of stimulation. On the other hand, when mixed together in a population cage for six months, the usual sustained fighting persisted. Blood pressure, tyrosine hydroxylase, and methyl transferase were greatly elevated in these vigorously competing animals.

The great increase in adrenal enzymes is a consequence of the activity of sympathetic nerves, which has been demonstrated by Thoenen et al. (1969). In our current work, these results were confirmed by unilateral and bilateral adrenal denervations which prevented the expected rise in the medullary content of tyrosine hydroxylase (Fig. 8-11) (Henry et al., 1972, 1976; Henry and Ely, 1976).

It takes only a few hours of stimulation to fully develop an increase of enzyme levels, and the return to base line following

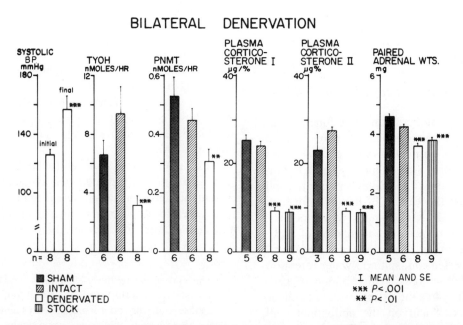

Fig. 8-11. Data from mice in this complex experiment are contrasted with that from stock controls (vertical shading) living as siblings in standard laboratory boxes and having neither surgery nor exposure to social stress. Previously isolated males who had recovered from bilateral adrenal denervation 10 days earlier (open histograms) were placed in a population cage containing females along with intact male controls (diagonal shading) and previously isolated sham operated males (stippled histograms). After seven days of vigorous social interaction, the blood pressure of the males, including those who were denervated, had risen from 125 ± 10 mm Hg to 155 ± 20 mmHg ($p < 0.001$). The series of histograms, from left to right, show that tyrosine hydroxylase (TYOH) in the adrenal medulla more than doubled in intact males, but remained unchanged in denervated males despite a rise in blood pressure, showing the enzyme's dependence on the activity of the sympathetic nerves to the adrenal medulla ($p < 0.001$). The next histogram shows that phenylethanolamine *N*-methyltransferase (PNMT) was also significantly affected by denervation ($p < 0.01$). Plasma corticosterone of bilaterally denervated males (measured twice in seven days) was contrasted with that of sham operated and of intact males undergoing stress, failing to rise above that of normal stock controls without stress ($p < 0.001$). Paired adrenal weights of denervated males remained at control levels (i.e., the same as for nonstressed stock controls), but those of sham operated and intact males in the population cage hypertrophied in response to social stress. These data point to a neural modulation with the stress of fighting not only of adrenal-medullary catecholamine synthetic enzymes but also of cortical steroidogenesis *(Henry et al., 1976)*.

stimulation is equally rapid. Yet high blood pressure persists for months in these chronically disturbed colonies with their frequent episodes of confrontation. Thus medullary hypertrophy serves to convert acute stimuli into long-sustained changes in the level of adrenal-medullary response. It may be assumed that the same stimulation in the sympathetic nerves to a hypertrophied medulla will lead to a greater release of catecholamines and so will accelerate the structural modification of the arterioles by an increase of the wall-to-lumen ratio that has been studied by Folkow's group (Henry et al., 1971; Folkow, 1975).

These data bear out the general theme that mechanisms causing arousal by intermittent and discrete emotionally stimulating events can lead to long-term functional changes in the neuroendocrine system, which in turn lead to chronic and irreversible pathophysiologic disturbances.

Changes primarily related to the pituitary adrenal–cortical response

Cushing's hyperadrenocorticism

Persistent disturbances of function may result from the sustained action of the pituitary adrenal-cortical as opposed to the sympathetic adrenal-medullary system. Gifford and Gunderson (1970) have presented evidence that the variant of hyperadrenocorticism, known as Cushing's syndrome, is a disorder of homeostatic regulation of a psychosocial origin. This disease is associated with hypertension, salt and water retention, and a characteristic redistribution of body fat which spares the extremities, but collects on the back and on the abdominal wall. These authors have connected this disease with pathophysiologic reactions to bereavement in persons having a life-long inadequate personality. They postulate that the victims suffer from a too readily disturbed homeostatic regulation of the hypothalamic–pituitary adrenocorticotropic hormone (ACTH) mechanism.

Gifford and Gunderson's evidence was based on combined psychiatric and endocrine studies made on more than 60 patients during a dozen years at the Johns Hopkins Hospital in Baltimore. They suggest that these patients were predisposed to the disease by experiencing extremes of overprotection or isolation during infancy and childhood, when they had often been deserted or maltreated. Later they often proved precocious, talented, and energetic. Their life histories told that a significant emotional loss had often been followed by a period of defensive hyperactivity and a denial of grief, and that this had immediately preceded the symptoms of hyperadrenocorticism. Patients showed a vulnerability to depression combined with pathologic defenses, including restlessness and overwork. Their personal relationships were flawed with conflicts and difficulties in identification. The authors considered these persons to be at risk because of their poor impulse control,

inconsistency of mood and self-esteem, and difficulty in keeping optimal closeness in personal relationships. The actual precipitating episode in this vulnerable group appeared to be a serious emotional loss. Here are two of the 10 case histories that they chose out of 60 as having both full psychiatric data and irrefutable evidence of Cushing's disease.

The first is that of a successful businessman who suffered repeated bereavements. He had the highest mean adrenal 17-hydroxycorticosteroid level of the series, and he was remarkable for the intensity of his aggressive drives.

> The patient was a thirty-eight-year-old and Jewish. He was the fourth of six children in a close-knit, very poor family. Always noted for his excessive ebullience, aggressiveness, and ambition, he became an accountant and eventually the owner of his own business. Both his own family and his wife's relatives looked up to him as their only successful member, and depended upon his generosity and leadership. At thirty-three, when his mother died, he applied himself more intensely to his work, and his business became even more successful. Three years later the pattern was repeated when his father-in-law died and his mother-in-law suffered a crippling injury. His own father died suddenly of a stroke and the patient (now aged thirty-seven, but the younger son) assumed responsibility for the daily mourning ritual. Seemingly as a denial of his profound grief, he transformed the ritual into a social occasion, indulging himself in food and conversation with his cronies. Near the end of the year, his favorite older sister died, and he began another inappropriate daily ritual, before the mourning period for his father was completed. An exhaustive physical examination of the patient three weeks before his sister's death had proved him entirely normal, but soon afterward physical and mental changes were noticed. His usual boisterous manner became exaggerated, and his aggressive disposition became belligerent and unpredictable.
>
> When admitted to a local hospital for renal colic one month after his sister's death, he was found to have hypertension,

diabetes, easy bruisability, and other signs of Cushing's syndrome. He continued to conduct his business from his hospital bed, by means of endless telephone calls and a continuous stream of visitors. When a urinary 17 KS level of 50 mg was found, he was transferred to the Peter Bent Brigham Hospital (Boston). His hyperactivity further increased, seemingly in response to loss of contact with his business affairs. He was agitated and garrulous, incessantly talking about grandiose business plans, and he reacted violently to being told he was diabetic. His manic psychosis was interpreted as a defensive reaction to the cumulative deaths of his closest relatives, a pathological denial of underlying grief, and fears of his own death. The right adrenal was removed and found to be enlarged and hyperplastic, but a surgical complication postponed removal of the left gland. He died of this complication four days later and autopsy was refused.

Another example is the following:

The patient was a married woman of thirty-eight, the younger of two daughters in a West Indian Negro family that emigrated to the United States when she was four. She was close to her mother and rebelled against the strict, punishing, penurious discipline of her father. She did well in school in spite of periods of brooding loneliness, and became an aggressive stubborn child who went to work at fifteen. Three years later her mother died after a self-induced abortion, and her father deserted the patient and her sister. By manipulating many men and working exceptionally hard, she supported herself successfully as an accountant.

At twenty-five she stopped working and married a lazy but faithful gambler. Disappointed with her inability to become pregnant, she returned to work and started an affair with an elderly man who bought her gifts. At twenty-nine, a year after an ectopic pregnancy and unilateral salpingectomy, she gave birth, by Caesarian section, to a child who died two days later. After a period of severe depression, she became involved in a series of intense, unstable sexual relationships. At thirty-four she left her husband and married another man, an alcoholic, homosexual drug addict who beat her sadistically and deserted her many times. Although distressed by her life, she felt compelled to satisfy her yearning for the exciting and bizarre, and moved all over the country involving herself in promiscuous and perverse relationships, continually searching for new experiences and exotic foods and drinks.

At thirty-seven her appetite and thirst became insatiable, and she noticed increasing emotional lability and an inability to concentrate. Over several months she developed hypertension, diabetes, oligomenorrhea, severe weakness, and the typical Cushingoid habitus. The diagnosis was made at a West Coast hospital, and after an unsuccessful trial of pituitary irradiation she developed paranoid ideas and fled to the East. On admission to the Peter Bent Brigham Hospital, psychiatric interviews and psychological testing showed an acute paranoid psychosis in a borderline hysterical personality, and a bilateral adrenalectomy revealed diffuse hyperplasia.

She was discharged after a stormy convalescence and readmitted a few months later with a clinical picture that suggested acute serum hepatitis. A year later, at the age of thirty-nine, she died quite suddenly, and autopsy showed a primary carcinoma of the liver, bile-duct type, with local metastases.

Disturbed adrenal-cortical function in high blood pressure

These extraordinary clinical histories are illuminated by the results of Wexler's many years of studying hyperadrenocorticism in breeder rats. He noted that severe arteriosclerosis occurs in repeatedly bred rats of various strains (Wexler, 1964a). Those bred four to six times differed sharply from virgins of the same age, i.e., 12 months. He speculated on the role of what he termed "interanimal stresses associated with breeding" (Wexler, 1964b). It appears that breeding conditions involved the chronic competition between the males for females and the possibility of frequent confrontations with resulting high intensities of psychosocial stimulation. The relevant behavioral data are lacking, but Wexler comments that the rats resemble patients with Cushing's syndrome in their high incidence of diabetes and in their having kidney stones, arteriosclerosis, accelerated aging, and hyperadrenocorticism (Wexler, 1964b). His studies also showed that the normal biosynthetic pathways for the synthesis of steroids, including aldosterone, were disturbed. These repeatedly bred rats proved to be deficient in an enzyme limiting the rate of cortical steroid synthesis (Kittinger and Wexler, 1965).

These studies correlate with the observations of Rapp and his associates who found that the Dahl strain of rats, which develop high blood pressure when fed a high salt diet, have an increase of the salt-retaining adrenal cortical hormone 18-hydroxy-desoxycorticosterone (18 OH-DOC) (Rapp and Dahl, 1971; Rapp et al., 1973). Since, unlike aldosterone, it is not under the control of renin in response to plasma sodium level, rats with high 18 OH-DOC lack proper feedback and continue to retain sodium despite an excess. The question arises as to whether the adrenal cortex might be at fault in this form of high blood pressure aggravated by a high salt intake.

The observations of Gunnells et al. (1970) and of Grim (1973, 1975) have led Grim to suggest that various disorders of the salt-retaining hormone (aldosterone), ranging from the adenoma to bilateral nonadenomatous hyperplasia, are variants of Conn's classic primary aldosteronism. The question also arises as to whether their incidence is in any way affected by the type and intensity of stimuli being delivered to the adrenal gland by way of the nervous system as well as by the hormonal pathway. The now convincing evidence for such innervation appears later in this chapter.

The significantly higher incidence of overgrowth or hyperplasia of the cortex that Russell and Masi (1973) found in 35,000 consecutive autopsies of persons who had suffered from essential hypertension suggests that this may be the case. Their data com-

pared many thousands of hypertensives with matched nonhypertensive controls. Russell and Masi found a highly significant excess of adrenal cortical abnormalities in all forms of hypertension ($p < 0.001$) as well as in essential hypertension ($p < 0.005$).

Various observations with colonies of mice experiencing sustained and excessive psychosocial stimulation have led us to the tentative hypothesis: that as they age, they gradually shift from a predominantly sympathetic adrenal-medullary response pattern to one associated with an increase in the pituitary adrenal-cortical mechanism. For example, the biochemical and behavioral changes observed in our socially competitive mouse colonies indicate that the adrenal cortex is being stimulated, for aging animals develop

Fig. 8-12. Tyrosine hydroxylase (TH) activity of an $n = 8$ random sample of males for each of the 10 mouse colonies described in Chapter 9 (Figs. 9-9 to 9-15). Abscissa and statistical details are also the same (as for Chapter 9) except that there is only one control, such as that shown in the blood pressure study (Fig. 9-10). This represents the value taken from an $n = 15$ sample of males that had been isolated for 10 months. Note the falling off of tyrosine hydroxylase activity in the older colonies.

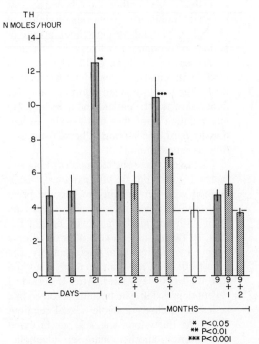

a significant irreversible adrenal hypertrophy. Thus we have observed permanent changes in the weights of the adrenals in our stressed colonies, shown in Fig. 9-13; see Chapter 9 for more details, including the design of the experiment in Fig. 9-9. Ten colonies were established with 16 males (four months old) that had been raised in isolation; an equal number of normal females complemented the population in the intercommunicating boxes of the type shown in Fig. 5-2. After periods of social interaction, as indicated on the abscissa, the colonies were either terminated (shaded columns) or returned to isolation (diagonal shading) for one or two months. Thus a nonlinear progression of age and an exposure to social interaction from two days to nine months is represented. Adrenal weight of mice exposed to only two months of

social stimulation returns toward normal during isolation, but the adrenal weight of those exposed to nine months of social interaction remains significantly elevated ($p <$ 0.001), showing little decrease, despite isolation (Fig. 9-13). Tyrosine hydroxylase (TH), which is reponsible for noradrenaline synthesis (Fig. 8-12), presents a sriking contrast to these figures, being elevated during the early stages of social interaction when there is much fighting. But in aging 13-month-old mice past the reproductive period, who do not fight much, judging from the absence of fresh bites, their TH level is scarcely elevated in keeping with the lesser arousal of the defense responses and the sympathetic system. Renin levels, which betray sympathetic activity, also rise in mice following their initial intense arousal during the first week of social interaction (see Fig. 8-13). However,

Fig. 8-13. Longitudinal study of plasma renin activity (PRA) and systolic blood pressure in control isolates and population cage mice. The latter had been previously isolated and then placed in the population cage at four months of age. The asterisks denote significant differences * = $p < 0.05$, ** = $p < 0.01$, and *** = $p < 0.001$. The number of mice in each group is inset in the histograms *(Vander et al. 1978).*

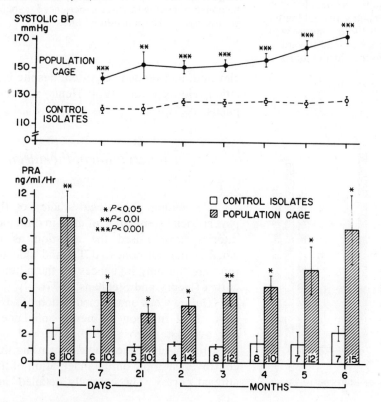

by the third month, their renin level is comparable to that of normal boxed siblings and of aging mice, but by the sixth month, as the kidneys fail, renin has risen again.

There is thus preliminary evidence of decreasing activity of the sympathetic adrenal-medullary system with aging since the level of the adrenal cortically mediated enzyme phenylethanolamine-*N*-methyltransferase (PNMT), which synthesizes adrenaline from noradrenaline, progressively rises and does not return to normal with isolation (Henry et al., 1974) (Fig. 8-14). When the fixed adrenal weight is considered with the increased level of the cortically dependent PNMT, it suggests that, as in Wexler's aging breeder rats, adrenal hypertrophy may be an expression of developing hyperplasia of the gland. Figure 8-15 supports these observations, showing that the plasma corticosterone of aging mice is also

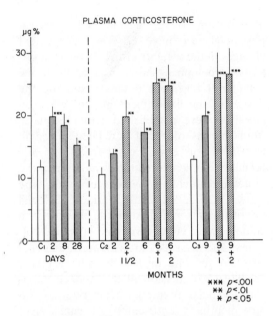

Fig. 8-15. Plasma corticosterone levels of all males in 11 socially disordered mouse colonies. Abscissa represents the statistical details; the controls follow the general design described in Chapter 9. There is a trend toward higher values in older colonies, and the return to isolation is accompanied by even higher values, suggesting that isolation stimulated the adrenal response of mice who have experienced a social environment, even a disturbed one.

Fig. 8-14. Phenylethanolamine *N*-methyltransferase (PNMT) activity of the same males in the 10 mouse colonies described in Chapter 9. Abscissa and statistical details follow the design used in Figs. 9-9 and 9-10, and there is only one control as in Fig. 9-10. In contrast with tyrosine hydroxylase, there is a trend toward increased PNMT activity in the older colonies. Asterisks denote significant differences ** = *p* < 0.01 and *** = *p* < 0.001.

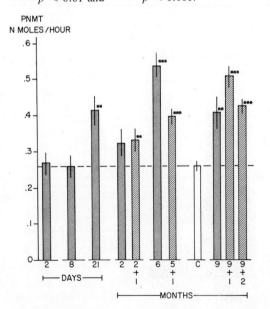

elevated, and remains elevated, despite isolation (Henry et al., 1974; Henry and Stephens, 1977).

Active innervation of the adrenal cortex

Continuing physiologic studies of the psychosocial stimulation of mice in our laboratories have raised the question as to whether the hormones ACTH and aldosterone are the only influences on the adrenal cortex (Henry and Stephens, 1977).

During work on the modulation of adrenal-cortical function by neural influences, our associate Kross (1975) reviewed the most recent anatomic studies regarding this controversial topic on the innervation of the adrenal cortex. The carefully detailed and independent observations of Mikhail and Amin (1969) and of Unsicker (1971) point unequivocally to a rich nerve supply. Furthermore, Paul et al. (1971) present biochemical evidence of the influence of the nerves, showing that the adrenal-cortical adenosine 3.5 monophosphate (cyclic AMP) production is reduced following splanchnic denervation. Ciaranello et al., (1976) have studied the regulation of both PNMT and dopamine β-hydroxylase. Their observations of the effects of denervation have led them to conclude that there is an autonomic regulation of adrenal corticoidogenesis. Indeed, they propose that steroidogenesis and the delivery of glucocorticoids to the medulla may depend on the action of a permissive receptor at the cortical cell synapse which allows the ACTH to regulate corticoid synthesis (Ciaranello et al., 1976). This is a

process in which cyclic AMP plays a critical role. The anatomist Mikhail had pointed to the rich nerve supply to the inner zones and suggested that this represents an important factor in the control of the gland in addition to ACTH (Mikhail and Amin, 1969). The biochemical evidence just cited supports his hypothesis.

Recently Henry et al. (1976) have shown that after seven days of vigorous fighting in a communal cage, formerly isolated mice that have had bilateral adrenal denervation did not have elevated plasma corticosterone. The difference between the experimental and the control animals was a matter of two to one ($p < 0.001$) (Fig. 8-11).

The effectiveness of the denervation was shown by the failure of tyrosine hydroylase to rise, and the rise in blood pressure showed that they were aroused by interac-

Fig. 8-16. This diagram summarizes the results of several experiments whose design follows that of Fig. 8-11, except that only one adrenal was denervated. In each experiment, six to eight formerly isolated male mice representing the three types of surgical procedures were placed with an equal number of females in a population cage where they experienced three days of intense arousal. Although the sham operated and the unilaterally adrenalectomized males showed the expected highly significant rise in plasma corticosterone, there was no significant change in the unilaterally denervated males. Thus the results are similar to those shown in Fig. 8-11 for bilateral denervation.

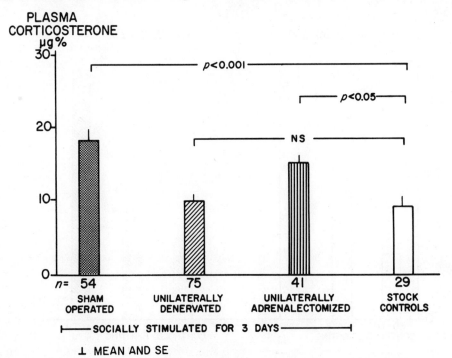

tion in the population cage. The integrity of the adrenal blood supply, despite denervation, was shown by the continued high PNMT assay and the sustained adrenal weight (adrenals in which the blood supply is damaged in the course of denervation atrophy).

The unexpected observation that corticosterone does not rise in mice that are fighting vigorously in a population cage led to a prolonged series of studies which have been reported in detail by Kross (1975) and briefly by Henry et al. (1976). Approximately 500 mice were studied in attempts to analyze the conditions more precisely. As Fig. 8-11 shows, following bilateral adrenal denervation, despite a highly significant rise of blood pressure from 125 ± 10 mmHg to 155 ± 20 mmHg ($p < 0.001$), plasma corticosterone levels failed to rise above those found in standard boxed controls. Bilateral denervation was difficult because of the position of the right adrenal and because its nerve supply parallels the artery. On the left, the nerves come in at an angle and are more easily separated. But in repeated experiments in which only the left adrenal was denervated, the corticosterone response to vigorous social interaction of formerly isolated mice was impaired, scarcely rising above that of normal unstimulated controls. If the left adrenal was removed, the effect vanished (Fig. 8-16). Further, it was found that unilaterally denervated mice respond normally to ACTH, producing a full rise of corticosterone (Fig. 8-17). Thus there is a

Fig. 8-17. A contrast between effects of the adrenocorticotropic hormone (ACTH) and three days of intense arousal due to social conflict on the plasma corticosterone levels in mice. The control group of unstimulated (boxed) mice with intact adrenal nerves run a normal 10 micrograms/percent. This value is doubled after three days of fighting and increases almost fourfold after ACTH is administered. Mice with unilateral or bilateral denervation (see Figs. 8-11 and 8-16 for more data) have no significant increase after three days of fighting, yet their response to ACTH is unimpaired.

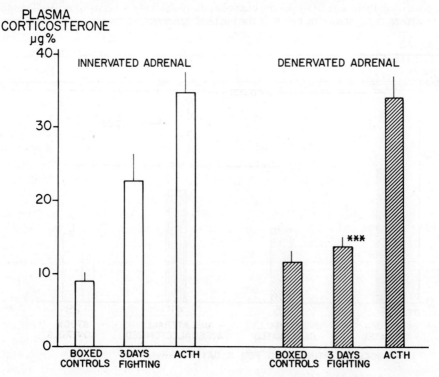

highly significant difference between the denervated and the control groups in their response to fighting.

Although further work is required, there is already sufficient evidence of an active innervation of the adrenal cortex which modifies hormonal control by ACTH and provides a mechanism by which subtle changes in steroidogenesis can develop, especially if these influences have acted over a long period. Taken with Wexler's evidence for breeder rats it suggests that chronic functional disorders of the adrenal cortex, such as hyperplasia, Cushing's disease, and Conn's disease may develop as a result of sustained psychosocial stimulation, influencing the gland by way of both nervous and hormonal pathways.

Adrenal–cortical hormones and myocardial damage

Selye presents evidence that, in addition to the foregoing more direct consequences of adrenal–cortical hyperplasia, cardiovascular disease may be precipitated by an excess of adrenal–cortical hormones. He found that when rats were simultaneously pretreated with glucocorticoids and mineralocorticoids, they became highly susceptible to the development of nonthrombotic myocardial necrosis (Selye, 1970). The triggering agent in this multifactoral situation was to expose the rats to forced exercise, a cold bath, or restraint. Obstructive coronary lesions were not found, but there was a decrease in myocardial potassium and an increase in sodium. This "electrolyte steroid cardiopathy" was characteristically evoked by administering an excess of a hormone possessing both glucocorticoid and mineralocorticoid potency together with trauma or restraint or an injection of the hormone noradrenaline or adrenaline. He reported that another important precipitating factor was the oral administration of triglycerides. Giv-

en these preconditions, he suggested that the simultaneous activation of the adrenal cortex as well as of the medulla would appear to potentiate the onset of myocardial damage.

These observations may throw light on the previously mentioned results of Corley et al. (1975) who observed functional changes and myocardial pathology in association with shock avoidance in squirrel monkeys. They found that the helpless partners, yoked to partners who could avoid shock, collapsed and died with bradycardia. This vagotonia appeared to be associated with the monkeys being shocked without having an opportunity of avoiding it, and was contrasted with the sympathetic arousal of their partners who could actively avoid shock (Corley et al., 1975)

It is relevant that Richter (1957) observed vagotonia in captive wild rats that died suddenly when forced to swim for their lives. Likewise, Carruthers and Taggart (1973) have shown that persons passively watching violence in films evidence vagotonia in addition to an increased secretion of adrenaline. Engel (1971) described related clinical observations. In discussing the life settings in which sudden death may occur, he found that the loss or threat of a loss of a person who was close was a major factor. Death may also occur during mourning or on the anniversary of such a loss. In addition, personal danger or threats of injury are effective. So, as in the studies with animals, the feeling of helplessness, the loss of an attachment figure, or the loss of control in a situation are the underlying factors, and Engel postulates that the parasympathetic is involved in hopelessness or depression. With a shift from the fight–flight response to the conservation–withdrawal response, he suggests that the excitation of both of these response systems may be particularly conducive to lethal cardiac events.

In summary: Sustained, mixed endocrine changes involving both sympathetic adrenal-medullary and adrenal-cortical activation may prove responsible for peculiarly damaging functional disturbances. The emotional aspects of these disturbances would be a combination of anxiety and depression.

Psychosocial effects and immune response mechanisms

Evidence from various sources indicates that emotional factors will affect the course of a disease by influencing the immune response. Some of this is reviewed by Amkraut and Solomon who point to the enormous complexity of the immune defenses and the many points at which the system might be affected. For example, in bacterial disease small changes in the immune process may permit potential pathogens to proliferate and penetrate the various barriers protecting the viscera. This may result from an unfavorable change in mucoid secretions. Once the infecting agent penetrates the barrier of the skin or mucosa, macrophages affected by the adrenal-cortical hormones may present antigens less effectively to the antibody-synthesizing cells, thus decreasing production (Amkraut and Solomon, 1975).

There is evidence that an emotional disturbance will affect herpes simplex infections. The disease may be kept in check by *T* lymphocyte monitoring of infected cells. These lymphocytes may then be disturbed by an altered hormonal balance. It is also possible that cancer in its early stages may be kept in check by cytotoxic antibodies. A decrease of beta cell activity or a lowering of the level of the immune complement may allow the tumor to break away and grow to proportions unmanageable by the immune system. They note that gross elevations of corticosteroids may lead to inactivation of macrophages, permitting the disease to spread. Furthermore, the development of antibodies can be reduced in stressful situations.

A good example of this is found in the recent work of Edwards and Dean (1977) who have shown that crowded mice have reduced humoral antibody formation to the potentially lethal challenge of a typhoid bacillus inoculation. When 30–60 white Swiss-Webster mice were crowded into a single "shoebox" cage, they had significantly lower levels of antibodies and fewer responded to antibodies than mice living two to 10 in a cage. Crowded, nonimmunized mice showed a marked increase in deaths from the pathogen. Edwards and Dean speculate that the unscarred, glossy-coated dominant mice retained their capacity to produce antibodies, despite crowding, whereas the

Fig. 8-18. Cyclophosphamide, which causes gastrointestinal upset, was given to rats with saccharine to induce a conditioned taste-aversion to the sweetener. Nonconditioned controls received only the cyclophosphamide. Three days later, the rats were injected with sheep cell antigens and their hemagglutinins were measured after six days. Nonconditioned rats had a significantly higher titer ($p < 0.05$) by two-tail t-tests than those who were conditioned to aversion and then received saccharine in their drinking water once (x1) or twice (x2) during the six days following the antigen injection. Thus behavioral conditioning partially suppressed the hemagglutinin response. The histograms represent the Mean and the vertical lines the Standard Error of the Mean *(Ader and Cohen, 1975).*

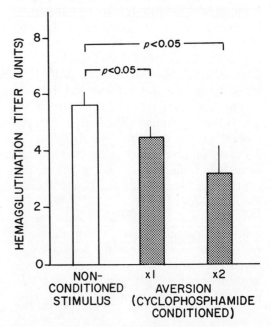

scarred and rough-coated subordinated mice were more susceptible to infection.

In a discriminating study Ader and-Cohen (1975) have analyzed the suppression of the immune mechanism in rats subjected to behavioral conditioning. In contrasting the effects of saccharine on rats with those of cyclophosphamide, a drug used in the treatment of cancer, causing a temporary gastrointestinal upset, they found that, typical of rodents, the upset led to an intense aversion to saccharine which had been given with the nauseating drug. The authors showed that hemoagglutinating antibody titre, which develops in response to an injection of sheep red blood cells, was high in all rats except in those with a gastrointestinally induced aversion (Fig. 8-18); the latter experienced a significant degree of immunosuppression. The data indicated that the phenomenon is not completely mediated by a nonspecific elevation of adrenocortical steroids. However, the door was left open for some steroid influence in subsequent work that demonstrated an elevation of corticosterone in aversively conditioned rats given saccharine (Ader, 1976).

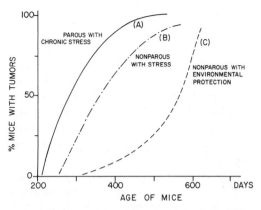

Fig. 8-19. Incidence and latent periods of mammary tumors in C_3H female mice under various experimental and environmental conditions. Group A parous mice were housed in steel boxes in a noisy communal room. Group B mice, similarly housed, did not become pregnant, despite exposure to males. Group C mice, housed without males in plastic boxes, were kept in a specially quiet room and received expert handling, and their conditioned air was drawn from the outdoors. Thus Group C mice were isolated from pheromones and pathogens and protected by husbandry practices from the arousal to which Groups A and B were chronically exposed *(From Riley, 1975. © 1975, the American Association for the Advancement of Science. Reprinted by permission.)*

Neuroendocrine mechanisms and mammary tumor formation

Recent work with mammary tumors in mice suggests that neuroendocrine arousal can change the incidence of tumors. Riley subjected C^3H female mice, carrying the usual mammary tumor-producing virus, to a turbulent environment of noisy steel cages in communal rooms, containing other species, in which there was much activity from the blood sampling and animal husbandry operations. A mortality of 80–100 percent was recorded during a period of eight to 18 months. However, Riley was able to greatly reduce deaths by having the mice placed in quiet plastic cages and carefully handled by experienced personnel in odor-free rooms with a low noise level (Fig. 8-19).

Riley suggests that the chronic arousal

of mice in noisy communal rooms was associated with increased plasma corticosterone levels. Cortisol increases the concentration of intracytoplasmic particles in (mouse) mammary tumors and corticosteroids stimulate the mammary tumor virus *in vitro*. At the same time, the stimulation might lead to a reduction in the critical protective lymphocytes from the thymus and other defense elements. These reductions in immunologic competence may indicate that the cells of early cancer are not held in check and could develop into lethal tumors (Riley, 1975).

In our laboratory we have observed a high incidence of mammary tumors in CBA mouse colonies that had been socially organized but whose social order had broken down. The social breakdown eventually led to the hypothesis that if the young born into a colony are removed much earlier than four weeks old when independent, the females become disturbed and their communal nurseries break up; this disorder spreads to the males who begin fighting. Once this happens, social order is not reestablished and the females, in effect, undergo the animal husbandry procedure of force breeding, since their newly born young are destroyed during the conflict. Our previous experience with socially disordered colonies of formerly isolated males and females has shown that, although the young are always destroyed at birth, there is no increase in mammary tumors over that normally observed in this same strain when used as breeders. Since tumors do not occur in colonized mice until the social system breaks down, it was suggested that the neuroendocrine changes associated with the imposition of social disorder on a previously ordered society induced a milieu favorable to their development.

In 1975 we described a pilot experiment in which a number of control observations were introduced (Henry et al., 1975c). Figure 8-20 presents the sequence of events during this study. All 99 weanings were taken at random from CBA stock. Scanning the figure from top to bottom: 15 females were isolated in jars for 16 months, but no tumors were observed. Twelve standard box-type cages (22 × 11 × 11 centimeters) were composed of four–seven female weanlings in each, living together as siblings; after 19 months, the incidence of mammary tumors in these virgin females was eight percent. Eight cages for breeding each had three females and one male confined to the cage at all times; these breeders were thus rapid-bred,

Fig. 8-20. The sequence of events in a pilot study of the spontaneous formation of mammary tumors in force-bred colonies of CBA mice. Tumors were observed in three of the five categories. Socialized females in the 12-box population cage at first exhibited normal maternal behavior that eventually broke down as their young were repeatedly removed at birth (force breeding); thereafter, none of the newborn survived the ensuing social disorder. There was a significant difference in the incidence of tumors between Study Siblings and Study Breeders and between the Socialized Colony and Colony Control Siblings (*p* = <0.001 by the Chi-Square Test) *(Henry et al., 1975c)*.

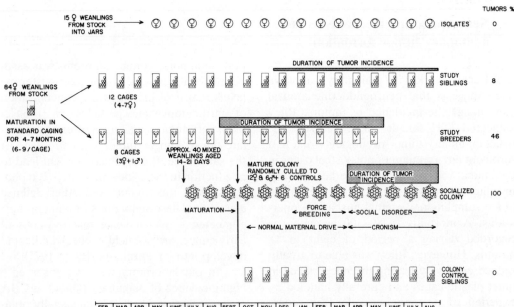

for the male was present for impregnation immediately after the young were born. After 16 months, the incidence of mammary tumors in the breeders was an unexpectedly high 46 percent; we believe this could be associated with early disturbance of the group, as described in our pilot study.

Forty of the four-week-old male and female breeder progeny were used to establish a population cage for the socialization of mice. After three months of colony life, the 40 were culled to 12 females and six males who formed a stable colony that matured and successfully raised its young. After the colony was six months old, all its young were systematically removed as soon as possible. The ensuing three months of force breeding resulted in disorder; fighting broke out in the colony and persisted thereafter. All the young were destroyed at birth by the females. The now ten-month-old females began developing mammary tumors and all had to be killed within five months. Meanwhile, six of the culled young females had been set aside as colony control siblings, remaining 11 months without developing mammary tumors to which their fellow colony members had succumbed.

Beatrice Cooley-Matthews (1977) has followed up on the study just described. She used force breeding, for, as Muhlbock (1956) reports, this procedure reliably induces an increased incidence of mammary tumors. Muhlbock's procedure of force breeding used one male and two or more females per box. The newborn mice are immediately removed, thus denying mothers the possibility of nursing. Cooley-Matthews' careful study has shown that when mice are housed one-to-one in male–female pairs, force breeding has no tumorigenic effect. But a pilot observation indicated that when they live in small groups, such as two or three males combined with four or five females, force breeding apparently leads to an increased incidence of tumors. Figure 8-21 shows the results of these preliminary observations.

No tumors developed in virgin controls

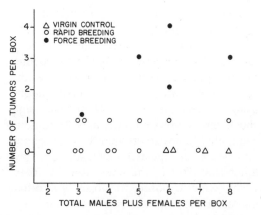

Fig. 8-21. The ordinate represents the number of mammary tumors developed during a nine-month period, beginning with one-month-old weanlings—male and female—from the same litter. The total number of mice in the box is shown on the abscissa. Open triangles represent four boxes of females (virgin controls); 13 open circles represent boxes of combined males and females (rapid breeding, since a male was always present); five solid circles represent similar boxes of mixed males and females from which the young were removed at birth (force breeding). The greater incidence of tumors in these grouped mice (see text) as compared with force bred male–female pairs suggest that social interaction is involved in the tumorigenic effect of force breeding.

during the nine months of observation. A modest incidence of tumors—never more than one tumor per box—developed in rapid bred mice (males continually present) living three to eight to a box (22 × 11 × 11 centimeters); but in force-bred mice (young removed at birth), also housed three–eight to a box, 13 of the 17 females, whose maximum age was 10 months, developed tumors. This observation merits further study, for the technique is simple and the work not only confirms Muhlbock's (1956) study but also our previously mentioned study of disturbed colonies of mice (Henry et al., 1975c), and points to social density as a determinant in the incidence of mammary tumors.

In important related studies, Newberry has induced the opposite effect in rats. He has shown that stress in the form of repeated daily exposure to a series of electric shocks or to daily immobilization within a wire tube would reduce the incidence of mammary tumors. Tumors were induced by injecting rats with dimethylbenzanthracene. Newberry has now twice made this observation, using different stresses, the first time using shock, and the second time, immobilization. Yet there is a possibility that the neuroendocrine status of repeatedly shocked rats may differ from that of the mice used by Riley which were exposed to noise and other unpredictable stimuli (Newberry et al., 1976).

As already noted in Chapter 7, recent work by Mikulaj and by Kvetňanský shows that although immobilization initially leads to an increased corticosterone response, if it is repeated daily, there is eventually a decreased response of the adrenocortical mechanism. At the same time, there is a progressively enhanced ability to replace catecholamines (Henry et al., 1976; Henry and Ely, 1976). What may be happening in the Newberry studies is that with daily repetition, the rat learns that aversive experiences are self-limiting and starts to develop reliable predictions. In keeping with the increasing confidence and the altering perception, the rat's neuroendocrine response may change from a predominantly pituitary adrenal-cortical response to a fight–flight sympathetic adrenal-medullary response. The susceptibility of such rats to the oncogenic virus may differ from rats having an increased corticosterone depressive response. It could be postulated that the latter endocrine pattern may predominate among mice in the experiments reported by Riley (1975) and by Henry (Henry et al., 1976; Henry and Ely, 1976).

The evidence that social interaction, which induces avoidance responses, may disturb immunologic competence as the result of various changes in the regulation of endocrines is becoming stronger. Even in the complex areas of infection and cancer, we are beginning to have clues of how functional changes, which follow on the heels of prolonged psychosocial stimulation, can lead to disease.

Summary

One of the gaps in the chain of events linking psychologic changes to the pathophysiology of high blood pressure has been recently bridged by remarkable work, showing how a gradual, seemingly innocuous increase in medial thickening can, for purely physical reasons, lead to a gross disturbance in the function of resistance vessels.

An accompanying gradual diminution of the responsivity of the baroreceptors adds to the problem of regulation. The fact that these changes occur insidiously and as a part of the normal functional hyperthropic response to increased nervous stimulation is of the greatest significance for the regulatory theory of psychosomatic disease. As Weiner (1975) has pointed out, if the concept that specific disturbances of physiologic regulatory mechanisms constitute the predisposing risk factor in these diseases is to carry weight, the details must be specified, and the sequence of events that lead to the imbalance must be determined.

As a result of neuroendocrine stimulation, important changes can also occur in the free fatty acid metabolism relating to atherosclerosis, but their long-term consequences have not been worked out as fully. Studies showing that similar mechanisms may underlie hyperadrenocorticism, and that disturbance of the immune response may lead to the formation of tumors are even less advanced. Nevertheless, they are already of sufficient weight to suggest that here, too, there are regulatory mechanisms, which, if disturbed, lead from normal reversible functional changes to irreversible disease.

9

Production of disease in animals by psychosocial stimulation

Evidence will be presented showing that if the bias produced by an emotional disturbance tilting the physiologic regulatory processes toward pathophysiology is sustained, it will eventually induce nonreversible pathologic disturbances, in other words, disease. Although the previous chapter dealt with disorders of the equilibrium from which recovery is possible, we now show that irreversible damage can occur. Much of this material, however, was collected without the measurement of intermediate functional stages—the focus of the preceding chapters—and therefore lacks direct evidence of a stage of neuroendocrine or local functional involvement. Yet the circumstances surrounding these cases permit assumptions to be made about the probable state, for example, of adrenal–medullary and cortical functions, but most importantly, they do not point to microorganisms as the cause of disease.

Effects of acute psychosocial stimulation

The consequences of intense excitement of the wild Norway rat have been described by Richter in his classic observations of sudden death. He points out that even the transfer of these animals from one cage to another, such as catching them in a dark bag and grasping them with the hand, commonly leads to fatal cardiac arrest. Yet tame domesticated rats subjected to the same procedure are rarely affected. Richter observed the electrocardiogram in another frequently fatal situation in which they were forced to swim for their lives in glass jars filled with water, after their vibrissae had been clipped. He noted that death came not by drowning, but with a brandycardia; he suggested its cause was vagal inhibition associated with acute emotional arousal. If the rats were trained by repeated brief exposures to the tank, they would quickly adapt, and their behavior would turn from ceasing to struggle to active aggression and sustained, vigorous escape attempts. Richter concluded from bradycardia and the occasional prevention of fatality by atropine that cardiovascular arrest was associated with intense vagal activity stimulated by the rats' perception of the lethal possibilities of their situation (Richter, 1957).

Similar circumstances were observed by Groover and his co-workers in Africa. Coronary vascular lesions and myocardial scars were found postmortem in seven out of 49 baboons trapped earlier and held for experimentation. The lesions were corroborated by electrocardiographic changes. As others have observed in the wild baboons, their vascular beds showed no signs of atherosclerosis. Groover et al. (1963) remarked on events that surrounded trapping and transporting these indigenous baboons in small cages and their subsequent handling at the laboratory with weighing, bathing, and tatooing. They speculated that the sum total of these experiences was strongly arousing; they noted that the required immobilization was achieved by a nontranquilizing agent, Sernyl, which does not dull the animals' perceptions of the environment.

Similarly, Corley and his associates made a recent preliminary study of 21 restrained squirrel monkeys. They were subjected to pressing a lever once each minute for turning off a light to avoid an electric shock (Sidman avoidance test) for approximately a week, alternating eight hours of testing with eight hours of respite. This test was shown to be associated with a significant incidence of acute myocardial degenerative lesions. The two control monkeys were free of histologic changes. Ten others restrained in chairs during the study showed minor ST segment changes in the electrocardiogram, suggestive of a lack of oxygen, and acute myocardial lesions involving histologic changes. These lesions showed up in microscopic sections stained with the dye, basic fuchsin, for which they have an affinity. All nine monkeys exposed to shock avoidance as well as to restraint showed a combination of marked ST segment changes with arrhythmias and severe myocardial fibrosis and fuchsinophilia. The authors concluded that restraint combined with shock avoidance had led to autonomic disturbances, which in turn resulted in myocardial pathology (Corley et al., 1973).

During his observations of the behavior of wild rats, Barnett (1964) reported on the death of vigorous males introduced into a cage having an already active social hierarchy with a dominant in residence. A dominant will attack an unwilling intruder who submits (as in the case of primates cited in Chapter 4) and is therefore not severely bitten. Despite this, the now subordinated intruder will frequently die within a few days.

More recently Barnett et al. (1975) have studied an Australian long-haired strain of wild rat, *Rattus villosissimus,* in groups of three to a large cage during their repeated, intermittent daily encounters with a male intruder for up to nine days. Groups of eight males and eight females previously strangers to each other were also maintained for 70 days in a large cage without intruders. Considerable fighting occurred in both groups, and renal pathology was observed, consisting of focal glomerular hypercellularity and dilated distal convoluted tubules. This condition was found in 21 of the 23 intruders and in all of the males that had been in the large cage for 70 days. Since none of the control groups had lesions, the authors concluded that renal pathology, especially glomerulonephritis, was a correlate of social intolerance, but probably not the cause of death. However, Von Holst, working with subordinated tree shrews, has evidence that the kidneys can be irrevocably damaged in this species.

An adult male tree shrew, *Tupaia belangeri,* was introduced daily to another male that was an experienced fighter. The latter immediately attacked, while the intruder submitted. The two males were then separated before injuries occurred, and the subordinate was positioned so that he could see the dominant without suffering attack. The emotionally roused subordinate lay still, watching the dominant's movements for more than 90 percent of his waking time. His tail hair remained erect, indicating a sustained sympathetic arousal. After two to 16 days, and despite eating and drinking, many of the subordinates fell into a coma and died. A rising blood urea was associated with histologic evidence of renal insufficiency, pointing to acute renal vascular changes as the cause of death (Fig. 9-1) (Von Holst, 1972).

Thus, in this species, psychosocial stimulation appears to result in sufficiently severe physiologic disturbances to lead to acute renal failure. Hoff et al. (1951) have observed the development of renal cortical necrosis following the stimulation of the frontal cortex of a cat, and Knapp and his associates have demonstrated that the continuous infusion of noradrenaline into the

renal artery of a dog for two hours will lead to irreversible renal failure (Knapp et al., 1972). It would seem plausible that a fatal reduction of renal blood flow might have occurred due to sympathetic adrenal arousal during Von Holst's experiment.

Effects of chronic psychosocial stimulation

The foregoing observations taken together provide evidence that disturbances, which may lead to death even in previously healthy animals, can be the result of an intensely emotionally arousing situation. But these are acute episodes and do not last long enough to account for the gradual deterioration and slow transformation from health to incapacity that is characteristic of a slowly developing disease, such as essential hypertension, with an accompanying renal or myocardial failure.

We have increasing evidence that sustained psychosocial interaction leads to cardiovascular disease. Weber and Van der Walt (1973) have demonstrated cardiomyopathy in crowded New Zealand white rabbits. Four were placed in a cage, 60 × 45 × 30 centimeters, for one week. They were then housed singly for one week, then crowded again, then housed singly, and so on. In the course of 10 months, 35 of 48 animals had succumbed, 10 dying the first week, 10 more during the first month, and the rest at intervals during the succeeding months.

The rabbits fought intermittently, biting one another, but not severely, and the authors concluded that the cause of death was not wounding or starvation, but chronic cardiomyopathy, a stress reaction, which terminated in cardiac failure. They observed severe myocardial necrosis and interstitial edema with patchy accumulations of acid mucopolysaccharides in the subendocardium and myocardium of rabbits that died

Fig. 9-1.   Blood urea nitrogen content in the highly territorial tree shrew. Sixteen subordinated animals, separated from the resident dominants by only a wire screen, were exposed daily to a brief repetition of defeat. Fatal uremia developed in two to 14 days *(Von Holst, 1972)*.

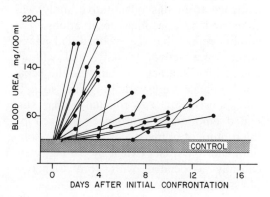

within a few days. Those that survived longer developed fusiform foci of myocardial fibrosis with collagen fibers and endocardial fibroelastosis.

As mentioned in Chapter 3, of the 100 adult male hamadryas baboons crowded together on Monkey Hill in the London Zoological Gardens, 53 died during the five-year interval of 1925–1930. Zuckerman (1932) cites atheromatous deposition of cholesterol and fat within the arterial walls as the principal cause of cardiovascular pathology, in addition to subacute and chronic bacterial infection of the abdominal and thoracic viscera. This unfortunate attempt to establish a colony that violated ethologic principles was enough to suggest that psychosocial stimulation plays a role in the induction of chronic disease.

The later observations of Lapin and Cherkovich (1971) in the Sukhumi laboratories in Russia with the same species of baboon have greatly strengthened this viewpoint. Although their experimental conditions were not rigorously controlled, they successfully measured hypertension and identified cardiovascular pathology histologically. Their work, which confirms the pathogenic potential of sustained social interaction, involved making changes in the living arrangement of dominant males as required by animal husbandry and experimental considerations and frequently violated their social relationships. For example, a male hamadryas baboon was separated from his females, with whom he had long been associated, and from his young. He was subsequently placed in full view of them in an adjacent cage. Since this particular species of baboon adopts immature females and develops an intense attachment to them, the displaced male showed intense agitation when another male was put into their cage.

During a period of several years, 57 baboons and macaques were involved in a series of such situations, each of which lasted for several months. Not all of these studies were aimed at deliberately producing disease, but rather in the attempt to develop experimental neuroses. There were 16 cases of hypertension as demonstrated by blood pressure recordings, 19 cases of coronary insufficiency as determined by electrocardiography, and six cases of proved myocardial infarction. This is a significant incidence of pathology, considering that arteriosclerotic changes were not observed in normal animals that were shot while living in the wild state. Lapin and Cherkovich (1971) concluded that hypertension and coronary insufficiency were connected with sustained emotional disturbances that had been induced in the animals.

In related work, Ratcliffe et al. (1969) have shown the importance of behavioral stimuli in the development of disease in swine. Forty were assigned to a stimulating environment at six to eight weeks of age. Of these, four males and four females were placed in isolation in large separate pens. In addition, four male–female pairs were set up. Finally, two control groups of 12, each with two males and one female, were used. All were housed in the same barn. After a year they were killed and their tissues studied. The heart muscle was graded for the incidence, extent, and severity of arteriosclerosis of the intramural coronary arteries by a special scoring technique. Both the male–female paired and separated swine had significantly more arteriosclerosis ($p <$ 0.005 for the paired set) than did the 16 males and eight females that had been in the two mixed groups. The pathophysiologic evidence from this quantitative study was supported by anecdotal observations. The authors report that the grouped and paired swine were active, friendly, and without competitive interactions, but that the separated animals were withdrawn and socially unresponsive. It was concluded that sustained emotional disturbances induced by the rupture of primary social bonds by isolation, and to a lesser extent by pairing, were causally associated with chronic pathophysiologic changes.

Lack of informational feedback and pathophysiology

The induction of gastric ulceration by the operant conditioning technique has led to important generalizations about the psychologic mechanisms involved. Weiss (1971a,b) worked with a less easily measured disorder than high blood pressure, but with one whose severity could be estimated by measuring the size of lesions in rats. Pairs of rats yoked together had electric shock applied to their tails. The shock either came without a warning or was preceded by a single warning beep or a series of beeps, alerting them to the impending shock. Only one rat could initiate and achieve an avoidance action by pressing a lever to escape shock. This rat developed less gastric ulceration than his helpless partner who was without a lever to press, but who was exposed to the same shock current because the electrodes affixed to his tail were wired in series (Fig. 9-2).

Furthermore, Weiss (1972) found that the presence or absence of a warning signal had an effect on the helpless rat as well as the rat in control; the warning signal reduced ulceration in both. One interpretation is that the warning signal tells the rat a shock is imminent; therefore, he can relax when it is not sounding. Without this signal, there is no way of knowing when the shock will occur, hence anxiety is sustained.

Throughout the years, Weiss's many ingenious experiments have led him to conclude that stress ulceration was a function of two variables: the number of coping attempts the rat makes, and the amount of relevant feedback these coping attempts produce (Weiss, 1972a,b). The lack of relevant feedback explains why the helpless, yoked rat developed more ulcers: Whenever he tried to cope, there was no response. But when the rat in control pressed the lever, there was a reassuring tone and the shocks stopped. Under these circumstances, with a

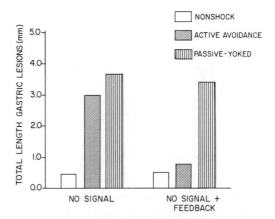

Fig. 9-2. Evidence that the predictability of a stressor influences the extent of tissue pathology. On the left, the median total length of gastric lesions of rats responding to nonshock, to unsignaled active avoidance of shock, and passive helplessness to shock when yoked to an active-avoidance partner. On the right, the situations are the same except that a feedback signal is given to the active-avoidance rat whenever he responded. The passive-yoked rat receiving no signal develops lesions to the same extent, but the lesions developed by the now cued active-avoidance rat are significantly less ($p < 0.005$) *(Weiss, 1971b).*

good feedback, little ulceration occurred (Fig. 9-2). Weiss showed that corticosterone in the plasma rose and noradrenergic activity in the brain declined when the rat learned he was helpless to control his environment (Weiss et al., 1975). Like Weiss, Seligman, who has studied the related problem of inescapable shock, finds that animals at the greatest risk are those lacking information indicating whether their coping efforts are successful and those unable to predict when the avoidance experience will occur (Seligman, 1975).

Weiss's studies are notable for their precision and for the illuminating generalizations to which they have led. The related work of Corley et al. (1975), discussed in Chapter 7, is important because it suggests that the responses of the helpless, yoked animal who collapsed unexpectedly with

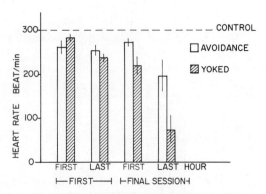

Fig. 9-3. Further evidence that helplessness is linked to pathology, showing the mean heart rate for six monkeys with shock-avoidance levers and for the six helpless partners yoked to them. The yoked monkeys experienced the same shock, but could not predict or avoid it. After a number of eight-hour shock-avoidance sessions, a bradycardia which at first had not been significant became severe, and the yoked partners collapsed and died in ventricular asystole. The shock-avoidance monkeys were far less affected. The vertical lines represent Standard Deviation of the Mean *(Corley et al., 1975).*

bradycardia (Fig. 9-3) may differ emotionally and therefore neuroendocrinologically, from those of one who can respond to the stimulus. They reported on six groups of "yoked chair" squirrel monkeys, studying their electrocardiogram, blood pressure, and myocardial pathology. A monkey who could avoid shocks (avoidance monkey) was yoked to one who could not respond to shocks that both received. Both animals were exposed to the Sidman avoidance test while seated in a pillory type of chair. They conclude that the avoidance monkey develops nonlethal myocardial damage because he is exposed to sympathetic (fight–flight) activation, and that the helpless monkey dies by a mechanism similar to that affecting Richter's rats, a parasympathetic-mediated "giving-up" response which is similar to "voodoo" death described by Cannon (1957) and sudden death in man described by Engel (1971). They argue that other experiments with the yoked procedure, such as Weiss's, have shown that the incidence of

ulcers in rats decreases if they know when shocks will occur. Helplessness or the inability to control or cope is the main factor related to pathology in the yoked animals. They have thus arrived at an experimental design which contrasts the sympathetic adrenal-medullary with the pituitary adrenal-cortical depressive response.

Chronic psychosocial stimulation and blood pressure elevation in mice

The foregoing studies leave little doubt that pathophysiologic changes of various types follow emotional disturbances. However, there are no experiments studying a number of neuroendocrine and histopathologic parameters over a period of time. Furthermore, most of the experiments imposed man-made stimuli and used limited numbers of subjects. Our prolonged series of psychosocial observations with the CBA strain of mice determine the effects of territorial restriction and disturbance of normal attachment behavior. Mice that had been disturbed by isolation (Fig. 5-4) were placed in a population cage with intercommunicating passages connecting the individual boxes to facilitate chronic conflict (Henry et al., 1967).

In experiments lasting from six to 12 months, there was a sustained elevation of systolic arterial pressure to approximately 160 mmHg in males from colonies with chronic social interaction; the pressure of females was also elevated, but only to 140–150 mmHg. Exposing castrates to potential social stimulation did not result in fighting or in a rise of arterial pressure. During these early studies, returning mice to a less stimulating environment resulted in a gradual subsidence of blood pressure toward the base line of 120 ± 12 mmHg. In earlier work, blood pressure was measured in mice maintained as siblings (male or female) in boxes throughout their lives; it was shown that even in extreme old age, their blood pressure remained at normal levels, i.e., two-month olds had a pressure of 123 ± 13 mmHg and healthy senile mice of 24–30 months, 129 ± 12 mmHg (Fig. 9-4).

These studies also demonstrated that early social development was critical even in mice. Mice born and raised as siblings in communal nurseries established by females had little social conflict while maturing in the

Fig. 9-4.   The distribution of systolic blood pressure in 300 young (two to four months), mature (10 to 16 months), and aged (24 to 30 months) male and female mice. They were separated by sex and lived six to a standard shoe box cage. The blood pressures of 100 from each age group were taken at random within a specific period of time *(Henry et al., 1965).*

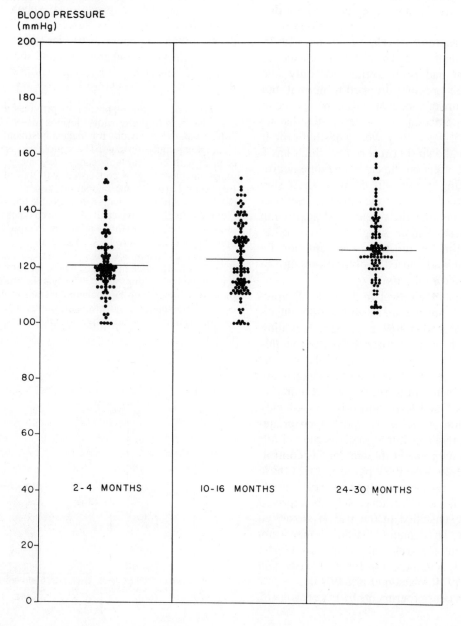

BLOOD PRESSURE
(mmHg)

intercommunicating box colony. These socialized mice had only a slightly elevated blood pressure, i.e., the females were normal and the males, approximately 140 mmHg. On the other hand, mice socially deprived by being weaned at only 10 days and trained to fight any mouse they met while still young were exceptionally aggressive. The blood pressure of the few surviving males attained a mean of 190 mmHg toward the end of the six-month interaction. This increase in blood pressure was not due to excitement during the actual blood pressure measurement (Henry et al., 1967). When a light ether anesthesia was used on mice that had been excited for only two days, their pressure dropped to normal, but the pressure of mice that had been exposed to social interaction for several months no longer fell when they were anesthetized. It was also shown that reserpine, which has a powerful effect on the catecholamine neurotransmitting system, will decrease these sustained ether-resistant elevations. The conclusion was that the threats and aggression with which a male sought to drive other males from his territory were emotionally disturbing and caused his blood pressure to rise (Henry et al., 1967).

Despite their level on the scale of evolution, mice are mammals with a fully developed mammalian limbic system, including the hippocampal complex. Evidence that this provides the organisms with a cognitive spatial map and so enhances and constantly updates the sense of territory was presented in Chapters 5 and 6. A mouse is also a highly social animal which will respond appropriately to symbolic gestures, such as the tail rattling of an opponent threatening his control. Wynne-Edwards (1962) points out that these warning threats exemplify the use of symbols in the defense of territory. Socially deprived mice are unskilled in the use of such sign language. They cannot put a dominance–subordination hierarchy to work and must constantly compete for territory (Ely and Henry, 1974; Watson et al., 1974).

In recent experiments by Ely et al. (1976,

1977) this same hierarchic deficiency arose because normally socialized mice whose hippocampus had been destroyed lacked the capacity to locate themselves in the complex maze of the population cage (see Figs. 5-1, 6-8). There was chronic social interaction with an ensuing considerable rise in blood pressure, but only in the population cages where mice had room for maneuvering and for attempting defense of territory. The controls in the standard shoe box cages, 23 × 11 × 11 centimeters, appear to have been too confined to fight out an agreement on the limits of their respective territories (Fig. 9-5); they had normal blood pressures and showed

Fig. 9-5. If the hippocampus provides a cognitive map of the territory, lesions might impair a mouse's capacity for social adjustment in a complex population cage. The systolic pressure of mice with bilateral hippocampal lesions (diagonal shading) was contrasted with that of two control groups: one unoperated (open column) and the other with neocortical lesions (stippled shading). Five each of the three types of mice were placed separately as groups in complex population cages where they have many opportunities to interact and in standard 23 × 11 × 11 centimeter shoe box cages where movement is restricted (six groups in all). The systolic blood pressure of mice with hippocampal lesions in the complex population cage was significantly higher ($p < 0.01$) than in the other five groups *(Ely et al., 1977).*

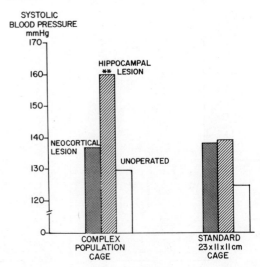

no evidence of intense social arousal with an elevated mean level of plasma corticosterone, but that of mice in the population cage was high to the point of indicating a strong arousal (Fig. 9-6).

Such studies of blood pressure in psychosocially stimulated mice led us to conclude that the closed social situation of the population cage inevitably leads to the repetition of symbolic stimuli day after day, month after month. If such a symbolic experience can be responsible for a physiologic response in mice, and if as the result of early experience and the structure of the habitat mice repeatedly confront each other, then they will be repeatedly exposed to emotional stimulation. These stimuli involve limbic activation with ensuing repeated hypothalamic arousal with the induction of fight–flight

Fig. 9-6. Corticosterone values of mice with hippocampal lesions whose systolic blood pressure was shown in Fig. 9-5. These mice with hippocampal lesions, living in complex population cages, have significantly elevated corticosterone values (*p* < 0.01) in comparison with those of the other five groups. This finding supports the blood pressure data and is compatible with the hypothesis that a mouse's difficulty in perception of territory leads to social instability with frequent emotionally arousing interactions *(Ely et al., 1977).*

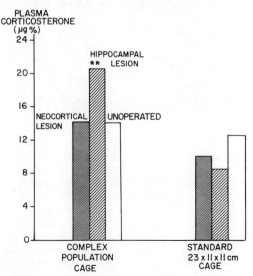

defense responses or activation of the adrenal-cortical system by ACTH or both. Evidence that the catecholamine-synthesizing enzymes (Henry et al., 1971a, 1972) and corticosterone are differentially involved in the response of mice to chronic psychosocial stimulation in population cages has already been outlined in Chapter 7 (Henry and Ely, 1976).

Psychosocial factors and arteriosclerosis in CBA mice

The question comes up as to whether degenerative changes eventually develop in the heart, blood vessels, and kidneys of mice that have been exposed to long-term psychosocial stimulation. Since all of our mice exposed to psychosocial stimulation in our laboratories over the years were routinely autopsied together with large numbers of normal controls, a considerable volume of histologic material was available. In one study, for example, 300 experimental mice were contrasted with 200 controls of the same age that had lived as siblings in stock boxes or in isolation in glass jars. Slides were coded and mixed at random to ensure blind grading and the following features, pointing to progressive arteriosclerosis, were observed. In normal vessels, regardless of age, the elastic fibers and intervening tissues together form the five to six wavy lamellae of a media that is abruptly set off from the adventitia (Fig. 9-7A). As high blood pressure persisted, we made the same observations as those made by Wexler (1964a) and Wolinsky (1972) in renal hypertensive rats and by Weber and Van der Walt (1973) in rabbits. Mucopolysaccharides and muscle proteins increased between the rings, thickening the wall (Fig. 9-7B). With more severe changes, there was fragmentation of the elastic rings, and the smooth muscle cells became radially oriented. They enlarged and vacuolated, forming a palisading arrangement. Subintimal pools, stained with Alcian

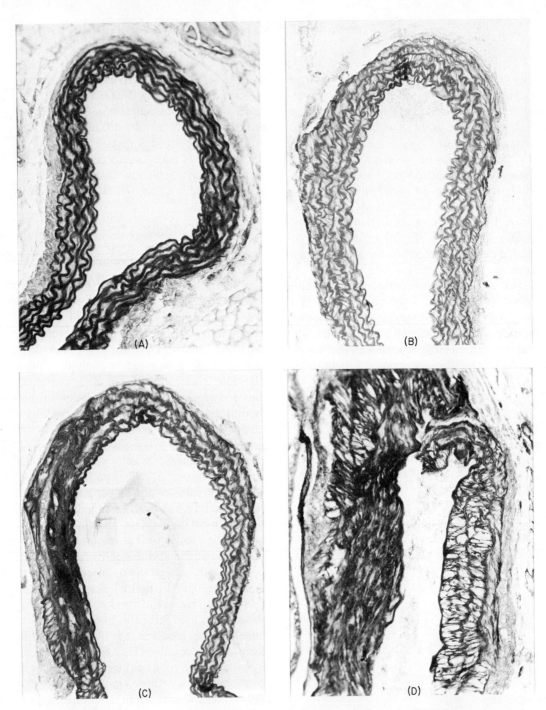

Fig. 9-7. Cross sections of aortas from variously socially stressed CBA mice. A: The distinct, wavy elastic fiber strands are continuous and unfrayed, and muscle tissues between the fiber strands are limited (PAS Alcian Blue × 250, normal). B: The elastic fiber rings of the aorta are more difficult to follow as they begin fragmenting, and the substance between elastic fiber rings has greatly increased, spreading them apart (PAS Alcian Blue × 150; Score 1+). C: The right side of the aorta shows a 1+ deterioration as elastic fibers become separated and hard to follow. The left side shows large pools, staining with Alcian Blue. The structure of the elastic ring is lost in these regions. A few palisading smooth muscle cells are seen at the lower left (PAS Alcian Blue × 150; Score 2+). D: An area of severe arteriosclerotic damage. Left: An invasion of spindle-shaped muscle cells has replaced the fibrous tissue rings. Right: These spindle cells enlarge and vacuolate with such severe palisading that the remaining fibrous rings are seriously distorted (PAS Alcian Blue × 250; Score 3+).

Blue, accumulated (Fig. 9-7C and D). Wolinsky describes the eventual substitution of fibrous proteins with collagen and elastin and the failure of such fibroelastic changes, accompanying long-term hypertension, to regress, despite the return of blood pressure to normal.

In the studies of mice, the result was a sharp shift in the scoring of both male and female aortas from hypertensive colonies. The most striking change was in the females in which the general categories + to 2+ and 3+ and above had no representatives in the control group, but scored 45 percent and five percent, respectively, in those that had been exposed to high blood pressure for six months or more (Fig. 9-8).

The heart muscle was scored for the amount and distribution of fibrous tissue around the vessels and between the muscle bundles. In the less affected hearts, there was almost complete freedom from stained material in these locations. The intramural arteries were clearly layered with easily discernible elastic rings. In the more severely damaged hearts, small scattered patches could be seen throughout the myocardium, and there was fibrous tissue around the vessels. The walls of the intramural arteries were thickened by an increase in the number

Fig. 9-8.   These histograms contrast the incidence of four types of pathologic changes in more than 300 male and female mice, four to 10 months of age, after exposure to social disorder in complex population cages. Heart fibrosis, changes in the glomerular mesangium, aortic arteriosclerosis, and lymphocyte accumulations in the kidney with areas of interstitial nephritis were the measures. Controls were siblings living in shoe box cages or isolated mice. Two persons were responsible for the scoring. The differences between groups were significant ($p < 0.01$) *(Henry et al., 1971b)*.

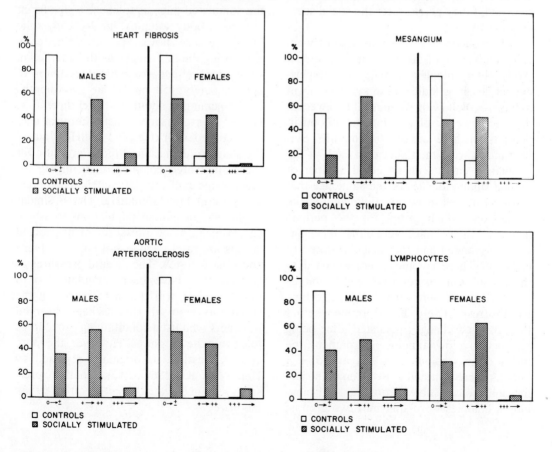

of cells. There was deposition of mucopoly-saccharide within and between the muscle cells. In hearts showing the most severe damage, the intramural vessels stenosed and vanished, blending with the investing fibrous tissue. Foci of fibrosis resulted in a patch-work of successive microinfarcts whose con-fluence led to lesions, extending through a large portion of the ventricular wall. In the males the percentage of moderately affected specimens increased about tenfold, from five percent to 50 percent. Females showed a similar dramatic increase in the incidence of myocardial damage (Henry et al., 1971b).

Rate of development of pathologic changes

It was important to determine how long pathophysiologic changes took to develop and to find out whether they become irrever-sible and if they persist after the social stim-ulus is removed.

Two successive year-long studies were completed; first of 10, then of 11 progres-sively older colonies of mice. The experi-mental design is indicated in symbolic form in Fig. 9-9. Following weaning at two weeks, the males were isolated until adulthood in pint jars for three and one-half months. Six-teen males were then placed in each of the population cages with an equal number of normal sibling females of the same age that had been raised in boxes. Following social interaction, which lasted for the periods indicated, the colonies were either terminat-ed or disbanded and the males returned to isolation. Three colonies were exposed to the social stimulus for two, eight, and 21 days and three more for two, six, and nine months, respectively. To determine whether the observed changes persisted after being returned to a low stimulus environment, the males of two colonies, 2 + 1 and 5 + 1 months, were returned to isolation in the jars for one month. Males from the two nine-month colonies were split into two groups; half were returned to isolation in glass jars, and the other half isolated individually in the original standard cages with ample living space. The colonies were started at stag-gered times so that autopsies could be per-formed simultaneously and tissues collected for a collaborating laboratory.

The 11-colony study followed the same design, however, an extra group was added to provide two months of isolation as well as one month of isolation following the six-month exposure to stress. The colonies were initiated with fully adult four-month-old mice, which made them 13 months old when the nine-month colony was terminated; since breeders are considered old at eight to nine months, this period represents much of their active life-span. Death from old age occurs between 24 and 30 months.

Figure 9-10 shows the blood pressures of the various colonies in the first 10-colony study.

Social interaction was not so severe in the stimulated mice as to cause a significant change in body weight (Fig. 9-11). Systolic blood pressure, however, showed a steady rise during the first weeks as the interaction slowly took effect, reaching a maximum of approximately 150 mmHg at two months and remaining at about this level thereafter. Higher pressures due to acute arousal may be recorded well over 200 mmHg. Indeed the standard deviation of blood pressure for these stimulated colonies is 20 mmHg, so that at a mean of 150–160 mmHg many pres-sures are at 170–180 mmHg. This is similar to findings in human populations in which casual mean blood pressures of unselected groups are rarely above 160 mmHg (Henry and Cassel, 1969). The arterial pressures of animals that have been stimulated for a month or less will return to normal if the stimulus is removed. This has been observed by others who used conditioning procedures to elevate the pressures. However, the more crucial question, as originally reported by Henry et al. (1967), was whether pres-sures remain elevated despite a return to iso-lation.

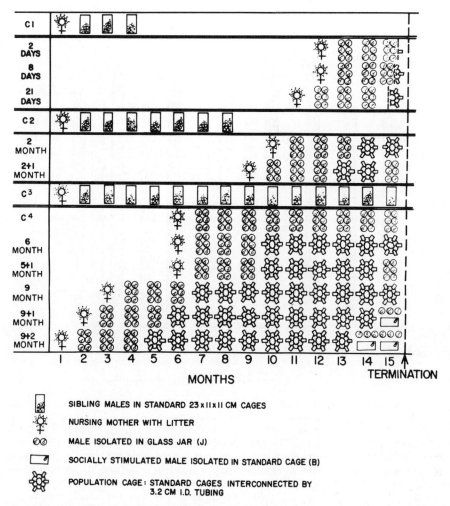

SIBLING MALES IN STANDARD 23 x 11 x 11 CM CAGES

NURSING MOTHER WITH LITTER

MALE ISOLATED IN GLASS JAR (J)

SOCIALLY STIMULATED MALE ISOLATED IN STANDARD CAGE (B)

POPULATION CAGE: STANDARD CAGES INTERCONNECTED BY 3.2 CM I.D. TUBING

Fig. 9-9. Overall experimental design for studying the rate of development of pathologic changes in mice. The symbols and legends below the main diagram indicate various animal husbandry procedures used during this study. C^1, C^2, and C^3 represent control groups of boxed siblings terminated at four, eight, and 10 to 15 months, respectively; C^4 remained isolated in jars for six months after the initial three and one-half month period. The two-, eight-, and 21-day groups represent colonies composed of 16 normal sibling females and 16 males that had been isolated for three and one-half months before being placed in the population cage for the foregoing brief periods. The 2-, and 2 + 1-month and the 6- and 5 + 1-month groups represent colonies made up like those just described. The + 1 indicates that the males were returned to isolation in jars for one month before termination of the experiment. Three colonies were exposed to the population cage for nine months. Half of the 9 + 1-month and 9 + 2-month groups were reisolated in jars (J) and half in standard cages (B). *(From Henry et al., 1975b. Reprinted by permission of the American Heart Association.)*

Blood pressures did not return to base line at the nine-month stage in the first set of 10 colonies, and the 11-colony study confirmed this observation; the data for this latter group is presented in Henry and Stephens (1977). The data on heart weights confirm these nonreversible changes. During the early stages, the increase was reversible and probably represented hypertrophy, but with the progression of arteriosclerosis in the coronary vascular bed, patchy myocardial fibrosis followed repeated microinfarction,

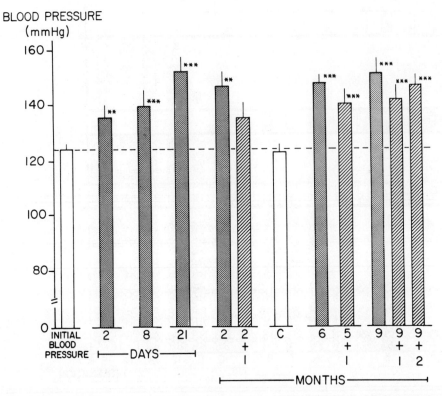

Fig. 9-10. Average systolic blood pressures of 10 socially disordered colonies of mice terminated after progressively increasing periods of social interaction (solid shaded columns). The diagonal shading indicates males returned to isolation. These shading distinctions also apply to Figs. 9-11 to 9-15. For the procedure adopted with each group, see Fig. 9-9. The open-column histogram (initial blood pressure) represents the mean initial blood pressure of all groups; column C represents the blood pressure of a control group remaining isolated in jars for six months after the initial three and one-half months. (This group is represented in Fig. 9-9 as C^4.) Vertical lines represent the Standard Error of the Mean: * = $p <$ 0.05, ** = $p < 0.01$, *** = $p < 0.001$ by the Two-Tailed Student's *t*-Test. The initial pressure value was control for the first five columns and *C* for the last five. *(From Henry et al., 1975b. Reprinted by permission of the American Heart Association.)*

and a nonreversible gain in heart weight occurred (Fig. 9-12).

The adrenal weights show the same trends, as confirmed in the second 11-colony study (Henry and Stephens, 1977). Thus the adrenals of these aging mice from competitive, restless colonies lacking a stable social hierarchy were significantly enlarged at later stages in life. Since 80 percent of the weight of an adrenal is cortex, this implies cortical hypertrophy in the older colonies (Fig. 9-13).

Pathologic changes in the aortas and hearts of mice of both the 10- and 11-colony studies were observed in order to determine when they ceased to regress. The early arte-

riosclerosis noted in colonies exposed to a few days of stimulation included an increase in mucopolysaccharides and an increase of smooth muscle in the lamellas, similar to that described by Wolinsky. Such changes can readily regress, and their reversible contribution to the wall-to-lumen ratio is compatible with the reversible elevation of blood pressure during the early stages. In older colonies, however, these changes became more severe, and by nine months, reversibility was lost (Wolinsky, 1972). The difference in scores between the vessels of older mice and those of the control group (C^2) was highly significant, i.e., $p < 0.05$ for one and $p < 0.001$ for the other (Fig. 9-14).

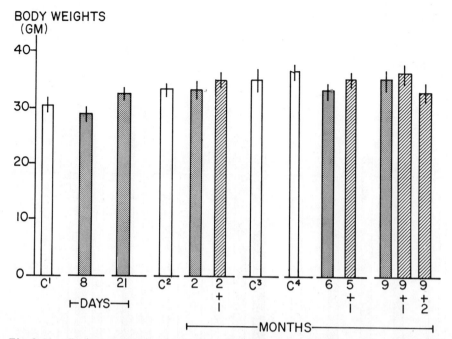

Fig. 9-11. Body weights of males in 10 socially disordered colonies of mice whose blood pressures are shown in Fig. 9-10. The experimental design is described in Fig. 9-9 and the same statistical comparisons as those in Fig. 9-10 were made, but no significant differences were observed. Weights for the two-day colony were not available. *(From Henry et al., 1975b. Reprinted by permission of the American Heart Association.)*

Fig. 9-12. Heart weights of males in 10 socially disordered colonies of mice whose blood pressures are shown in Fig. 9-10. The experimental design is described in Fig. 9-9 and the statistical comparisons are the same as those in Fig. 9-10. *(From Henry et al., 1975b. Reprinted by permission of the American Heart Association.)*

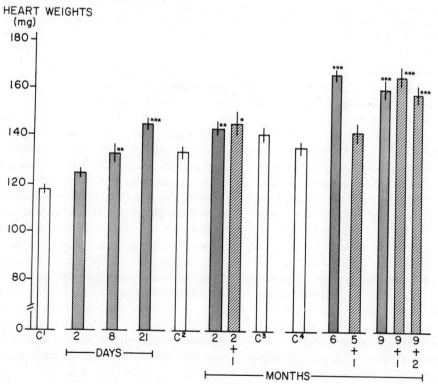

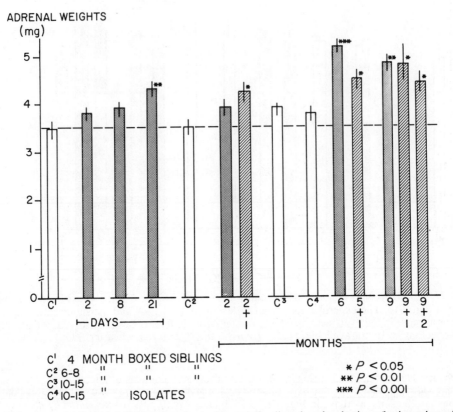

Fig. 9-13.   Adrenal weights of males in 10 socially disordered colonies of mice whose blood pressures are shown in Fig. 9-10. The experimental design is described in Fig. 9-9 and the statistical comparisons are the same as those in Fig. 9-10. *(From Henry et al., 1974. Reprinted by permission of the American Heart Association.)*

The myocardial damage score subsided in mice isolated for one month after five months of colony life (Fig. 9-15). This fall paralleled the return of heart weights to normal (Fig. 9-12). In the nine-month colonies both heart weights and fibrosis scores remained elevated, despite the return to isolation. As in our previous studies, these changes significantly exceeded those found in the controls (boxed siblings of the same age) ($p < 0.001$). Thus the critical time for irreversibility to set in appears to be in excess of six months. It can now be seen why operant conditioning, thus far, has not produced permanent pathophysiologic changes. In the first place, even in the accelerated life cycle of the mouse, the stimulus must persist for six months before these changes become irreversible with the depo-

sition of fibrous proteins, elastin, and collagen in the lamellae (Henry et al., 1975). The severity of the stimulus must also be considered. Our studies of arteriosclerosis uncovered a great variation in the extent of lymphocyte invasion of the kidneys in different members of a single colony. Even in groups showing great social disruption, some individuals showed only minimal changes and others much more. This occurred despite uniformity of diet and homogeneity of genetics. On the other hand, there were sharp differences between mice according to their roles in the social hierarchy. These differences occured even in disordered colonies. Thus a whole range of changes can be expected to occur in mice just as in a human society whose members may appear to be equally stimulated; for, as already noted

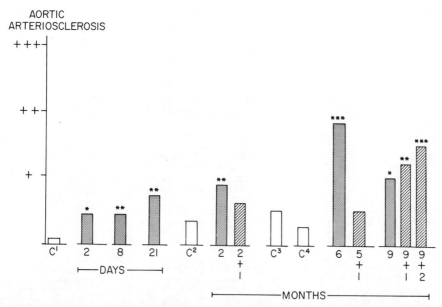

Fig. 9-14. Incidence of aortic arteriosclerosis in males of 10 socially disordered colonies of mice whose blood pressures and heart and adrenal weights are shown in Figs. 9-10 through 9-13. The experimental design is described in Fig. 9-9 and the statistical comparisons are the same as those in Fig. 9-10. Ordinate: + separation of elastic fiber rings, + + fragmentation of rings and palisading, + + + spindle cell invasion with gross distortion of rings. *(From Henry et al., 1975. Reprinted by permission of the American Heart Association.)*

Fig. 9-15. Incidence of myocardial fibrosis in males of 10 socially disordered colonies of mice whose aortic arteriosclerosis evaluations are shown in Fig. 9-14. The experimental design is described in Fig. 9-9 and the statistical comparisons are the same as those in Fig. 9-10. Ordinate: + scattered fibrous tissue between muscle bundles, + + small scattered patches throughout the myocardium, + + + confluent lesions forming a patchwork of microinfarcts extending a considerable distance in the ventricular wall. *(From Henry et al., 1975b. Reprinted by permission of the American Heart Association.)*

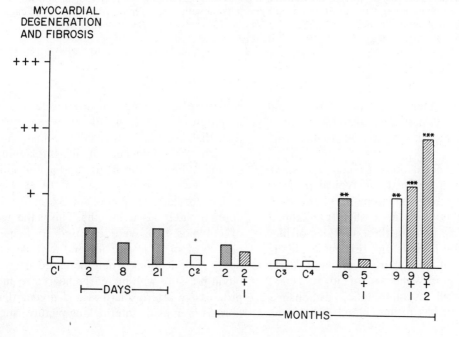

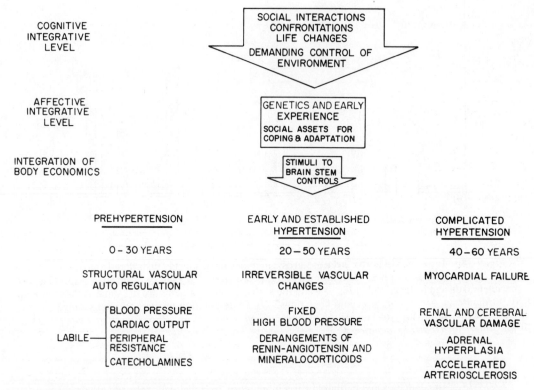

COGNITIVE
INTEGRATIVE
LEVEL

SOCIAL INTERACTIONS
CONFRONTATIONS
LIFE CHANGES
DEMANDING CONTROL OF
ENVIRONMENT

AFFECTIVE
INTEGRATIVE
LEVEL

GENETICS AND EARLY
EXPERIENCE
SOCIAL ASSETS FOR
COPING & ADAPTATION

INTEGRATION OF
BODY ECONOMICS

STIMULI TO
BRAIN STEM
CONTROLS

PREHYPERTENSION	EARLY AND ESTABLISHED HYPERTENSION	COMPLICATED HYPERTENSION
0 – 30 YEARS	20 – 50 YEARS	40 – 60 YEARS
STRUCTURAL VASCULAR AUTO REGULATION	IRREVERSIBLE VASCULAR CHANGES	MYOCARDIAL FAILURE

LABILE — ⎡BLOOD PRESSURE
⎢CARDIAC OUTPUT
⎢PERIPHERAL
⎢RESISTANCE
⎣CATECHOLAMINES

FIXED
HIGH BLOOD PRESSURE

DERANGEMENTS OF
RENIN-ANGIOTENSIN AND
MINERALOCORTICOIDS

RENAL AND CEREBRAL
VASCULAR DAMAGE

ADRENAL
HYPERPLASIA

ACCELERATED
ARTERIOSCLEROSIS

Fig. 9-16.   Essential hypertension develops as a result of the interaction of two chains of events. The first is shown in the upper part of the diagram by a large cognitive arrow representing the pressure of events as the individual searches for desiderata, deals with life changes, and attempts to control his environment. The affective "gain control" block, below the arrow, represents his genetic endowment, early experience, and social assets, which modify the stimuli to brain stem controls. The lower part of the diagram shows the role of time, as the induced changes progress from labile prehypertension with structural vascular autoregulation through fixed hypertension with cardiac hypertrophy to complicated hypertension with organ damage. *(From Henry, 1976a. © 1976, Harcourt Brace Jovanovich. Reprinted by permission.)*

in earlier chapters, the social status and assets of any particular individual determine the intensity of his neuroendocrine response.

In his recent book *Clinical Hypertension,* Kaplan outlined the typical progression of hypertension in man. Figure 9-16 presents this view in a slightly modified form. During the first three decades of life, hypertension is labile and reversible; this is the state of prehypertension and early hypertension. By the age of 30–50 years, although still asymptomatic, established hypertension has begun; blood pressure is consistently elevated and arteriosclerosis is in progress. But from 40–60, when more than half of the expected life-span has passed, the incidence of life-threatening complications of the heart, aorta, and kidneys has risen sharply (Kaplan, 1973). The equivalent half life-span of a CBA mouse is approximately 12–15 months. This is the age of colonies that were exposed to longer periods of social interaction and were developing complications. Their increased arterial blood pressure with increased heart size and progressive arteriosclerosis and myocardial fibrosis creates an interlocking picture, suggesting that certain aspects of murine psychosocial hypertension model the human condition.

Psychosocial stimulation and renal damage

The kidneys of mice living in socially disturbed colonies are frequently grossly pitted and scarred and are often small, blanched, and have an adherent capsule. There is evidence of a gradual replacement of the healthy organ by fibrous tissue; such changes are typical of chronic nephritis and renal failure in man (Robbins and Angell, 1976).

In a recent series of studies we found elevated blood urea and blanched kidneys in more than 50 percent of the males, but not in

Fig. 9-17. Increasing blood urea in colonies of mice that had been exposed to social stress for two, six, or nine months by the animal husbandry procedures described in Fig. 9-9. Both males and females were used. Vertical lines represent the Standard Error of the Mean: * = $p < 0.05$, ** = $p < 0.01$, *** = $p < 0.001$. *(From Henry, 1976a. © 1976, Harcourt Brace Jovanovich, Inc. Reprinted by permission.)*

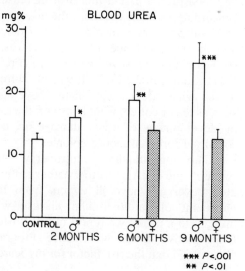

females. Blood urea tests (Fig. 9-17) showed that by the age of two months males began developing renal damage that progressed steadily to such serious renal failure at nine months that the average blood urea level of survivors was 25 milligrams/100 milliliters. Females escaped renal damage, presumably because their social stimulation was far less intense (Henry, 1976a); their normal kidneys suggested that the cause of uremia was not renal infection, since there was no reason for the difference. On microscopic study they showed a range in the incidence of lesions. Typical details of scoring for lymphocyte accumulation and tubular damage are presented in an earlier study by Henry et al. (1971b). During the early stages, i.e., 1+ and 2+, there is an increase of perivascular infiltration followed by peritubular infiltration by the lymph cells. The more severe cases (3+), when renal failure had elevated the blood urea, showed considerable destruction of the kidney tubules with replacement by fibrous tissues, if the condition had developed slowly and was chronic. Figure 9-8 presents the distribution of these lesions in a large number of mice that had been exposed to approximately six months of social interaction. Half the males and females have lesions in the 1+ to 2+ range; few males and even fewer females have the 3+ lesions (Henry et al., 1971b).

One might wonder whether these changes were the consequences of infection, especially since many of the more subordinated mice had bites on their tails and haunches. A bacteriologic study by Dr. A. P. Shapiro of the University of Pittsburgh, however, showed that this was not so. The possibility always exists that although the lesions are primarily of ischemic origin, secondary infection of the damaged areas may occur (Henry et al., 1971b).

In a separate study, Shapiro et al. (1968) noted that mice exposed to the social interaction of crowding show more areas of round cell infiltration than isolated mice. Crowded mice also show progressive deterioration of the glomeruli of the type that

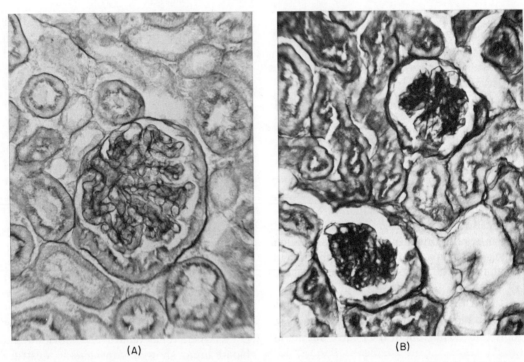

(A)   (B)

Fig. 9-18.   A: Normal glomerulus in a 12-month-old CBA mouse. Notice the well-defined capillary network with blood vessels of a relatively uniform size and the well-defined space in Bowman's capsule lined with cuboidal epithelium. The mesangium is scanty, and the basement membrane around Bowman's capsule is well rounded (PAS Alcian Blue × 420, normal). B: The most extreme form of glomerular damage (3+); the capillary structure has virtually disappeared. The mesangium is extremely dense, and the lining of Bowman's capsule is atrophic. The basement membrane is wavy and the overall size of the glomerulus is reduced (PAS Alcian Blue × 420; Score 3+).

Christian et al. (1965) have observed in socially stimulated rodents. As the legend to Fig. 9-18 indicates, in the more severely damaged mice, the mesangium becomes dense, the lining of Bowman's capsule atrophic, and the overall size of the glomerulus reduced. The difference in glomerular scores for disordered mice as opposed to the controls of a colony is shown in Fig. 9-8.

Acceleration of pathologic changes by caffeinated beverages

The effects of caffeinated beverages have thus far received very little attention from the viewpoint of catecholamine release

and their possible pathophysiologic effects on blood pressure. Yet this is of increasing concern as we come to realize the major role of blood pressure as a risk factor in determining the incidence of arteriosclerosis, strokes, and congestive heart failure (Freis, 1971; Kannel et al., 1972). It was of interest to see what effect a caffeinated beverage, such as tea or coffee, would have on the rate of development of renal damage in our socially disordered mouse colonies.

The long-standing controversy surrounding the question as to whether caffeinated beverages have ill effects from the viewpoint of cardiovascular disease was brought to a peak by a report of the Boston Collaborative Drug Surveillance Program (Jick, 1973) that the risk factor for myocardial infarction viewed retrospectively appeared to be twice as great for heavy coffee drinkers. Tea appeared to be exempt. Subsequently, it turned out that tea as consumed in the United States has one-third the caffeine content of coffee. For an intake of 8.5 milligrams/kilogram of caffeine that Gilbert (1976) suspects as being critical for both addiction and health consequences, a 70-kilogram man need only drink four to five eight-ounce (250 cubic centimeter) cups of standard brewed coffee at 140 milligrams of caffeine per cup. This is significantly less than the daily fluid requirement. But to ingest this much caffeine daily would require a gallon of tea as Americans use it (tea bags steeped briefly in hot water).

Hennekens et al. (1976) have recently reviewed the issue of coffee drinking and death due to coronary heart disease. Their basic data confirm that of the Boston group, but the problem is whether the authors were justified in correcting for factors, such as obesity, lack of exercise, and especially smoking. If, as Thomas (1973) suggests, a certain type of nervous personality was responsible for these characteristics as well as for coffee drinking, then the basic influence would be personality. Since both smoking (Thomas, 1973; Carruthers, 1976; Cryer et al., 1976) and the ingestion of caffeine (Bellet et al., 1969) increase plasma catecholamines and since emotional responses do so, also, it would not seem feasible to disentangle these factors by statistical analysis. What is needed are prospective studies on populations that do not smoke and whose degree of emotional arousal can be controlled.

In their work on coffee consumption and coronary heart disease in middle-aged Swedish men, Wilhelmsen et al. (1977) report that the coffee consumption of myocardial infarct patients appears to increase during the months immediately preceding development of the lesion. They ruled out bias due to a possible decrease in coffee consumption because of disease in the controls. (This cannot be excluded in the Boston study because the controls were hospitalized patients.) Wihelmsen and his associates suggest that some type of psychologic change occurring as a premonitory mechanism in advance of a myocardial infarct is responsible for the increased con-

Fig. 9-19. The blood urea of 11 colonies of mice, exposed in sets of three, to five to six months of social stress in population cages. There is a suggestion of a break point at 300–400 micrograms/milliliter caffeine. This corresponds to 75–100 milligrams/250 cubic centimeter cup, i.e., weaker than the recommended manufacturer's brew of 125 milligrams/cup. The symbols *T, C, D,* and *W* represent stressed mice in population cages drinking tea, coffee, decaffeinated coffee, and water; whereas, *t, c, d,* and *w* represent boxed siblings (controls) on the same series of beverages. Normal blood urea is 10 milligrams/100 milliliters. The increased levels of blood urea in *t* controls are believed to occur because mice on tea fought in their boxes. Vertical and horizontal bars represent the Standard Error of the Mean.

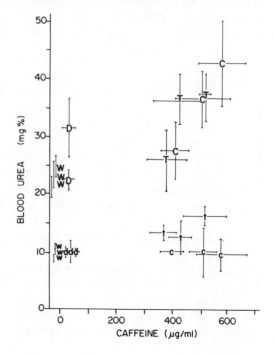

sumption of coffee. Chapter 1 outlined the evidence that during the year preceding a myocardial infarct, individuals are often under more pressure and are more anxious as the result of an increase in life changes (Theorell and Rahe, 1975; Rahe, 1976). In attempting to meet these pressures, the Type A personality may well increase his consumption of caffeine.

We have been able to avoid some of these human epidemiologic problems in controlled experiments with mice. We have compared nonstress groups with groups exposed to high levels of psychosocial stress in population cages, both groups having received either water or decaffeinated coffee, or tea or coffee with a high caffeine content. The confounding variables of smoking, obesity, and exercise could thus be eliminated. Thus far the results are preliminary and are summarized in Fig. 9-19 and the details are explained in the legend. The data show that psychosocial stimulation greatly enhances the incidence of renal failure in mice ($p < 0.01$), but, in addition, the increasing levels of blood urea in colonies consuming higher concentrations of caffeine in the beverage suggest the drug has an added effect and accelerates the damage induced by social interaction.

Mice consuming tea or coffee do not develop higher plasma caffeine levels than humans, but this chapter has shown that when mice are exposed to social stress, they will develop renal failure in association with arteriosclerosis. This does not occur in the control mice in boxes. The preliminary data also indicate that caffeine in excess of 8.5 milligrams/kilogram/day, i.e., four to five 250 cubic centimeter servings of coffee daily, accelerates this stress-induced renal failure. The latest work of Wilhelmsen's group from Göteborg is compatible with the suggestion that an increase in coffee or tea consumption by persons exposed to the mounting stress of increasing life changes may be part of a crescendo of neuroendocrine arousal culminating in myocardial infarction.

Summary

Acute psychosocial stimulation can lead to the death of an animal when it is made helpless or cannot escape from an aggressor's threats. The collapse may come by acute heart or kidney failure. Chronic stimulation will also lead to death; here arteriosclerosis of the large vessels as well as of the heart and other organs can be a cause of the fatal outcome. An important factor in producing lesions such as peptic ulcers is the animal's perception of being helpless to induce desired changes. Colonies of mice in sustained conflict over territory develop a progressive increase in blood pressure and heart weight together with arteriosclerosis throughout the vascular bed. About six months of competition in a standard population cage will induce permanent arteriosclerotic deterioration. The changes in these "middle-aged" mice are of classic arteriosclerosis, but nonreversible enlargement of the adrenal cortex and progressive renal damage with death in uremia also occur. If sufficient caffeinated beverages such as tea or coffee are consumed daily to give more than eight to 10-milligrams of caffeine per kilogram, the risk of renal damage increases in socially stressed mice. In man this would correspond to four to five cups of strong coffee daily.

10

Pathophysiologic consequences of human social disturbance

The previous chapter touched on the last step in a chain leading from environmental events to disease and considered that psychosocial stimulation induced disease in animals. This chapter is concerned with the evidence that subtle disturbances of human social relationships can be reliably associated with the onset of disease, such as coronary arteriosclerosis, high blood pressure, and even cancer.

In 1960, Kissen, a clinician, in discussing his own approach to clinical and epidemiologic research in psychosomatic medicine used Halliday's definition of psychosomatic disease: "a bodily disorder whose nature can be appreciated only when emotional disturbances, that is, psychological happenings, are investigated in addition to physical disturbances, that is, somatic happenings" (Kissen, 1960).

Kiritz and Moos (1974) have presented a view of the physiologic effects of social environments which cover an ethologic and social science approach to these emotions and to the factors controlling them. They discuss the functions intervening between the external environment and the emotional arousal of the internal milieu, i.e., the inborn and acquired factors that determine an individual's perceptions. In a close relationship to the concept of social assets, the authors point out that the cohesion or affiliation shown when group members agree and cooperate with one another while performing a difficult task reduces their physiologic response to the stress; for example, their fatty acids are reduced in comparison to when they are not cooperating. Hence, it is protective to have a strong affective relationship toward the members and goals of one's social environment. An example is the unexpectedly low plasma corticosterone found by Bourne in soldiers in Vietnam who had high morale and were dedicated to their mission (Chapter 7). Kiritz and Moos conclude that although environments characterized by the higher levels of involvement will usually lead to increased hormonal activity, the critical factor is the precise nature of a person's perception of the situation. They cite Hofer et al. (1972a, b) in their famous studies of the parents of leukemic children (also mentioned in Chapter 7) whose corticosterone levels were dependent on their defenses. They were able to avoid grief and the accompanying hormonal changes by maneuvers, such as denial, and even by a certain psychopathic lack of involvement.

Tough and easy cultures

We have shown that disturbance of the early experience of an individual leads to inadequate behavior patterns for meeting the needs of the group. This deficiency results in failure to maintain normal social relationships. One reason the breakdown of social structure has a continuing adverse effect is that it disturbs the maternal care of the next generation (see Fig. 5-5); consequently, social disorder is self-perpetuating. A normal, stable, hierarchic social system in which persons stick to their proper roles permits a smoothly functioning territorial drive with all of its elaborations in the complexity of human culture. When parents and their young form a normal attachment to one another, the society is easier to live in and desiderata are more readily attained by all members provided the group has access to the necessary physical resources. From a sociobiologic viewpoint, one would expect that a uniform and cohesive human social system enjoying a common history and ancestry would be easier to live in than one suffering from cultural incongruities and individual and ethnic rivalries.

The anthropologists Arsenian and Arsenian made a comparative study of the mental hygiene of various cultures in the late 1940's and found that some are tough on their members and others easy; this difference extends to minority and class groups within the culture. Indeed, the authors imply that, in this context, the United States in the 1940's was tougher on Negroes than on Caucasians in that it was harder for Negroes to attain desiderata. They point out that a culture determines how man's most basic physiologic needs are to be satisfied. For example, is safe drinking water—virtually free— to be obtained by merely turning on a tap or

must one walk half a mile to a deep well? The paths toward desiderata differ greatly. The goal may be wealth sought by so many in a modern state, and the paths may range all the way from wage labor to the stock market. In a society of food gatherers, however, wealth simply does not exist. Furthermore, the accessibility of goals varies. If dominance is prized, but there is room for only few at the top of large groups, the difficulty of attaining these positions by competition may be enormous, especially if there is race or class prejudice against the individual.

If a society is small, has few grades, and accepts several positions in the hierarchy as equivalent, the tensions are low; but if there are virtually no grades, as among the food gatherers, the tensions are lower still. According to Arsenian and Arsenian (1948), an easy culture provides both a number and a distribution of goals so that all persons can find ready access to them and can attain at least some of the highly valued objects. But in a tough culture, although the goals are numerous and the individual is encouraged to aspire toward them, their clarity, accessibility, and distribution are such that only a few can attain them, thus leaving the vast majority with unassuaged tensions. These anthropologists conclude that a tough culture leads to nervous people because tensions are high. Suicide, neurosis, and crime are frequent because the access to desiderata is so difficult that the rules are ignored and social breakdown occurs. Not only do differences between the various minority groups exist within a single culture, but the route toward assuaging some of their needs, such as hunger and thirst, may be more readily followed than that leading toward other needs, such as sexual tensions.

Cardiovascular disease in Roseto

Contrasts between a relatively easy and a tougher enclave in the United States were brought out by Bruhn et al. (1966) in their comparative study of the social differences between the Pennsylvania towns of Roseto and Bangor.

The exclusively Italian–American Catholic families in Roseto are cohesive and patriarchal; their society is mutually supportive and gregarious with clearly defined male and female roles. In Bangor, an ethnic mixture of English, German, and Italian, the family is more individual, the religion Protestant, and the male and female roles overlap. Some years ago it was suspected that these social factors were involved in the sharp and highly significant difference in death rate from myocardial infarction (Fig. 10-1). Roseto's death rate was one-half that of the neighboring communities. An investigation indicated that diet was not responsible (Stout et al., 1964), for a careful survey was made of the dietary preference for and the consumption of 31 general food items used by 250 of the 314 original Roseto inhabitants studied. A dietitian reviewed 'the

validity of the data from each questionnaire and found that 41 percent of the 2700-calorie diet came from fat. Lard instead of olive oil was used for cooking, and both men and women were about 20 pounds overweight, compared with the U.S. average.

According to anthropologist Carla Bianco, the crucial difference between the inhabitants of Roseto and those of neighboring communities, such as Bangor, was their reinforcement of mutual trust and cohesion upon arrival from Italy. Perceiving themselves as culturally isolated in an alien land, they reinforced those elements of their traditional culture that gave them a sense of security and self-appreciation. Bianco says that the people are still antagonistic toward the chief values and symbols of American society and still retain highly traditional attitudes toward family, education, work, law, and authority. These attitudes were perpetuated during earlier years because of hostile neighbors so that

Fig. 10-1.   An unusually low death rate from myocardial infarction was observed in Roseto, a traditional Italian–American community in Pennsylvania, between 1955 and 1961. Its inhabitants, who derive from Roseto (province of Foggia) in southern Italy, eat a high-fat diet. The ethnic mixture of residents in Bangor, Pennsylvania, a town of the same size only a mile away, was not considered traditional. The difference between death rates (both sexes) in both towns was significant ($p < 0.001$); the authors considered it compatible with the difference between the life styles of the two communities. *(From Stout et al., 1964. © 1964, American Medical Association. Reprinted by permission.)*

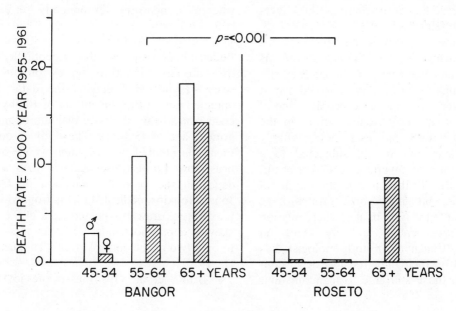

the community of Roseto, Pennsylvania was actually more homogeneous and traditional than the parent village of Roseto, in the province of Foggia, in southern Italy (Bianco, 1974).

In their study of Roseto and Bangor, Stewart Wolf and his associates (Bruhn et al., 1966) have pioneered an important natural experiment with their statistically tenable series of continuous observation of several hundreds of persons in these contrasting communities for more than 10 years. Meanwhile, the patterns of culture in Roseto, under the combined influence of the mass media and education at the high school and college levels, have gradually shifted toward the mainstream of American life. Consequently, according to prediction, the mortality rate from myocardial infarction will rise with this shift. Wolf's (1976) preliminary data suggest that this shift may now be taking place. Should the predictive power of the hypothesis be successful, it will point even more strongly to the role of sociocultural factors in causing coronary heart disease. Wolf also reported on the remarkable freedom from diseases of stress among the people of Borneo who are now on the verge of a massive culture shift due to the impact of their newly rich oil economy in the hinterland. He predicts an increased incidence of heart disease here also when the full effects have been felt (Wolf, 1976).

Another people poised on the verge of a cultural change are the Yanomamö Indians of Brazil and Venezuela. Although they still have normal blood pressure into old age, it can be predicted that these people—one of the last of the truly isolated tribes in the world—will show changes as they inevitably become acculturated and subjected to a Western form of government (Oliver et al., 1975). Normally they live in the depths of the jungle, but now some groups have moved out to the river banks, where mission stations are located, and are living on handouts. Chagnon, an anthropologist, has remarked on their impaired morale in contrast with those still able to maintain their sovereignty as independent tribesmen (Chagnon, 1974).

Freidman and Rosenman's type A versus type B behavior pattern

Starting out in the 1950's, Friedman and Rosenman (1974) have carried out predictive studies of major importance in the field of psychosocial stimulation and disease. They evaluated members of our society on a sliding scale, ranging from the extreme behavior pattern, Type A, to the opposite, Type B. Type A behavior is an action–emotion complex exhibited by an individual engaged in a relatively chronic and excessive struggle to obtain an unlimited number of things from his environment in the shortest time or against the opposing efforts of other persons or things. Thus the continual struggle consists of attempting to do more and more in less and less time, often while in a state of undue conflict with a person or persons. The authors stress that Type A persons do not despair but "soldier on alone," thus differing from anxiety-prone persons who feel overwhelmed and seek help from others. They suggest that a Type A confidently advances to grapple with his challenges, whereas a neurotic despondently retreats before his.

However, a 1975 study by Caroline Bedell Thomas suggests the susceptibility of the coronary victim to depression under stress. Figure 10-2 depicts the data she obtained during the student life of 10 physicians who sustained myocardial infarction at a mean age of 45 years. The ordinate contrasts the number of these men whose records showed traits (observed) with their incidence in the general population of 1337 Johns Hopkins medical students from which the 10 were drawn (expected). Six of the 10 showed depression under stress as opposed to only two of the control group (Thomas et al., 1975).

Bruhn et al. (1974) associate joyless

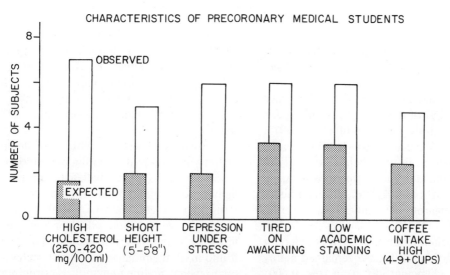

Fig. 10-2.   The open histograms (observed) present the incidence of six precoronary traits found in 10 former medical students who eventually sustained myocardial infarction at a mean age of 45 years. The stippled histograms (expected) represent the incidence of these traits for every 10 persons in the main medical student body of approximately 1337. *(From Thomas et al., 1975.* © *1975, Johns Hopkins University Press. Reprinted by permission.)*

striving with myocardial infarction. They speak of an effort-oriented person who struggles against odds but with very little sense of accomplishment or satisfaction. Because the work continues endlessly without the reward of emotional fulfillment, they describe it as a Sisyphus reaction pattern, for Sisyphus, King of Corinth, banished to Hades, was required to push a huge stone up the side of a hill. Each time he was near the top, it would roll down again, requiring him to continually labor without success.

Friedman and Rosenman (1974) see the Type A behavior pattern as a response to the contemporary Western environment; they think it develops because our society rewards those who think, perform, and communicate more aggressively than their peers. Our increasing urbanization and technology lead to an ever more urgent need to synchronize interdependent services. The pattern emerges only when challenges in the milieu arise, eliciting this response in susceptible individuals. They believe that if these challenges were absent, the Type A pattern might be less evident and that there is a socioeconomic basis for such behavior.

Typically the Type A is a robust, vigorous, keen well-set man with brisk body movements who clenches his fists in ordinary conversation. His explosive, hurried speech patterns drive him to the irritating habit of finishing or condensing the speech of others. The typical Type B, however, lacks the sense of time urgency, is patient and not compelled to display his achievements. He works without agitation and accepts restrictions of the environment cheerfully.

About 10 percent of the urban population have the extreme Type A behavior pattern and higher than average cholesterol, plasma triglycerides, and serum B lipoproteins (Rosenman et al., 1976). When given the adrenocorticotropic hormone (ACTH), their urinary 17-hydroxycorticosteroids are lower than those of Type B (Friedman et al., 1969); although when challenged, their excretion of noradrenaline is increased, whereas that of Type B does not respond (Friedman et al., 1975). This biochemical dichotomy is analogous to that of a dominant animal versus a subordinate one, as discussed in Chapter 7.

The 1975 report of the Western Collaborative Group Study initiated by Rosenman and others in 1960–1961 reviews their eight and one-half year follow-up of 3500 men, 39–59 years old, employed by 10 California companies. Clinical coronary heart disease occurred in 257 of the employees during this prospective study (Rosenman et al., 1975, 1976). Type A behavior was not associated with differences in age, height, or weight. When simultaneous adjustment was made for all other risk factors, i.e., parental history, use of cigarettes, blood pressure, serum cholesterol (Fig. 10-3), and triglyceride level, the association between Type A behavior and coronary heart disease remained highly significant, changing only from $p < 0.0001$ to $p < 0.003$. Hence the predictive relationship of behavior pattern to coronary heart disease could not be explained away by other risk factors; it remained unchanged, threatening the Type A person with an approximately twofold incidence of myocardial infarction and angina pectoris (Fig. 10-4) (Rosenman, 1971). Rosenman states that

Type A's advance to overcome their challenges, yet there is a deep sense of insecurity which drives them to unrealistic attempts to dominate in all situations. Inevitably they will fail, except briefly, to appease this insecurity despite an ever-increasing number of successes (Freidman and Rosenman, 1974; Rosenman, 1976).

Hostility together with free-floating anxiety are compatible with a description in ethologic terms of a challenged dominant fighting to maintain his position or of a rival struggling for dominance. Assuming this is so, the Type A person will then have close links with behavior patterns of dominants found in all mammalian societies—behavior by no means unique to man. It is our impression that the social systems of formerly isolated animals striving for dominance parallel the Type A behavior pattern in human society as described by Friedman and Rosenman. These animals are extremely active, hostile, and agitated; although when young their plasma corticosterone is normal, as they age their blood pressure is elevated,

Fig. 10-3. Clinical coronary heart disease in 257 of the 3500 men 39–59 years old studied during an eight and one-half year prospective study. The Type A behavior pattern was strongly related to the incidence of coronary heart disease and persisted whether the cholesterol level ($p < 0.001$) (milligrams/100 milliliters of plasma) was low <220, medium 220–259, or high>260. The authors concluded that the predictive relationship of the behavior pattern to coronary heart disease cannot be explained away by other risk factors such as cholesterol. *(From Rosenman et al., 1975. © 1975, American Heart Association. Reprinted by permission.)*

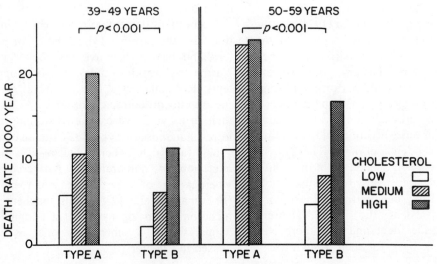

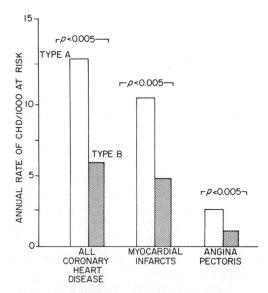

Fig. 10-4. The annual rate of coronary heart disease (CHD) in 1354 subjects during a prospective study lasting eight and one-half years. The incidence of all forms of coronary heart disease in the Type A subjects is significantly higher ($p < 0.005$) than in the Type B *(Rosenman, 1971).*

and catecholamine synthesis increases. A dominant monkey or a dominant mouse has a lower adrenocorticotropic hormone (ACTH) response than a subordinate one, similar to the response in a Type A man (Sassenrath, 1970). And the picture of inadequate social integration in a mouse colony of former isolates has similarities to those following a breakdown of cultural traditions in a human society (Henry and Ely, 1976). Thus a stable, socially integrated, hierarchic society of animals that grew up together as siblings is closer to the structure and behavior of a traditional human society with an established social order.

The following account of Type A behavior written with rueful insight and publicly avowed determination to reform by John Getze, business and financial writer for the Los Angeles Times, exemplifies confrontation even between strangers in a social environment that fosters the attitude of striving for dominance.

"Competitive driving" is the circumlocution I use to describe the way my car tends to speed and weave through traffic whenever I'm behind the wheel. On some subconscious level, I feel I'm always in a race.

Slower-moving vehicles are obstacles to be mastered, or—when there's no alternative but to reduce my own speed—hounded by aggressive maneuvers such as tailgating.

Along with my wife and son, I was returning from a weekend at the beach. It was early afternoon and traffic on the freeway, which had been light from Oceanside to Mission Viejo, quickly began to thicken as we passed through Irvine Ranch.

Frustrated when our speed dropped below 55, I began to change lanes in an attempt to advance.

During one such move, my car came within a few feet of a small camper's rear bumper. But when the anticipated "hole" failed to open up, I switched back into the fast lane within half a mile, deciding there was no use trying that kind of maneuver; traffic was too heavy in all lanes.

A few minutes later, I noticed the same small camper directly behind me. I thought nothing of it until its male driver moved up within inches of my bumper. Suddenly I was the target of a deeply competitive driver.

Realizing that he was giving me a taste of my own medicine, I went along with it for at least a mile. If I could dish it out, I was also willing to take it—but only up to a point. After several minutes, I grew tired of the game and angry with my antagonist's persistence. So I used a trick a friend had taught me: tapping the brake pedal so that the brake lights came on but the car does not slow down.

It worked magnificently, I thought. Frightened by my apparent braking, the driver of the small camper jammed on his brakes, producing a short swerving skid. He fell back several car lengths, regrouped, then sped up behind me again. Instead of tailgating me, however, the driver switched into the next lane and came alongside. I leaned forward to confront the face that had tormented me, expecting a brief shouting match.

The young driver of the camper was angry beyond words, so he had chosen a different weapon. Instead of his red face, I was looking at the black barrel of a gun. It was pointed out the driver's window, directly at my wife. I felt my adrenalin surge from fear, but I could not believe he actually intended to shoot. I lowered my speed, allowing the camper to move ahead of me.

The subsequent events are hazy in my memory. I remember that he cut in front of us, slammed on his brakes and reduced his speed—and mine—to less than 10 m.p.h. Behind us, I heard the screeching of tires as the long line of traffic registered the effects of our duel. I felt aghast that, no matter how ridiculous his response, he was only reacting to my own aggressive tactics (Getze, 1976).

Monastic life and coronary heart disease

Caffrey (1966) made an important study of different monastic groups, capitalizing on the fact that American Benedictine monasteries during the early 1960's had different groups of monks, who, while following the same rules of the Benedictine Order, had vastly different life-styles. One was the Benedictine Brothers who dedicated themselves to prayer and meditation and worked in small industries. They ate the same type of food at the same tables with ordained priests. The Benedictine Priests lived in the mainstream of American life, maintaining churches, seminaries, schools, colleges, and parishes; consequently, they had great demands on their time and energy and experienced much psychosocial stimulation.

Caffrey also evaluated Trappist Monks who subsist on a low-fat milk and vegetable diet and live a placid life behind monastery walls, submitting to a vow of silence. He contrasted their eating habits and life-style with that of the Benedictine Brothers with their high-fat diet and placid, prayerful life and that of the Benedictine Priests with the same high-fat diet, but with an active, socially demanding life at a highly competitive tempo.

From his study of about 1300 men in 10 Trappist and 17 Benedictine monasteries, Caffrey hypothesized that the groups differing in the incidence of coronary heart disease may also differ in the number of Type A personalities. Whereas 64 of the 862 Benedictine Priests had had a myocardial infarction, only six of the 203 Benedictine Brothers and four of the 284 Trappist Monks—none of whom, neither Priests nor Brothers, have contact with the outside world—had been so afflicted. This represents a highly significant difference ($p < 0.0001$) between the incidence of myocardial infarction in socially active Benedictine Priests and in other more cloistered Benedictine Brothers and Trappist Monks.

Three separate raters showed that many more Benedictine Priests than Benedictine Brothers had an extreme Type A personality ($p < 0.0001$). Benedictine Priests, although sensitive, were more extroverted and more strongly oriented toward interpersonal manipulative skills, a direct contrast to the sober, industrious attitude of the Benedictine Brothers. Caffrey regards Benedictine Priests as modern men, responding with a Type A personality to society's demands on them (Caffrey, 1966). Their high incidence of myocardial infarction can be expected in view of the difficulty they experienced in reconciling the promise of an ordered, predictable, sheltered monastic existence with the reality of their competitive and demanding people-oriented working life in the school and parish.

Contrasts between traditional Japanese and American cultures

At this point, we turn to the new and important work by Marmot on acculturation and coronary heart disease in Japanese–Americans (Marmot, 1975; Marmot and Syme, 1976). This remarkable study contrasts the behavioral patterns and incidence of coronary heart disease in Japanese–

Americans who are acculturated to the competitive, individualistic American way of life with those who remain closely tied to a more traditional Japanese culture.

In explaining why he and his associates were not content with the majority opinion that the leading cause of coronary heart disease is dietary, Marmot comments that Kannel, one of the organizers of The Framingham Study, said, "It is paradoxical that in free-living affluent populations no one has convincingly demonstrated a difference in nutrient composition of the diet between persons who develop coronary heart disease and those who do not." "Nor," he says, "has there been a demonstration, *within* such populations, of a connection between the nutrient content of the diet and serum cholesterol values from one person to the next" (Kannel, 1974). Marmot quotes Keys, a strong proponent of the dietary hypothesis, as saying that less than half the coronary heart disease incidence in American men is explained by even the combination of all traditional risk factors (Keys et al., 1972).

The hypothesis of Marmot's study with Syme and others is that the missing factor may be the effectiveness of a social support system. Marmot et al. (1975) began by confirming Gordon's (1967) observation that the gradient in mortality from coronary heart disease per 1000 rises from 1.8 in Japanese to 3.2 in Hawaiian–Japanese to 9.8 in American–Caucasians. This gradient holds for each of the complications such as angina and myocardial infarct. Although there is some evidence that the Type A behavior pattern may be a Western phenomenon, it is far less evident in Hawaiian–Japanese than in American–Caucasians—an interesting fact in view of their lower incidence of coronary heart disease.

Another question is the matter of rapid social change. Tyroler and Cassel (1964) showed that rural mountaineers who work in factories have an increased incidence of coronary heart disease. They draw the distinction between a traditional society which supports a man socially and culturally by presenting him with the stable patterns of a familiar world and a transitional society which confronts him with challenging situations of discontinuity or incongruity due to rapid sociocultural changes. Another consideration may be that despite the rapid changes at work, there may still be an important protection to the individual in being surrounded by a stable, traditional social group at home who provide emotional support.

The social support in Japanese culture forms the core of Matsumoto's (1970) important review which stimulated the Marmot study. This quality of social life was first clearly brought out in relation to coronary heart disease by his hypothesis that the absence of social stress, not diet, is responsible for Japan's lower rate of coronary heart disease—only one-eighth that of the United States—even though Japan is a fully modern, urbanized, and industrialized state by Western standards. He points out that in well-integrated societies, anxieties and tensions are kept within appropriate limits by the techniques used by certain social groups. Other societies, i.e., Arsenian and Arsenian's tough cultures, do not have as efficient stress-reducing techniques.

What are the differences? In the West, persons are regarded as individuals more than in Japan where their behavior reflects a greater expression of attachment and interdependence. Japanese children receive more emotional support from their parents and, in general, the culture encourages attachment behavior. For example, once a company hires the average Japanese man, he is rarely dismissed. Seniority is a major criterion for advancement, and changing jobs from company to company is rare. Moreover, the enterprise is paternal and provides supporting company stores, churches, and sports facilities. Unlike his American counterpart, the Japanese takes his leisure with his fellow workers. His relationship with them is clearly differentiated from that with his family with whom he spends less time than the American. On the way home from work,

Japanese men chat with one another in tea shops in a relaxed atmosphere designed for releasing tensions and regaining composure and serenity. Group cohesion goes a step further at various drinking places where female company is provided to support their egos. Bath houses are yet another spot where, as Ruth Benedict says, "they value the daily bath for cleanliness' sake as Americans do, but they add to this value a fine art of passive indulgence which is hard to duplicate in the bathing habits of the rest of the world" (Benedict, 1946).

Marmot follows up on Matsumoto's theme which points to the commitment of the individual to the group as a dominant feature of Japanese society. Personal obligation and duty are regarded as more important than individual fulfillment. The community is the locus of value. The leaders of various groups, culminating with the emperor, have an especially important place in this symbolic value system. The company replaces the old feudal aristocracy in modern industrial Japan. It is now responsible for the major portions of social and communal life, and it succeeds in providing powerful emotional support. Individuals stay with the company for life; their commitment to superiors and co-worker friends is very important to them. The company offers security, a familiar situation, and a guaranteed job advancement.

There is an important difference, however, between the highly structured Japanese society with its reliance on order and hierarchy and the American society's faith in freedom and equality. The Japanese is more concerned with taking his proper station in life than the American and his goals are sought in cooperation with his peer group. His social structure protects him against the challenges of the unfamiliar and against those for which the changing technology did not prepare him.

Advancement along socially prescribed lines in Japan and a lack of competition within the group differs from the Type A behavior pattern of highly individualized striving, ambition, and competitiveness in the United States. Marmot and his associates noted these differences and questioned whether our American culture might not promote more coronary heart disease than the Japanese culture. They hypothesized that for any particular subgroup of Japanese–Americans in California—the greater their exposure to Western culture, the greater their chances of having coronary heart disease. Conversely, they argued, the more the subgroup clung to the traditional Japanese values of loyalty and commitment to the group, the less the stimulus. This type of group orientation might provide stability and emotional support and cut down on the competitiveness between group members, despite industrialization and a rapidly changing advanced technology.

The original Japanese settlers in California formed tightly knit ethnic enclaves by choice and because of the external pressures of racial prejudice (Marmot, 1975). Close and supportive and committed to group values, they provided much help in settling the new arrivals. This segregated community preserved the Japanese family structure prior to World War II. Children had a strong sense of duty to the older generations because of their strong family backgrounds. The Buddhist and Christian churches were also an important focus of Japanese community life in providing education, social groups, and meeting places.

After World War II, the American-born Japanese worked hard and gained success in the wider American middle class society they had entered, but even here they supported family unity. Despite the economic achievements of the Japanese, the two cultures still differ: The contemporary American middle class, predominantly Type A, sets a high value on efficiency, output, and productivity, in contrast to the Japanese traditionalist emphasis on style and mode of interaction. Today, although they have discarded their native language and many of their old customs, they still seek the ethnic structure and cradle-to-grave service offered by their culture (Marmot, 1975).

Coronary heart disease in acculturated Japanese–Americans

A study was made of the prevalence of cornary heart disease in 3800 Japanese–Americans living in eight San Francisco Bay Area counties. Each subject completed medical, demographic, and cultural questionnaires from which four indices of acculturation were compiled to measure cultural upbringing, cultural assimilation, social assimilation, and social and cultural attitudes. Laboratory procedures and a standard 12-lead electrocardiogram were also included in the investigation. When classified according to cultural upbringing, the most acculturated group of Japanese–Americans was shown to have 2.5 times more coronary heart disease than the most traditional group. This value was undiminished by controlling successively for Westernization of diet, smoking, serum triglycerides, serum cholesterol, blood pressure, relative weight, or serum glucose (see Figs. 10-5 and 10-6). When classified according to cultural upbringing and to the degree to which they were disassociated from the ethnic group, there was a fivefold difference between the most and the least acculturated groups. The least acculturated group had a prevalence comparable to the low rates observed in Japan, and the most acculturated group approximated the high rates observed in American–Caucasians. These differences in disease rates are not explained by differences in coronary risk factors.

Marmot concludes that although the differences in dietary habits in Japan and in the United States may be importantly related to the differences in the incidence of disease, they alone do not explain them. The evidence suggests that closely knit stable

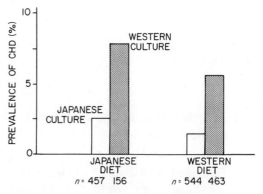

Fig. 10-5. Prevalence of definitive coronary heart disease (CHD) in men according to their cultural upbringing and social assimilation, controlling for risk factors. Japanese (open columns) and Western (shaded columns) cultures show a highly significant difference regardless of dietary preference *(Marmot, 1975)*.

subgroups whose members enjoy the support of their fellowmen may be protected against otherwise highly socially stimulating situations in a rapidly changing society. This important study focuses attention on the social assets of the individual and suggests

Fig. 10-6. Prevalence of coronary heart disease (CHD) in Japanese–American men 45 years or younger. Those whose upbringing in the United States was still traditionally Japanese-oriented appear in the open columns; the nontraditional whose upbringing led them to identify more with the Western culture appear in the transverse-shaded columns. The data are controlled for cholesterol; the difference at higher levels is highly significant *(Marmot, 1975)*

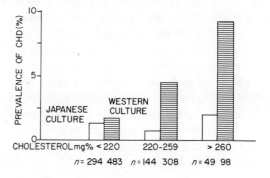

that they protect against the arousal of the neuroendocrine system by the stimulus of life changes (Marmot, 1975; Marmot et al., 1975; Marmot and Syme, 1976).

Myocardial infarction in former medical students

Caroline Bedell Thomas and her associates provided some startling information recently on their remarkable long-term prospective study of medical students beginning with their admission to the Johns Hopkins School of Medicine in Baltimore. In a detailed psychologic evaluation of the 1337 students, who were originally registered in classes that had graduated between 1948 and 1964, they found that the hypercholesteremic students were older, shorter, and heavier and had younger mothers; they had less depression and anxiety and less overall nervous tension under stress.

A group of 103 men with cholesterols in excess of 250 milligrams/100 milliliters, whose mean age was 47 years, were controls for the 10 persons who had had an acute myocardial infarction at a mean age of 45 years. Precoronary subjects were also hypercholesteremic while still in medical school, but differed in temperament; they had more anxiety, anger, and depression, especially under stress. They were more tired on awakening and had lower academic standing than the controls without myocardial infarction (Fig. 10-2).

Thomas et al. (1975) conclude that the combination of hypercholesteremia and a personality profile denoting sensitivity and vulnerability to stress best characterizes the 10 subjects who sustained myocardial infarction at an early age. Thus they agree with Friedman and Rosenman who also found that the combination of personality characteristics and high cholesterol levels is a better predictor of future coronary heart disease than either alone.

Bereavement and myocardial infarction

Holmes and Rahe's (1967) work indicating that there can be a relationship between recent life changes and illness (see Chapter 1) casts light on a 1969 study of Parkes and his associates on the increased deaths among widowers. They followed up on 4486 widowers, 55 years and older, for nine years after the death of their wives. During the first six months after bereavement, 213 widowers died—40 percent above the expected rate of married men of the same age (Fig. 10-7). Coronary thrombosis caused the most deaths. After the first year, however, the mortality rate fell to that of the married men and remained at about the same level. An evaluation of all the possibilities led the authors to suspect that the emotional effects of bereavement with the concomitant changes in psychoendocrine functions are responsible for the increase in deaths, and they conclude that there is a need to develop methods of diminishing these changes (Parkes et al., 1969).

Gutmann's description of the aging male's shift away from activity and independence, cited in Chapter 2, may be relevant in the context of bereavement and the increased incidence of coronary heart disease in recent widowers, but not widows. The bereaved man whose changed social situation forces a return to a pattern of active self-sufficiency and competition must fight a growing disinclination for new activities. His depression may help to defeat his new efforts and lead to a loss of control. Adrenal-cortical activation may then be added to the arousal of the adrenal-medullary system. This combination may be particularly unfavorable for an arteriosclerotic cardiovascular system. If Gutmann is correct, the bereaved older woman does not bear the added burden of an opposing biologic trend as she faces new adjustments (Gutmann, 1977).

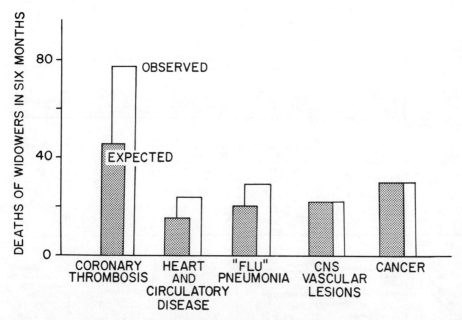

Fig. 10-7.   Mortality rate based on 4486 widowers during the first six months of bereavement (open columns) as a proportion of the expected mortality rate for married men of the same age (shaded columns) taken from 1957 statistics for England and Wales. Coronary heart disease surpassed other causes of death (see abscissa). Figures for stroke and cancer were unchanged *(Parkes et al., 1969).*

Blood pressure and cultural change

Although a correlation of the incidence of social stimulation with coronary heart disease presents a case for considering the deficiency of social assets as a major risk factor, a similar but subtly different body of evidence exists for high blood pressure. Cassel (1975) recently reviewed the epidemiology of hypertension from a psychosocial viewpoint; he pointed out that we are still without a clear understanding of the mechanisms underlying the rise in blood pressure—a characteristic of aging in so many societies.

In an earlier survey, Henry and Cassel (1969) reviewed the evidence that there are cultural groups throughout the world whose blood pressures are low and do not change with age; moreover, coronary and hypertensive heart diseases and strokes are rare. The fact that such a large number of these groups

exist—Shaper (1974) refers to about 40— and that these groups are not confined to any special race, such as Negro or Caucasian, and that they are found on every continent and include all races of man, makes it unlikely that their normal blood pressure is an expression of some genetic immunity peculiar to race.

An illustration from the Henry-Cassel review (Fig. 10-8) demonstrates the point by presenting blood pressure data from cultural groups around the world, showing those in which blood pressure did not rise with age, those with a moderate rise, and those in which it was steep. Eighteen pressure curves arranged into six vertical columns, each containing three examples, show (from top to bottom) the rate of blood pressure rise with age. From left to right, the first two columns show Americans and Western Europeans, and Russians, Poles, and Czechs; the next two, Amerindians, followed by persons of Negro descent; and the

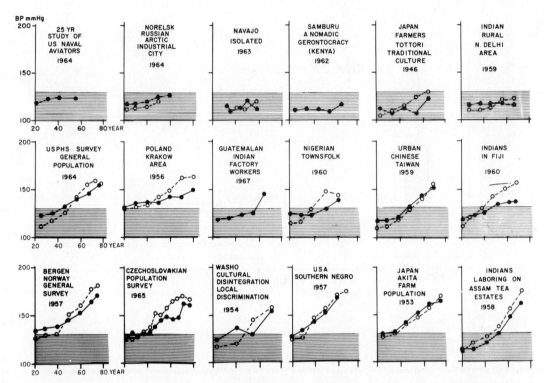

Fig. 10-8. Blood pressure change with age can be found in all races. In general, blood pressure is lower when the culture is stable, traditional forms are honored, and group members are adapted to their roles by early experience and secure in them. Open circles: females. Closed circles: males *(Henry and Cassel, 1969)*.

last two, Japanese and Chinese, and finally Indians, both residents and nonresidents of India. The origin of the survey appears in each of the blood pressure diagram captions and the source is cited in the review article. By contrasting the top, middle, and bottom rows of Fig. 10-8, we find that in general the thesis of psychosocial stimulation holds.

The U.S. naval aviators were a select group of 1000 men who entered flight training during World War II. Only men thoroughly adapted from youth to the demands of a technologic society were chosen by careful testing. We may hazard the guess that the population of Norelsk is also composed of persons well adapted by early experience to life in an Arctic industrial environment. The elderly isolated Navajo had elected to stay in their ancient homeland

and continue their traditional culture. The Samburu, who are related to the Masai, are a well-integrated and traditional group of pastoral nomads living in the desert of northern Kenya. Ruled by elders and still retaining a warrior caste, they live in an isolated ecologic niche, relatively undisturbed by the social and technologic revolution surrounding their world.

A low set of blood pressures with no significant rise with age is seen in the data from a small farming village near the northern coast of Japan. It is believed that these people had retained much of their traditional culture and, at the time of measurement, had not been exposed to the same intensity of change that has since swept over the cities and countryside of Japan. A similar picture emerges after evaluating the blood pressure of villagers in the countryside near New Delhi made nearly 20 years ago.

In the first two columns from the left, the contrast is clear between the two curves (top) which show no major increase in blood pressure with age and the two curves (bottom) for the Norwegian city of Bergen surveyed in 1957 and for an extensive survey of the general population of Czechoslovakia in 1964. The two middle columns show the next curve with the highest pressures which represent data on the disintegrating, formerly migratory Washo tribe evicted from their homeland in the Lake Tahoe area because of sociocultural events and economic pressures and living in squatters shacks outside Carson City, Nevada. Similarly, the constant blood pressure of the Samburu Negroes of Kenya may be contrasted with a detailed 1957 survey of the blood pressure of Negroes in the southern United States. The two columns at the right show the elevation of blood pressure among elderly persons living on the increasingly unprofitable farms in Akita, the northern province of Japan, contrasted with that of the traditional farming group in nearby Tottori province 20 years earlier. Finally there is a sharp rise of blood pressure among expatriated Indians of a generation ago, living in Assam as indentured laborers. They lost many of their caste affiliations and much of their traditional Hindu culture as they worked on the rigidly controlled tea plantations.

Interpolated between these six extremes are other measurements representing groups with intermediate levels of social stress. The general population of the United States is perhaps finally adapting to what is for them a 100-year-old technologic revolution and developing new traditions to deal with this science-oriented culture. The two diagrams representing data from the area around Krakow in Poland and from a factory town of Indian workers in the highlands of Guatemala, as disparate as they seem, have in common their depiction of rural people who, while adapting to cultural change, still

had strong traditions from the past. The Nigerian townsfolk and the urban Chinese of Taiwan represent people who are retaining some traditional ties while seeking to adjust to great changes within their lifetimes. The expatriated Indians of Fiji represent men and women who have found a good measure of social satisfaction, yet live in racial conflict with the native Fijians. Born on the islands and adapted to their new status as members of this pleasant community, they have lost, for better or for worse, the complex caste structure in which their traditions as socially integrated and religiously oriented Hindus would have been embedded two generations ago.

The conclusion was that a man living in a stable society and well-equipped by his cultural background to deal with the familiar world around him will not show a rise in blood pressure with age. This thesis holds whether he is a modern technocrat who became a fighter pilot early in life or a Stone Age Bushman who is a skilled hunter–gatherer living in the Kalahari Desert. However, when radical cultural changes disrupt his familiar environment with a new set of demands for which past acculturation has left him unprepared, his social assets are then critical. Should they fail to protect him, he will be exposed to emotional upheavals and ensuing neuroendocrine disturbances that may eventuate in cardiovascular disease.

In a recent review, Cassel (1975) asks whether normal blood pressure which does not change with aging and is still found in small often unacculturated groups will rise with the inexorable encroachment of industrialized Western culture into their protected ecologic niches. He discusses three types of situations. The first is a comparison of similar people living under different degrees of cultural contact: the inhabitants of Puka Puka and Rarotonga. The small group living on the uniquely traditional, still isolated tiny Polynesian atolls of Puka Puka have normal blood pressure and have been repeatedly compared with the more heavily acculturated transitional group on Rarotonga, which lies several hundred miles down the Cook Island chain and is the administrative capital of the archipelago governed by New Zealand. To the casual observer, the mechanisms at work leading to neuroendocrine upset cannot be perceived at this beautiful mountainous resort. But Rarotonga is the focal point for cultural exchange and migration between the various Cook islands and the now largely modernized Maori population in New Zealand. The inhabitants are exposed to the conflict between the demands of their still-surviving Stone Age-Polynesian tradition, farther up the island chain, and of the industrial, democratic Western culture now governing them. Their blood pressure is consistently higher than that of their contemporaries on Puka Puka (Fig. 10-9) but then so was their salt intake, 130 versus 60 milliequivalents of sodium chloride. Prior's group concluded that further research was needed to find out whether this difference in salt is important (Prior et al., 1968).

The differences between two groups in New Guinea, found by Maddocks (1967), are of interest. The territory of the Chimbu was discovered only in the 1930's and remained a subsistence economy at the time of measurement in the 1960's. The inaccessible, mountainous terrain cut by gorges supported a high population density made possible by the cultivation of sweet potato gardens perched on precipitous hillsides, making a strong pair of legs the greatest personal asset. The inhabitants at that time had not yet adopted Western ways; they followed their own way of life and were busily integrating shovels and sewing machines into their traditional subsistence economy. They were ruled by their own officials who held tribal positions, but worked for the Australian government in Port Moresby. Chronic warfare had been stopped and medical care and schools were started. Few European traders visited their

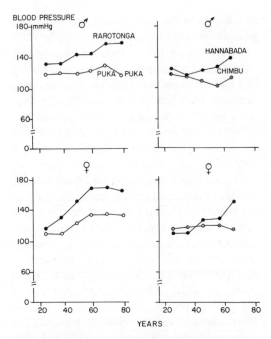

Fig. 10-9. On the left, the systolic blood pressures of Polynesians living under different degrees of cultural contact are contrasted: males ♂(above) and females ♀ (below). In Rarotonga (solid circles), the capital of the Cook Island chain, the inhabitants can earn wages. Puka Puka (open circles), remote and inaccessible, has a subsistence economy. On the right, in similar studies in New Guinea, the Hannabada natives (solid circles) live in a suburb of Port Moresby where they work for wages. The natives of the rugged Chimbu highland (open circles) maintain a traditional subsistence culture *(Cassel, 1975).*

villages, and the Chimbu, whose blood pressure does not change with age, flourished under a peaceful regime imposed by Australia (Fig. 10-9) (Brown, 1972).

The Hannabada, by contrast, were formerly fishermen. They lived in villages built over the sea, joined to the land by footpaths, at Port Moresby. Although they had long associated with Europeans, their standard of living was nevertheless poor. Yet they did have electric lights, a piped water supply, and owned some cars and trucks; the men and many of the women earned wages as clerks, typists, or artisans in Port Moresby (population 32,000). Consequently, they lived in the cash economy of the West and were caught up in its culture. Many had adopted European food and their salt intake was threefold the five grams or less taken daily by the Chimbu (Lea and Irwin, 1967; Maddocks, 1967). Here again, it remains to be seen whether salt intake is an important factor in their having higher blood pressure (Fig. 10-9).

Cassel (1975) has also discussed the differences in blood pressure surveys made on the islands of Palau and Ponape in the Carolines. These two islands, now incorporated into the U.S. Trust Territory of the Pacific, represent an important natural experiment. During the past century both have been successively under European, then Japanese, and finally under United States' control. Since the end of World War II, three different ethnographic studies on Ponape, which is only 12 miles in diameter and has a population of 15,000, showed that the traditional ways of life continued to persist. Moreover, the survey in 1947 showed that the blood pressure of males was low and without significant increase up to the age of 60 (Murrill, 1949). During the last quarter of a century, however, social and cultural changes have taken place as a result of contact with Americans. The missionary zeal with which not only Christianity but also Western technology was promoted has been mitigated by an anthropologically led respect for such surviving enclaves of ancient cultures.

Nevertheless, 86 percent of those living in Kolonia (population 1500), the little administrative center and capital of Ponape, are significantly acculturated into Western habits and values. This holds true for only half of those living in remote areas. The extent of acculturation in the different districts was determined in terms of change from the original ethnographic studies of the island. A sociocultural interview composed of 55 items collected data on language, diet, education, and culture. As Fig. 10-10 shows, a recent blood pressure survey on Ponape

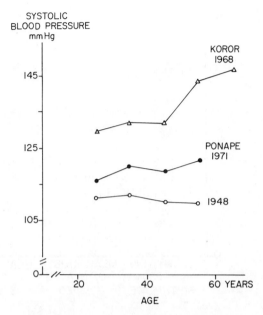

Fig. 10-10. Contrasting the rise in blood pressure with age in 1968 in Koror, the capital of the Palau Islands, Western Carolines, in Micronesia with that of the general population of the more traditional South Sea island of Ponape in 1948 and also in 1971. The curve for 1948 represents conditions before the American occupation had started to take effect after World War II, and the 1971 curve represents a survey after 23 years of American administration *(Cassel, 1975).*

revealed slightly higher blood pressures than those taken some 20 years earlier, but no clear-cut rise with the degree of modernization (Cassel, 1975).

By contrast, Labarthe et al. (1973) have obtained definitive results on Palau. Some of the sociocultural indices of modernization are shown in Fig. 10-11. A considerable difference exists between Koror, the capital, and the isolated village of Ngerchelong which retains its original culture. The measures cited were supported by further observations contrasting the village with the capital—its automobiles, quality of housing, density of population, access to commercial food, mass media, and cash economy. In all these, Ngerchelong scored low, clearly

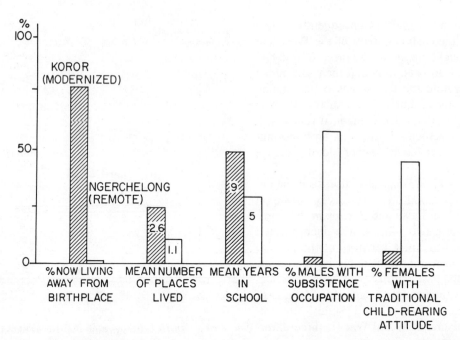

Fig. 10-11. In the first, fourth, and fifth pairs of histograms, left to right, the ordinate contrasts the percent of the populations in Koror and in a remote area who are now living away from their birthplace, working in a subsistence occupation, and have a traditional attitude toward child rearing, respectively. The mean number of places lived in and the mean number of years in school are printed inside the second and third sets of histograms. The data show a difference in acculturation between the two populations *(Labarthe et al., 1973).*

remaining traditional. As can be seen in Fig. 10-10, the blood pressure of Palauans in Koror was significantly higher than that of Ponapeans. It also suggests a sociocultural effect that the reported dietary patterns in Ngerchelong were not in agreement with the biochemical results. Despite a higher caloric intake with a greater contribution of saturated fats to the total calories in the coconut-eating villagers of Ngerchelong, the males were less obese and had lower serum cholesterol than those of Koror. Labarthe and his associates concluded that among adult male Palauans modernization was associated with health indices that in other populations are related to the risk of cardiovascular disease.

One may ask why modernization, thus far, has had so little effect on the blood pressures of the Ponapeans as opposed to the Palauans. For one, Koror had a huge World War II population of many thousands of Japanese colonists, soldiers, and sailors; also the Palauan islands were more heavily colonized with vigorous immigrant farmers during the period of Japanese control from the 1920's to the 1940's than the distant Ponape. As a consequence, the Palauans may have gone much further in identifying with Japan and in abandoning their traditional culture than the Ponapeans. Later, with the transfer of authority to the Americans in 1945, the reversal of their newly adopted culture that was now demanded of them may have led to serious ambiguities. The double loss, first, of traditional forms, then, of the new culture, and the consequent uncertainties as to values and goals would be the most severe in the capital and its environs.

The classic, sleepy Pacific island of Ponape seems to have escaped these intense seesawing acculturation pressures. The 1970 Ponape blood pressure survey with its now commencing upward tilt with age and overall 10 mmHg elevation over the 1948 values may represent the beginning of a change which has progressed a good deal further in Koror (Fig. 10-10).

Another example Cassel discussed was a study of migrants emerging from their ecologic niches into modern societies. He cites Shaper's (1972) observation of the blood pressure of nomadic Samburu warriors of Kenya measured at different times after they enlisted in the army and the blood pressure of warriors who remained with the tribe. The systolic blood pressure of warriors living their traditional life-style is remarkably low, scarcely rising above 110 mmHg, even in those 60 years old, but that of army recruits showed a significant rise. Importantly, the recruits' blood pressure did not rise after their first six months in the army when their weight gain had been considerable, but only after two years of military service when their

weight gain was actually less. But gradually their blood pressure rose still further—until after six years of military service, it was significantly higher than in their age-matched controls (Fig. 10-12) (Cassel, 1975). Thus it was not the general improvement in nutrition that led to the blood pressure rise. A tribesman's normal diet contains only two to three grams of salt daily, whereas the army diet is said to provide over 15 grams of salt. Again, as in the previous examples, the question is whether the change in salt intake is sufficient to increase blood pressure or whether the change in social stimuli also plays a role.

The problem is similar to that found in coronary heart disease. It is our theme that it is not possible to focus on single causes of disease and that neuroendocrine upsets following social stress can at least accelerate the development of long-term pathophysiologic changes. Stress can arise from the

Fig. 10-12. On the left, the blood pressure of nomadic Samburu warriors who entered the Westernized army in Kenya (diagonally shaded columns) show little change after the first six months, but with the years diverges more and more from the control group (open columns) who remain with their tribe. On the right, the body weight increases during the first six months of army life, but then remains almost constant (shaded columns), suggesting that nutrition and body weight did not determine blood pressure: * = $p < 0.05$, ** = $p < 0.01$, *** = $p < 0.001$ *(Shaper, 1972).*

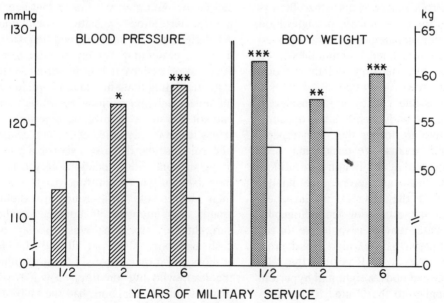

migration of a society or from its transition to a different value system. A change in values leads to situations where previously sanctioned behavior, especially that which is acquired during the sensitive learning period in youth, can no longer be used. Although the opportunity to express himself in the manner to which he is accustomed no longer exists, the individual still cannot help attaching great value to this behavior. The ensuing confrontations with his conscience and with his fellows lead to repeated emotional crises and consequent arousal of the neuroendocrine system. Chapter 8 describes the mechanisms which alter the level of blood pressure. Coronary heart disease and high blood pressure are only two of a number of diseases affected by psychosocial variables; both are contemporary epidemics and there is much convincing data based on effective and well-controlled research.

Psychosocial factors, salt, and hypertension

In contrast with Cassel's views presented earlier, Shaper (1974), Freis (1976), and Page (1976), have independently discussed the role that various other factors may play in the development of high blood pressure. They all agree that unacculturated people living in isolated communities often do not have hypertension and their blood pressure fails to rise with age.

Four possible causes are considered: the difference in body weight since unacculturated people are leaner than Westerners; general health because Westerners may benefit by adequate diet and health care; differences in psychosocial factors; and, finally, salt intake, since they suspect that the generally greater salt intake of technologically developed states may be responsible for the contrasting prevalence of high blood pressure. Freis agrees with Page that the relationship between body weight and hypertension that applies to the United States does

not seem to apply to unacculturated peoples. The available evidence, he contends, does not support the concept that their lack of hypertension is due to their leaner body habitus.

Lot B. Page reviews the question of their general health, the hypothesis being that low blood pressure is an abnormality and that when adequate diet and modern health care become available, a normal age-related increase in blood pressure is revealed. He gives his own observations of the excellent health and nutrition of people with low blood pressures living in the Solomon Islands. Shaper has commented on the vigor of the nomads in Kenya and the Bushmen of the Kalahari Desert, both of whom have low blood pressure. It is concluded that debility and chronic infections do not play more than a minor part in keeping blood pressures low. Further, the people of the Gilbert Islands and Ponape have had adequate medical services for decades thus disproving the suggestion that their normal blood pressure was due to an early selective mortality among those who might have developed high blood pressure (Henry and Cassel, 1969).

The two remaining hypotheses the authors seriously considered are psychosocial factors and high salt intake that accompany acculturation. Freis attaches only modest weight to the former, pointing to the difficulty of defining it in quantitative terms. Page, also, assigns it less importance than salt, suggesting that such factors would only influence short-term blood pressure trends and not pressure over prolonged periods. He refers to his own studies of the antecedents of cardiovascular disease in six tribal groups living in contrasting locations in the Solomon Islands where anthropologists graded their degree of acculturation to include length and intensity of contact, medical care, literacy, religion, Western diet, and cash economy (Page et al., 1974). The authors noted that out of six groups studied, the Lau, who live on tiny, crowded man-made islands in a lagoon, had the highest of the very modestly increased blood pressures. They ranked third in acculturation, but were by far the highest in salt intake because they use salt water for cooking. Page and his associates concluded that the dietary intake of salt correlated best with the intrapopulation trends of blood pressure. But this judgment depends on the accuracy of the anthropologists' low scoring of the Lau acculturation level.

The famous "Man-Made Islands of the Pacific" are sanctuaries of traditionalism. At least one of these lagoon islands is open to tourism and includes inspection of its sacred places (Kent, 1972); this is not surprising because the architecture of these artificial islands, such as Sulu Vou that the Lau have built, is impressive from the viewpoint of picturesque social integration (Fig. 10-13). There is a possibility that traditionalism and

a conscious archaism with a relatively sophisticated rejection of Western lifestyles, including Christianity to which they have been exposed for generations, played a role in giving the Lau a low score for acculturation. Such archaism can be misleading and could still be associated with political unrest and emotionally arousing cultural conflicts.

The Yanomamö Indians are interesting from this same viewpoint since they combine a very low salt intake with an intact sovereign culture almost untouched by Western technocracy. They have lived in isolation for hundreds of years in the relatively unexplored jungle between Brazil and Venezuela. Up to now, their blood pressure had been normal throughout life and their renin level appropriately high for their low salt intake. Oliver and his associates attrib-

Fig. 10-13.   This artificial island built on a hand-built platform of coral rocks is one of many in a lagoon off the southeast coast of Malaita in the Solomon Islands. The architectural design has playgrounds, places for dancing, sacred areas, and men's clubhouses *(Ivens, 1930).*

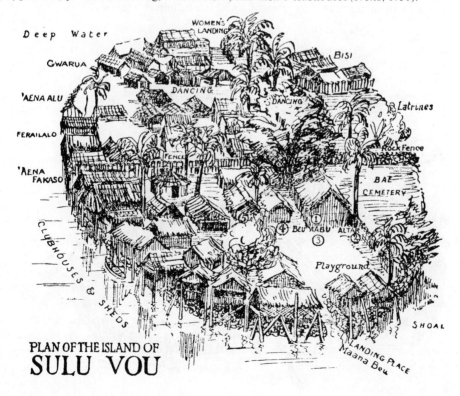

PLAN OF THE ISLAND OF
SULU VOU

ute their normal pressure to the low salt intake. But these people also enjoy an unchallenged, ancient cultural tradition, and their handsome settlements are illustrated in Fig. 10-14 (Oliver et al., 1975).

Chagnon, an anthropologist, has lived with the Yanomanö Indians and has studied them for years. He does not question their adaptation to their environment, and admiringly describes their elegant circular villages which are designed with living space for individual families on the periphery and a plaza for social interaction in the center (Fig. 10-14). Although less sophisticated than Lau villages, The Yanomanö design still meets the needs of their socially integrated group. Chagnon describes the mental state of the villagers who abandoned their tribal lifestyle and were becoming acculturated by missionaries, viewing them as a deteriorated people (Chagnon, 1974).

Freis challenges the psychosocial proposal which he regards as saying that the absence of hypertension in unacculturated peoples is due to a lack of economic stress, racial or ethnic tensions, urban life-style, noise, and a fast pace of life. Arguing that it is really the salt that is responsible, he points to Lowenstein's comparative study of the Mundurucú and the Carajá tribes in the Amazon basin. The Mundurucú had been converted to Christianity by missionaries who had also introduced them to table salt (Lowenstein, 1961). Although still living under relatively primitive conditions without the noise and the fast pace of life, they showed a rise of blood pressure with age, and some had hypertension. The Carajá, on the other hand, spurned all contact with civilization including table salt; they exhibited no change in blood pressure with age and no hypertension.

Fig. 10-14. The warrior Yanomamö are a still largely undisturbed tribe of Indians living in the tropical rain forest on the inland border between Venezuela and Brazil. They have been isolated for many hundreds of years and build simple circular villages, as shown, enclosing a central open space which serves as a common ground for all types of social interaction *(Chagnon, 1974).*

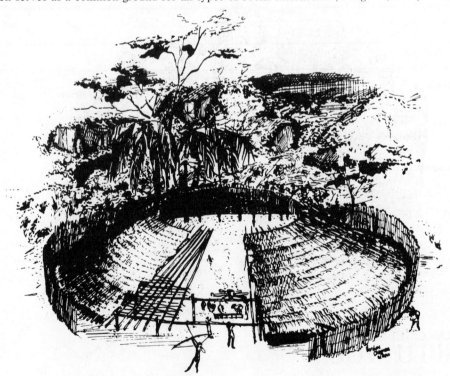

But the pressure differences of the Mundurucú were modest, i.e., 110 versus 130 mmHg systolic. Once active warriors of the savannah, the predatory Mundurucú raided the neighboring tribes whose women their war chiefs enslaved. Forty-five years ago, the group Lowenstein studied moved 400 miles away and settled on a river bank near a Franciscan mission. Tamed, they had given up their war chiefs, polygamy, and aggressive raids; their nuclear families now live in individual houses.

The always more peaceful, sedentary Carajá still live in large family groups, 20–30 in a hut, and they have long been in their present location. They are still pagan and still practice their old rites and dances. Despite their close proximity to Caucasians and their familiarity with them, they have maintained their culture relatively intact. It is plausible that the Mundurucú, in addition to using salt, have experienced more socially stimulating events leading to life changes over the decades as they struggled to exchange their old values for Christian ethics.

Freis draws the dangerous conclusion that because there is more hypertension in the United States among Negroes of the rural South than among those who migrated to the large cities of the North—that urbanization is not an important influence. But there may be more incongruity and social disturbance among those left behind in the country, bereft of the religion and mores of their old cultural canon and with few resources for coping with the new secular technocracy. They are exposed to the blandishments of radio, television, telephone, and rapid transportation but without the resources to profit by them. The city dweller enjoys more support from a city culture which is rapidly adapting to the electronic revolution. Freis also cites data from Scotch's report on the relation of sociocultural factors to hypertension among the Zulu.

Since the urban Zulu exhibit hypertension, but not the rural Zulu who do not use salt, he viewed this as evidence in support of the salt hypothesis. On their reservations, status is given to the aged as repositories of tradition in the extended family, as pointed out by Scotch (1960, 1963). Although the men work hard during the planting season, they have fewer demands made on them during the rest of the time. Women have a more sustained workload, but a large family does not pose the same economic problems in this agricultural community where the ancient traditions of the tribe persist. The chief rules on disputes and the specter of the white man outside of the reservation could almost be forgotten. The Zulu living in the apartheid section on the outskirts of Durban in South Africa in the late 1950's found their tribal customs distorted and engulfed by change. The youth sought formal education and were eager to become acculturated into European technology, but were frustrated because they could not attain this goal. Meanwhile, the extended family was gone and the old found neither honor nor respect in the overcrowded homes of their sons where they were unwelcome guests.

Scotch, himself, concluded that the critical factor responsible for the difference in blood pressure was psychologic tension resulting from an unsatisfactory relation between the traditional patterns of behavior and the socially frustrating living conditions on the fringes of the white segregationist-dominated city.

The work of Prior contrasting the atoll dwellers of Puka Puka with the more acculturated inhabitants of Rarotonga was cited as further support of the salt hypothesis: the Rarotongans used twice as much salt and hypertension was common, whereas, the Puka Pukans used only 60 milliequivalents per day (Fig. 10-9). But the difference between the uniquely sustained, traditional Polynesian life-style of the atoll dwellers, living without clocks beside their lagoon, and that of the Rarotongans, who after 60 years of repressive, autocratic missionary government (1845–1905) now have a cash economy and telephones and live in the headquarters for the administration of the Cook Islands by New Zealand, must also be put into the equation, and Prior's group withheld a decision, although agreeing that the data were compatible with the salt hypothesis (Prior et al., 1968).

A final example of the importance of weighing all factors and not salt alone is found in the Marshall Islands whose residents, Dahl notes, have a moderate incidence of high blood pressure at the level found in the general population of the United States (Fig. 10-15). Dahl (1960) regards their pressure as appropriate for their moderately high salt intake. The Marshall islanders studied in 1958 formerly lived on the Rongelap atoll that had been exposed to radiation from an atomic cloud in 1954. They were precipitately removed from Rongelap, quartered briefly at the naval base at Kwajalein, then moved to Majuro atoll for three years until the contamination had subsided enough to permit their return home in 1957 to a newly built Westernized village. The cultural changes to which they had been exposed did not include urbanization, noise, or a fast pace of life (Hines, 1962). But despite the restraint and consideration on both sides fol-

lowing the accident, the natives' frustration and irritation with the imposition of life changes from being arbitrarily removed from their familiar lagoon and quartered in the camp of an alien culture and still later subjected to restriction even after their return can only be surmised.

Finally, as Henry and Cassel (1969) point out in their discussion of psychosocial factors in essential hypertension: In 1960, Buddhist farmers in Thailand were using 20 grams of salt per day, yet their blood pressure remained normal throughout their lives. The blood pressures of the U.S. naval aviators and of the citizens of Soviet Norelsk also remain normal despite their culturally determined levels of salt intake of about 10 grams per day. The massive U.S. Framingham Study of various factors concerned with the development of cardiovascular disease has shown no evidence of a relationship between urinary sodium excretion and blood pressure level (Dawber et al., 1967). There is no doubt that a high salt diet is compatible with persistent low blood pressure. The question remaining is whether high blood pressure simply cannot develop in the presence of a lifetime of a truly low intake of salt, i.e., less than 2 grams/adult/day.

Fig. 10-15. The average daily intake of salt among various peoples differs greatly. In general, unacculturated people living in primitive circumstances lack salt as an additive and have a far lower intake. But salt intake reaches high levels in Japan, especially among the farmers of the northern province of Akita. As the figure shows, higher levels of salt intake are often accompanied by an increased incidence of essential hypertension *(Dahl, 1960).*

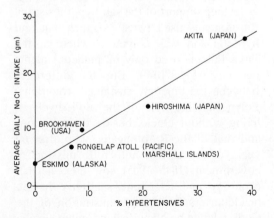

Cancer of the lung and psychosocial parameters

In the context of the relatively untouched area of psychosocial aspects of tumor formation, the remarkable studies of Kissen should be cited. Starting his career just after World War II as a chest physician, he investigated the role of emotion in the etiology of pulmonary tuberculosis. The approach he adopted became a model for his later work (Kissen, 1958). Kissen confirmed earlier observations that patients with tuberculosis had an "inordinate need for affection," and showed that bereavement or other deprivation of attachment bonds in childhood, such as parental death or separation, together with what he called "a break in a love link," i.e., a broken romance or marriage, enforced separation, bereavement, or an unfulfilled desire for a family, occurred more frequently in the history of tubercular patients than in that of nontubercular controls. He concluded that this sensitivity to and need for attachment explained certain psychosocial aspects of the disease.

Massive exposure of populations to a rupture of their love links is a commonplace tragedy of wars, revolutions, and forced migrations. Similarly, when earlier cultural systems, such as those of Eskimos, Polynesians, and North American Indians, have clashed with a modern technocratic culture, a disruption of their social systems with the consequent rupture of their normal attachment behavior has occurred, and their susceptibility to tuberculosis is a familiar one (Kissen, 1958).

Next Kissen made controlled clinical observations of lung cancer. From 1958 to 1967 he conducted structured clinical interviews with nearly 1000 patients admitted to the hospital with only an unidentified chest complaint. They were questioned before the final diagnosis was made; Kissen avoided all information regarding the diagnosis. Eventually about 50 percent of the patients were found to be suffering from lung cancer. He established that significantly more lung cancer patients had had adversities in childhood, such as an unhappy home with the death of a parent; they also had more adversities as adults, such as financial troubles, problems at work, or disturbed interpersonal relationships (Kissen et al., 1969). He further determined that they had had a contrasting lower-than-normal incidence of childhood behavioral disorders, such as bedwetting, stammering, or temper tantrums; these are childhood disorders correlated with neuroticism. The patients thus had less evidence of emotionality in childhood. His appraisal fits in with his later determination, in collaboration with Eysenck, that patients with lung cancer were somewhat extroverted, being outgoing, uninhibited, sociable,

and markedly lower in neuroticism than normal controls; in other words, they were normally aggressive and normally sociable (Fig. 10-16) (Kissen and Eysenck, 1962).

What was significantly different in patients with lung cancer was their poor outlet for emotional discharge ($p < 0.01$) (Fig. 10-16). This meant not merely shrugging off an emotional conflict; it was a facility for "absorption and unconscious containment," according to Kissen. Consequently it came under the psychoanalytic connotation of denial and repression. Patients with lung cancer, for example, would give an account of a marital problem or a bereavement with extraordinary objectivity, and it was very difficult to coax them away from factual statements to those with a more emotional ring. It was almost as though they had a mental block that kept everything rational and avoided the intrusion of limbic-based

Fig. 10-16. Showing the lower rate of neuroticism in male patients with lung cancer. This is consistent with the observation that they have a diminished outlet for emotional discharge. General lability, overresponsiveness, and liability to neurotic breakdown were measured by using Eysenck's inventory. Patients and controls were divided into groups with and without psychosomatic disorder (right and left columns, respectively). Those on the left had slightly higher neuroticism scores than the controls with cancer ($p < 0.01$). Vertical lines on the columns represent the Standard Deviation of the Mean *(Kissen and Eysenck, 1962).*

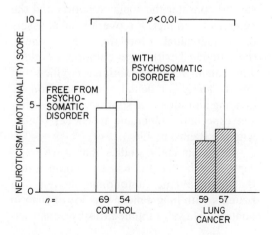

affect. By contrast, the same type of loss of an attachment figure would be emotionally described by a control patient as the bereavement that, in fact, it was (Kissen, 1967). But it took skillful and prolonged interviewing to bring out the psychologic loss to the cancer patient despite his facade of openness. As can be seen from Table 6-1 of Chapter 6, Kissen was reporting on people with alexithymic characteristics (Sifneos et al., 1978). Type A personalities show similar findings. Questions as to the possible role of chronic inhibition of transcallosal communication between the dominant and the nondominant hemispheres have been raised in Chapter 6.

The poor outlet for emotional discharge characterizing patients with lung cancer was dramatically related to their mortality from the disease. Whether they did not smoke or whether their daily use of cigarettes was moderate (one–four) or high (25 or more) greatly affected the incidence of the disease, increasing it tenfold for those who smoked the most cigarettes. But their emotional set also affected the incidence. Those with the most favorable emotional discharge had only one-quarter the incidence of lung cancer compared with those having the greatest difficulty in expressing emotion (Fig. 10-17) (Kissen, 1965).

Kissen's conclusions were the now familiar ones: It is not the life situation, nor the life changes alone that are critical. As Bahnson and Bahnson point out, it is necessary to consider the social supports and the personality, in fact, the overall social assets of the individual. From this point of view, the individual with poor emotional outlets, who cannot resolve emotional conflicts but has a facility for denial and repression by denying himself social support, renders himself especially vulnerable to cancer (Bahnson and Bahnson, 1964).

In preliminary studies that were interrupted by his death, Kissen demonstrated that sympathetic autonomic activity in patients with lung cancer was lower than in controls. He substantiated this by construct-

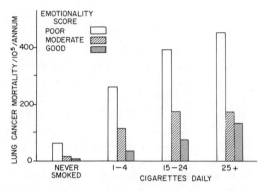

Fig. 10-17. The annual incidence of fatal lung cancer for a population of 100,000 is plotted for persons who never smoked and for those who smoked one to four, 15 to 20, or more than 25 cigarettes a day. The histograms also indicate the influence of the outlet for emotional discharge: poor (no shading), moderate (diagonal shading), and good (dotted shading). Persons with a poor outlet have more than four and one-half times the mortality rate for lung cancer compared with those having a good outlet and two and one-half times the rate of those with a moderate outlet. *(From Kissen and Rao, 1969. Reprinted by permission of the New York Academy of Sciences.)*

ing a scale of 11 items, each referring to a different system associated with autonomic activity (Bahnson, 1969). Kissen's work with Rao showed that daily patterns of steroid excretion differ in patients with lung cancer. The urinary excretion of 17-ketosteroids and 17-hydroxycorticosteroids of 48 patients was contrasted with those of 48 controls immediately after their admission to the hospital and for seven days thereafter. The cancer patients showed an increased day-to-day fluctuation of steroids. Both the sum and the ratio of the two groups of steroids differed significantly ($p < 0.01$). The results were confirmed in a second group of 34 cancer patients and 64 controls. The controls showed an increase in the excretion of steroids during the first two days, followed by a gradual fall as they adapted to the situation. In addition to larger fluctuations, cancer patients do not show so large an initial increase and thereafter show a smaller decrease than the controls (Fig. 10-18). Although it will be the task of future studies

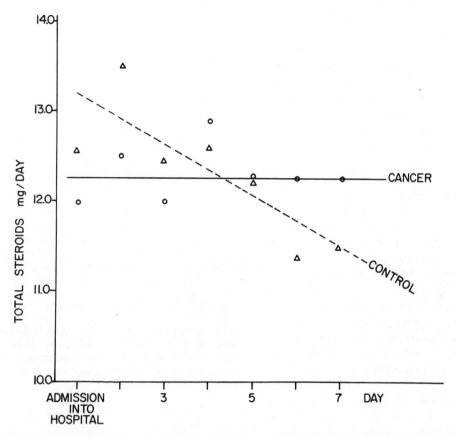

Fig. 10-18.   The mean excretion rate of 17-ketosteroids and 17-hydroxycorticosteroids in the controls are more elevated when they are admitted to the hospital than in patients with lung cancer. As the week goes on, however, the controls show a steady decrease, but the cancer patients do not (Fig. 10-17) *(Kissen and Rao, 1969).*

to shed light on these observations, they do suggest that patients with lung cancer differ from controls in their neuroendocrine responses; instead of subsiding normally after the initial perturbation of being admitted to the hospital, they do not respond enough at first, but then develop a higher level of arousal. It is a testable hypothesis that the higher level of arousal leads to a pattern of hypothalamic response that decreases the individual's immune resistance. The biochemical changes to look for would be lowered catecholamine levels and elevated adrenal corticoidogenesis with abnormal levels of gonadotropins and other tropic hormones (Kissen and Rao, 1969).

Psychologic attributes of breast cancer

In their recent work on the psychologic attributes of women who develop breast cancer, Greer and Morris (1975) employed structured interviews and psychological tests patterned after those that Kissen used with lung cancer patients. Their subjects were admitted to the hospital with a lump in the breast which could be either an early operable cancer or benign. Greer and Morris, who had no knowledge of the provisional diagnosis, also interviewed husbands or other relatives to verify the patients' accounts of their own emotionality. In line with Kissen's approach, they assessed the degree to which patients concealed or expressed their emotions, including anger and their social adjustment in terms of marital, sexual and interpersonal relationships, work satisfaction, and leisure activities.

Of 160 women in a consecutive series, at surgery 69 were found to have cancer and 91 a benign disease of the breast. There were no significant differences in marital status, social class, age, psychiatric disorders, social adjustment, I.Q., hostility, extroversion, or even neuroticism. The occurrence of previous stress, such as the loss of an attachment figure during the past five years, was the same in the two groups. What did differ was the degree to which the subjects suppressed or broke out in an explosion of anger or other feelings. Those who had not openly shown anger more than once or twice in their lives were the extreme suppressors. The exploders, however, had frequent outbursts of temper and very rarely concealed their feelings (Fig. 10-19). The authors found significantly more of these two extreme response patterns in subjects with cancer and a preponderance of normal response patterns in those without it. A feature of the study was that it represented a consecutive series and all women were treated exactly alike during the interview; thus there was no separate control group. The study merely compared in retrospect the psychologic attributes of those who eventually turned out to have a malignancy with those who turned out to have a benign lump. During the interview, just as in Kissen's lung cancer series, no one knew what the diagnosis was, so all the subjects were under equal stress.

Thus the life-long behavioral pattern of the extreme suppression of emotion (more common) or of exploding with emotion (more rare) characterized the future cancer victims, but the authors did not find any correlation between breast cancer and extroversion, neuroticism, or depression. A sociobiologic explanation for the extreme suppression of emotionality may be that the

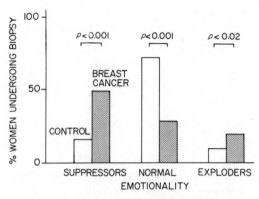

Fig. 10-19. Showing an association between breast cancer and behavioral pattern. One hundred sixty women admitted for a biopsy of the breast were divided into three groups from the viewpoint of their emotionality: the suppressors, the normally emotional, and the exploders. The majority of women with nonmalignant biopsies (73 percent) had normal emotional expression, but 68 percent with malignant biopsies had scored preoperatively as either suppressors of emotion (48 percent) or exploders (20 percent). Only about 30 percent had normal emotionality scores *(Greer and Morris, 1975).*

individual experiences social relations from a subordinate's submissive viewpoint with a consequent vulnerability to the hypothalamic and limbic patterns of depression. And perhaps the individual with a problem of controlling his explosive emotions considers social relations from the viewpoint of an angry dominant. His abrasive repeated flare-ups will eventually result in social difficulties with rejection and defeat. Thus despite starting from the opposite end of the scale, the exploder will also be vulnerable to the biochemical pattern of depression, even if his original behavior did not express that emotion.

In the context of emotions, the prospective studies of Caroline Bedell Thomas with John Hopkins medical students are, again, very much to the point. In reporting on the psychologic characteristics of 30 students who eventually in later life suffered from malignant tumors (out of the 1337 she has studied for so long), she found a striking lack of closeness to their parents, suggesting that they were alienated and lonely in childhood. Furthermore, she considered that the results were compatible with LeShan's hypothesis of the etiology of cancer (LeShan, 1966), i.e., the damage of a child's developing ability to relate to others had resulted in a vulnerability to hopelessness and despair in adulthood when a central relationship was lost (Thomas and Duszynski, 1974). The event might be the death of a spouse, a forced job retirement, or children leaving home. During an interview by the *Medical Tribune,* Dr. Thomas comes to the conclusion on the basis of her personal experience with medical students together with research data that the cancer victim is much gentler, sweeter, and quieter than the more aggressive coronary patients. But, as she comments, the unfortunate side of the profile is the continuing deep-rooted alienation and isolation of the patient in adult life (McBroom, 1975).

pattern. There is now a persuasive weight of human epidemiologic evidence connecting coronary heart disease, hypertension, and cancer to problems of psychosocial adaptation.

Summary

Several carefully controlled studies of large population groups numbering in the thousands have been completed and have yielded statistically significant results. They vary from the Pennsylvania community of Roseto, American Trappist and Benedictine Monks, and The Western Collaborative Group Study of Type A and Type B personalities to Japanese–Americans with varying degrees of acculturation: Together they are powerful evidence of the importance of sociocultural factors in determining the incidence of coronary heart disease. Large-scale blood pressure studies have recently shown the importance of a shift in traditional values and implicate a deficiency of social assets in the disorders of the regulation of blood pressure. Finally, quantitative pioneering work has shown that patients with lung cancer have difficulty in freely expressing emotions; others using the same approach to study breast cancer have found a similar

11

The prevention and treatment of detrimental effects in the psychosocial environment

Natural defenses against stressful events

This chapter poses the question as to what mobilizes the defenses standing between distressful life changes and emotional arousal with its accompanying neuroendocrine disturbances. In formalizing a schedule of life changes, Holmes and Rahe (1967) and more recently Rahe (1976) have defined a series of categories, such as work, home, family, personal, social, and financial. For example, a major health change demanding defenses could be massive burns or quadriplegia from a broken neck. Or a work change could be a new job, bringing a man under the control of an excessively dominating personality and an unfamiliar social order. Or the death of someone close, such as a spouse, could induce severe changes in home and family life. A change in personal or social affairs could be the decision to become engaged to marry—an abandonment of other intimate relationships—whereas, a change in financial status could be the loss of salary following loss of employment.

Horowitz (1976) in his book *Stress*

Response Syndromes points out that a person's reaction to acute episodes of loss or challenge, such as those already mentioned, is initially denial, which is an aspect of the conservation–withdrawal response. This protects the individual and gives him a chance to come to grips with the crisis. The action he takes can assume various forms, depending on his personality and intelligence. Katz et al. (1970), also mentioned in Chapter 7, analyzed the responses of a group of women to the shock of an impending biopsy of a tumor in the breast. Experienced and skillful interviewers evaluated them on the extent to which their defenses failed, differentiating denial from rationalization; stoicism (what will be, will be) from prayer and faith (I try not to think of it and trust in God); and differentiated these defenses from displacement and projection by which others were made responsible for the predicament. The extent to which such defenses failed determined the intensity of the ensuing affect which ranged from fear to hopelessness and despair. The affect as evaluated by the interviewers was significantly related to the level of hydrocortisone produced (see Fig. 7-17).

This initial response to severe loss or

the threat of it resembles the reaction Bowlby (1973) describes in the separated child and Harlow et al. (1971) in the separated monkey. Following the initial period of protest and denial, the loss is recognized and is accompanied by the depression: a full-blown conservation–withdrawal response. Finally the animal or the man caught in the crisis begins to explore the possibilities and begins to piece together a fresh pattern of living with which to cope with the new state of affairs.

At first there is an introspective movement, then the organism ventures outward. The outward movement of coping is discussed in the context of the group; a review of the conservation–withdrawal-related relaxation response follows. The relaxation response, which originated as an offshoot of behavioral biofeedback research, now approaches the threshold of objective study as a therapeutic measure. We conclude with a discussion of the role of the traditional, revered cultural canon or religion as a social asset which protects the individual from isolation, enabling him to cope as a member of the social group, yet, at the same time, through prayer and ritual, providing a pathway by which he can maintain contact with the biogrammar rooted in the vital core of his brain mechanism. By maintaining an equilibrium at higher levels in the brain, the neuroendocrine regulatory mechanisms are protected from disease-producing disturbances.

gains time for repetitive working and reworking of the situation; and with this reworking, its implications are slowly evaluated, both intellectually and emotionally. At some point, the healthy responder will cease to deny and start to seek information about the best way of tackling possible new roles in the new situation that "in his heart" (i.e., with his right hemisphere) he knows he must face. A person trained by a secular educational system to rely on intellectual understanding and rational mastery will use every available resource to find out and attempt to predict and plan, but another type of person, responding to a religious culture, will share responsibility with an autonomous part of his personality, which he may perceive as a higher power capable of offering inspiration.

Different situations demand different solutions, and Antonovsky (1974) speaks of homeostatic flexibility, meaning the ability to accept alternatives. He refers to the good coper's richness and complexity of self-images in which sees himself as husband, father, singer, gardener, doctor, grandfather, etc. This variety helps the victim to survive a loss by increasing the chances that some role or roles will remain open to him. Further, the capacity to accept conflicting values, such as technologic versus religious, as legitimate alternatives has a distinct advantage over an inflexible attitude that resentfully rejects other values. Those who can recover the most rapidly to the point of going about their affairs normally without emotional blunting are at an advantage.

Individual coping behavior: conservation–withdrawal and group-oriented responses

In their study of coping behavior, Hamburg and Adams (1967) point out that, as time goes on, depending on the extent of native intelligence and resourcefulness of the individual, a threat is met with complex positive approaches. The critical response, described earlier, by which threat is minimized, and perhaps denied recognition,

Psychosocial assets and the group

To achieve success, the coping qualities of a person are enormously dependent on the ties that bind him to others, forming a critical part of his social assets. Both Antonovsky (1974) and Hamburg and Adams (1967) point to the great need of a person in crisis for a continuity of interpersonal relationships. Nuckolls et al. (1972) have studied the relationship between social stress, as measured by the cumulative life change score of Holmes and Rahe (1967), and psychosocial assets, relating it to the prognosis of pregnancy. A series of social assets were evaluated, extending from the subject's feelings and perception about self to the relationship and duration of marriage. Intimacy, happiness, and the concordance of age and religion were important. The degree to which a woman was supported by an extended family was determined by estimating her confidence in receiving emotional and economic support from parents, siblings, and in-laws. Her social resources were probed by determining her adjustment to the community, her patterns of friendship, and the support she could depend on from the community.

Pregnancies were considered complicated if any of a wide variety of threats to the mother or infant was present. More than half (96) of 170 patients at a large military hospital had complicated pregnancies. Neither life change scores nor social asset scores were significantly related to complications if they were evaluated alone. When the values were combined, however, if the life change score was high before and during pregnancy, women with favorable social assets had only one-third the complications of those with low assets (Fig. 11-1). But if there was no high accumulation of life changes, there was no significant relationship between assets and complications.

This study shows (as noted in Chapter 1) that it is insufficient to evaluate the effect of life changes alone, but by adding social assets, a tool of remarkable analytic power develops. A study by Brown et al. (1975) on the effect of social class on the incidence of depression among young women in London reached the same conclusions. They found that women whose husbands were laborers were far more at risk than those married to white-collar workers. Brown and his associates measured experiences of threatened or major loss, such as eviction, debt, children in trouble, husband in jail, separation, or serious illness, finding that the lower class women had significantly more of these epi-

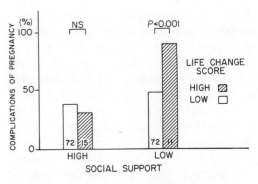

Fig. 11-1. Women with high life-change scores before and during pregnancy have an excessive incidence of complications if their social support is low, but a high level of social support protects against the influence of life changes (*Nuckolls et al., 1972*).

sodes in their lives, especially when young children were at home; but then they went on to show that a critical factor protected them from depression—this was the support and quality of the interpersonal relationships they enjoyed.

Brown and his associates devised a four-point scale for evaluating the extent to which a woman could talk to someone about her problems. A score of *A* was given only if she had an emotionally intimate relationship with someone in whom she could confide each day, such as her husband or boyfriend. This relationship usually reinforced her self-esteem as wife and mother. Occasionally the relationship was with another woman with whom she lived; in most cases, however, the relationship was heterosexual. A score of *B* was given if a woman saw and confided in her mother, sister, or friend once a week, a *C* for a confidant seen less than once a week, and a *D* for no confidant at all. Severe losses and major difficulties associated with depression were found primarily in women lacking the *A* score. A high degree of intimacy gives a woman almost complete protection, but even a large number of friendships are of little value if they are mere acquaintances. Three other factors mediate the effect of severe events in life and place a woman at greater risk: losing her mother before the age of 11, having three or more young children at home, and lacking employment and the associations that go with it.

Brown and his co-workers thus identify a close intimate relationship as an important asset; they cite Weiss's work showing the human need for certain relationships. Weiss (1969) emphasized the importance of close intimacy found in a good marriage; such a relationship protects against loneliness, a forerunner of depression. Other social assets are the camaraderie of colleagues and friends and the opportunity of being important to others and contributing to their nurturance, as when children are involved. The reassurance of personal worth in being able to do socially valued work or to competently maintain a home also ranks as an important asset.

Weiss discusses the need of assurance from relatives for long-term assistance if required and of guidance from representatives of society, for example, doctors and priests. The strength of a well-functioning extended family community, such as a kibbutz or a stable tribal village or a hunter–gatherer group, is that differing social needs can be met through various relationships, giving a broad protection against emotional disturbances.

In a disturbed society it can be profitable to be disturbed. In fact, Hinkle (1974) voices the suspicion that persons who weather long periods of isolation (such as solitary confinement) and undergo torturing hostile pressure without yielding may have a rigid character structure lacking in homeostatic flexibility. It may be that alexithymia with its blindness to feeling makes an indifferent environment more tolerable.

Social support as a moderator of life stresses

Cobb (1976) has recently discussed social support as a moderator of life stresses and his analysis is illuminating. He sees it as yielding information falling into three classes. The first leads the subject to believe he is loved and cared for. This is conveyed in situations involving mutual trust and is expressed in a dyadic relationship between persons who express their attachment to one another by meeting each other's needs. Harlow et al. (1971) describe this behavior in the rhesus monkey mother–child and peer–peer relationships as love in its various categories. The importance of such mammalian attachment behavior has been detailed in Chapters 2–4.

In the second class of information, social support leads a person to esteem himself as the result of public expression of group approval and is thus related to a favorable position in the social hierarchy. This is an aspect of the control of territory and with it goes the publicly recognized right of access to desiderata enjoyed by the dominant members of a group. Conversely, a loss of control accompanies defeat, subordination, and withdrawal of group support and esteem. The ensuing self-perception of helplessness with increased corticosteroids and depression is discussed in Chapter 7 in the context of hippocampal function.

The third class of information from social support is the perception of social congruity derived from a shared network of information and mutual obligation in which each member participates, and the common knowledge is shared and accepted by all. Cobb subdivides the information, first, into traditions of social hierarchy and how the social structure evolved, calling this the "essence of history"; next, into goods and services available to any member of the group on demand. He includes, here, the accessibility of services required only occasionally, i.e., equipment, specialized skills, technical information.

One may well ask what are the threats and dangers to social support and what is the mutual defense against them (Cobb, 1976). Cobb is thinking in terms of our contemporary society, but his definition of the network of information and mutual obligation and control over the environment is broader than this. It is related to the concept of cultural forerunners that bind together even animals, especially the primates, such as baboons and apes. In man, the hunter–gatherer, it flowers in increasingly complex and effective patterns of cooperation and mutual support as the result of specialization of activities and skills. We discuss the cultural canon of a society as a psychosocial asset later in this chapter.

Cobb, who begins his review by citing the work of Nuckolls and others mentioned earlier, discusses further evidence that social support affects the length of hospitalization and the rate of recovery from illness, minimizes the effects of retirement and bereavement, and helps one to endure the threat of catastrophe. The important new development is that we can now assemble hard evidence that adequate social support can protect people in crisis from a wide variety of pathologic developments. Cobb pioneered in the work on social support by studying the effects of job termination. One hundred men whose jobs were abolished were visited by public health nurses before and after their jobs were terminated and periodically up to 24 months after the plant closed. Figure 11-2 shows striking evidence of a tenfold increase in arthritis with two or more swollen joints on moving from the

Fig. 11-2. In a study of social and medical variables in 100 men whose jobs were abolished, Cobb reports a tenfold increase in arthritis with two or more swollen joints on moving from the highest to the lowest quartile of social support *(Cobb, 1976).*

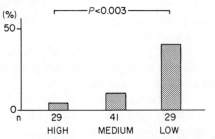

highest to the lowest quartile of social support ($p < 0.0001$).

Combat studies of group-coping mechanisms

Bourne's (1970) two remarkable studies from Vietnam confirm that active, outer-directed coping efforts made within the milieu of a supportive social group form an effective defense against neuroendocrine disturbance. In the first study, 17-hydroxycorticosterone (17-OHCS) levels were assayed once every 24 hours in seven medical corpsmen flying dangerous combat rescue missions in a helicopter ambulance (Fig. 11-3). There was no difference between their 17-OHCS levels on flying and nonflying days (Bourne, 1970). This held true even for the days when enemy fire was met; in half of the measurements, the highest levels were obtained on nonflying days when there was no danger. Furthermore, very little variation occurred, although the danger was high on some days, and the men were off duty on others.

Indeed, the mean 17-OHCS level for each man during the entire 17 days of the study was below that expected of a civilian population at home not under combat stress. This suggests that the fear induced by combat flying with threat of death and mutilation or capture can be countered by changes in perception, so that the pituitary adrenal-cortical mechanism is not aroused. Bourne reports that when the men were interviewed most denied that their job involved any real danger, although the casualty rate flatly belied this. He suspected that a strong support group was an important social asset. One defense was a deep sense that their job was worthwhile, induced by the gratitude of the men they rescued. This feeling combined with a sense of personal worth was socially validated by the frequent medals and the added pay they received.

Another defense was pseudorational,

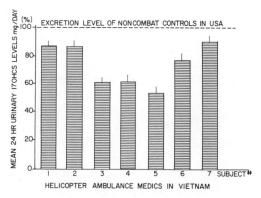

Fig. 11-3.   Mean 24-hour urinary 17 hydroxycorticosteroid (17-OHCS) excretion level of seven medical corpsmen on helicopter ambulance duty collected during a 17-day period is contrasted with anticipated 17-OHCS levels based on studies of recruits and of the general population in the United States. All subjects were exposed to several hazardous combat rescue missions in Vietnam. The vertical lines represent Standard Error of the Mean. Their excretion is significantly less than would be anticipated, pointing to effective psychologic defenses. *(From Bourne, 1970. © 1970, Little, Brown and Company. Reprinted by permission.)*

relying on a reassuringly small statistical chance of disaster based on a formula of dubious calculations, compounded of the number of flights flown, casualties in the unit, and time left to serve in Vietnam. But the irrationality of this defense was made clear by one man's refusal to venture into Saigon on the statistically remote danger of being killed by a land mine. Bourne concluded that reason was being bent to fit the needs of the occasion; if fear was legitimate then even a minor danger, such as being on the streets of Saigon, would be avoided and the subject was, in fact, unduly cautious. But if there was no acceptable escape, and fear (i.e., neuroendocrine arousal) would have been socially unacceptable, fear was effectively suppressed. Thus the men's perception of the social situation was important in determining their hormonal response.

Bourne's second study was of men in the Special Forces (Green Berets) in a camp surrounded by the enemy and constantly

exposed to the threat of attack. On the day of the anticipated attack, the responses of the officer and of the radio operator who worked closely with him were different from those of the five enlisted men assayed at the same time for urinary 17-OHCS (Fig. 11-4).

The findings were consistent with those of the helicopter ambulance medical corpsmen. The enlisted men of the Special Forces had effective defenses minimizing the threat of death or mutilation. They reacted to the stimulus by externally directed action and tended to avoid affective responses. They spent little time in introspection. Their response was to engage in furious activity,

Fig. 11-4.   A study of urinary 17 hydroxycorticosteroid (17-OHCS) excretion in experienced enlisted men in a Special Forces (Green Berets) camp isolated in Viet Cong-controlled territory. Twenty-four hour collections of urine were made for one officer and six enlisted men for three days, i.e., before, during, and after threat of attack. The radio operator and the officer, who were picking up and executing orders from a command post 40 miles away, had significantly higher levels of 17-OHCS than the enlisted men ($p < 0.03$). *(From Bourne, 1970. © 1970, Little, Brown and Company. Reprinted by permission.)*

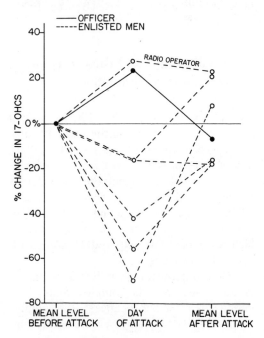

and their competence in building defenses and maintaining equipment gave them plenty to do. Bourne contrasted them with the officer who was being strongly influenced by radio messages from the higher command (Fig. 11-4). The problem was that the orders coming through might not be relevant to the present situation, so the officer had to compromise between satisfying his superiors and not disturbing the experienced sergeants with orders they would regard as inappropriate. Bourne notes that the officer's duties did not permit him to keep busy with emotionally satisfying manual chores at camp. He considered that the demands made on this young officer to maintain his role as an authority figure over older, experienced enlisted men was a tension producing influence that could have elevated the 17-OHCS.

Bourne's results show that the degree of adrenal-cortical arousal evoked by an event, even in the arousing circumstances of active warfare, is determined by a man's subjective assessment of the event. A most important asset is the group consensus as to how a stimulus should be perceived. The social evaluation of the group with which the subject identifies determines the intensity of his neuroendocrine response (Bourne, 1970).

Small groups and the control of psychosocial stimulation

Bourne's work deals with the special circumstances of war and the mutually supportive behavior of men in groups working in a military organization that is attuned to the problems of morale and the avoidance of incongruity. But the individual living in isolation and lacking the social support of an organization is hard pressed to maintain the high level of effort required to cope with severe life changes.

Culture protects the individual by incorporating him into its complex folds, but, during great social changes, the culture along with its religion loses credibility and no longer fulfills individual needs. The stability of tradition handed down from father to son during the sensitive learning period is critically important for instilling cultural beliefs. Today a large part of the world's population is caught in the throes of cultural change, a type of "Future Shock," (which is the title of Toffler's book on the subject) due to the scientific and technologic revolution. In these circumstances there is an especially acute need of social support in small groups and of the experiential knowledge that such self-help or encounter groups provide (Toffler, 1970).

In a recent paper Kaplan et al. (1977), like Cobb, perceive support as critical in determining a person's vulnerability to stimuli induced by life changes, but very little is known about its physiologic mechanisms and effects. He and his co-workers are concerned with finding out how a person's attachment needs can be met by the social networks operating in the framework of our contemporary culture. An 18th Century monastery of silent celibate Trappist monks or a well-integrated Stone Age hunter–gatherer group lived in a social system in which their patterns of behavior effectively protected them from excessive stimulation. By the same token, Kaplan and his associates are seeking ways of socially supporting persons in our contemporary technocracy who are suffering from conflict and ambiguity of roles, blocked aspirations, and cultural discontinuities. They believe that by concentrating on strengthening social supports it may be possible to protect such persons from excessive arousal, despite disturbing social situations.

The theme of social support is validated by the available evidence. The presence and attachment of other persons close to the individual help him to cope, as we have been discussing (see also Chapters 3 and 10). The mechanism of social support includes the extent to which a person feels security or attachment and has control of the environment, according to Kaplan and his associates, who enumerate the need for approval, affection, trust, and intimacy. There must be a chance to understand what is going on and to be able to come to a clear and consistent view of the difference between one's self and others having an opposing outlook. One needs to perceive one's self as a member of a group which gives support by consensus, dependable backing in common tasks, and tangible approval for tasks well done.

They discuss the value of a self-help peer group which attempts to manage and reduce personal distress through mutually supportive efforts, despite the erosion of the extended family and the religious community through technocracy. Persons need to know who to call in a crisis. They need frequent and regular association with persons to whom they can relate warmly, freely discussing distressful events with the assurance of receiving warmly supportive responses. The cocounseling community they describe attempts to provide a close, easily reached group of persons who are available to give such support (Kaplan et al., 1977).

In related work, Thomasina Borkman discusses the role of the various self-help groups in achieving these goals. She draws a sharp distinction between "experiential knowledge," which forms their primary strength, and "colder expertise" based on professional knowledge, which is the foundation of most of the "helping" professions, such as medicine. The potential client must believe or take on faith the professional's claim that he can handle the problem. In the distinction drawn between the two types of approaches, the experiential is pragmatic, is oriented to action here and now, and is holistic, but the professional is theoretical, systematic, and scientific. This suggests the distinction between right and left hemispheric perception. In view of this probable right-hemispheric bias, it is not surprising that self-help groups describe experiential knowledge as truth learned from personal experience rather than acquired by logical reasoning. These groups support the faith of their members by the validity and authority of

a special knowledge gained from sharing common experience. Furthermore, they will venerate a leader who has resolved their problems by drawing on his own experience. Thus their emphasis is on obtaining concrete, observable results that work subjectively because they are derived from group experience instead of from theoretical, systematic, scientific help of the professional. The philosophy of self-help groups, oriented to action here and now, is that members learn and are changed by doing (i.e., action). Finally the experiential approach encompasses what the individual perceives from an overall, common sense point of view.

For example, a surgeon performing a radical mastectomy for cancer might primarily consider the biologic and pathologic condition of the patient, but Reach for Recovery, a self-help group for postmastectomy patients, shows concern beyond the woman's actual surgery: in the prognosis of the disease, her changed body image and its implications in sexual expression, the presentation of a normal appearance to others, and the financial and familial effects of the illness (Borkman, 1976).

Alcoholics Anonymous, Parents Without Partners, Child Birth Without Pain Education Association (the Lamaze Technique), The Council of Adult Stutterers, Weight Watchers, and Gamblers Anonymous are only a few of the better known self-help organizations. There are groups for parents who abuse their children, for parents of drug addicts, and for sex offenders, divorced Catholics, and adoptees. The fact that such groups exist for priests and nuns who have left religious life and for others exposed to alienating experiences leads to the concept that these small groups are necessary because contemporary society has lost its religious convictions and does not have a coherent cultural canon.

One of the most impressive of these was the Marriage Encounter groups started in Spain in 1965 by Father Gabriel Calvo, a Catholic priest (Koch and Koch, 1976). The movement originally centered on the church, God, and the community, but lost these specifics on being transplanted to American soil. Nevertheless it appears to have a tantric capacity to tap the sacramental aspects of the love relationship. About 40 couples spend a weekend at a hotel attending a well-planned series of meetings. Husbands and wives are required to regularly write down their innermost feelings throughout the weekend and to exchange these love letters; then, to accept each other's emotions poured out on paper in a private dialogue. Although the meetings are nondenominational, a priest, pastor, or a rabbi is always present. Perhaps by providing an environment of religious and community social support, this particular self-help experiential group gives participants a sense of social approval and increases bonding between husband and wife by relating episodes in their personal lives to the biobehavioral roots of male–female attachment behavior. The emphasis on feelings in the marriage relationship is especially significant in counteracting an often impersonal (alexithymic) social milieu.

We have already mentioned that Brown et al. (1975) and Weiss (1969) show the value of an intimate, usually sexual, relationship as a protection against depression. Their work suggests that encounters between friendly individuals, such as those in the anonymous groups we have discussed do not have the value of a truly intimate relationship, for this is usually between persons of the opposite sex. Marriage Encounter may owe some of its effectiveness to this feature.

During the past two centuries, Western society has passed through a period of intense preoccupation in achieving scientific rational expression and technologic mastery. It may be that the proliferation of self-help groups and the growing recognition of a need for social support are forerunners of new compensatory religious movements. As discussed later, a culture that is supported by a dynamic, intrinsic experiential religion incorporates socially supportive functions into its structure. There is probably less need for independent self-help groups among those which Gordon Allport calls "intrinsic cults," such as Roman Catholic Trappist Monks, Society of Friends (Quakers), Mennonite (Amish) Church, Seventh-Day Adventists, and The Church of Jesus Christ of Latter-Day Saints (Mormon) (Evans, 1971).

Relaxation response and biofeedback in the control of hypertension

The preceding analysis of social assets that are required for maximum stability in meeting life changes shows that men need the support of a stable community. If a highly structured social group, such as the military, the church, or the kibbutz, is not available, there is further possibility that small social groups can help meet some particular problem weighing heavily on the individual, be it alcohol, divorce, or paraplegia. While the activities of such groups are directed toward mutual assistance, insofar as they are experiential, they involve the right hemisphere and connections of the limbic system and the biogrammar of attachment and territorial behavior. But can a person's need for better contact with his feelings and with his biogrammar be met within the loose framework of our culturally mixed society?

A technique of relaxation response, developed from physiologic studies of the effects of feedback on autonomic events, is being explored from this viewpoint. Although of scientific and secular origin, relaxation is closely associated with prayers and meditation that form an intrinsic part of the cultural pattern of world religions. Harvard physiologist Benson's introduction of the relaxation response into a secular framework has been termed "noncultic" because he believes a physiologic method can be used without accepting the patina of religious myths and symbols with which relaxation has been embellished by the various faiths (Benson, 1975). He regards the relaxation response as the physiologic opposite of the fight–flight response induced by threat and therefore of great value in reducing anxiety. When taught with biofeedback, monitoring instruments are used to detect and amplify internal physiologic information which is thus made available to the ordinarily unsuspecting subject.

Dr. Chandra Patel, a physician in general practice in the London suburb of Croydon, has made an impressive study of the effects of relaxation on hypertension. In Patel's (1973) first report, she described the effects of combining yoga with a biofeedback method in which a galvanic skin response of the finger was a measure of relaxation. Patients, who lay on a couch in a quiet room, were told to pay attention to their breathing, making sure it was smooth and regular; then, they were asked to become as limp as possible, and attempt to relax physically. They were instructed on how to avoid tension in the muscles of the face, neck, chest, and abdomen. Working along the tested lines of Jacobson's (1970) progressive relaxation technique, patients were encouraged to repeat phrases such as, "My arms are feeling very heavy and relaxed."

Physical relaxation was stressed during the initial training (Patel, 1973). However, after a few weeks, when patients had learned to relax physically and had used the biofeedback technique to tell them how they were doing, they had to learn mental relaxation. Although they became oblivious of the outside world and unaware of their limbs, they found it difficult to ignore the movement of their own breathing. At this point, Patel resorted to yoga methods, instructing them to focus attention on breathing as the object while concentrating on inspiration and expiration. In a further application of yoga (mantra) they kept repeating a word such as "relaxed" with every expiration (Benson, 1975). Patients were free to select their own object or idea for this concentration, but

sleep was to be avoided; however, it presented no problem because concentration kept them mentally alert.

Patel recently reported on the results of a nine month follow up on 40 hypertensive patients taking drugs to control their illness; their mean age was 57 years. Twenty of the randomly selected patients were treated by practicing combined yoga and biofeedback relaxation exercises, and the other 20 (controls) by resting on a couch during the half-hour sessions at the clinic, three times a week for three months. Thereafter, although those being treated did not receive additional yoga training, they were encouraged to relax and meditate. Thus the effects of increased medical attention and repeated blood pressure measurements were not different in the controls (Fig. 11-5). The results are impressive: the average systolic blood pressure at the end of the study for those practicing relaxation and meditation was reduced by 20 ± 11 mmHg and the diastolic pressure by 14 ± 8 mmHg ($p < 0.001$). The total drug requirement fell by 40 percent. But the blood pressure and drug requirement

Fig. 11-5. Twenty hypertensive patients on drug therapy received further treatment by being trained in combined yoga and biofeedback relaxation exercises; they were contrasted with 20 controls also on drugs for hypertension, but not on relaxation therapy. The drug requirement and the blood pressure measurement were both lower during a nine-month follow-up of the patients who practiced relaxation and meditation, but remained unchanged in the controls *(Patel, 1975a).*

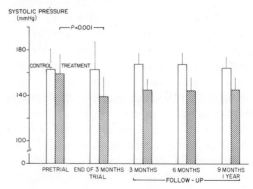

for the control patients remained unchanged (Patel, 1975a).

In answer to the question of the practicality of a yoga technique with a biofeedback: it is no more demanding to discipline one's self twice each day to 20 minutes of relaxation and meditation than it is to be a devout religionist. However, since hypertension has no symptoms and improvement provides no relief from discomfort, there is little reason to continue such a noncultic practice without special motivation. Patel was successful in getting patients to practice twice each day at home, and some features of her program indicate the extent of involvement demanded. For example, patients made frequent subjective checks of their tension and quickly relaxed several times a day. They were taught to react to red traffic lights, ringing telephones and doorbells, and arousing personal situations with quick relaxation lasting 30 seconds to three minutes. Dr. Patel reports on the indirect effectiveness of this type of relaxation. The rise in mean blood pressure was measured after the patients had climbed a nine-inch step 25 times or immersed their hands in 4°C water for 80 seconds; both measures were significantly lower ($p < 0.02$) in trained versus untrained subjects (Patel, 1975b).

The results of her methods with yet another group of hypertensive patients were reported in Patel's paper written in collaboration with W. R. S. North of the Epidemiology Unit at Northwick Research Hospital, London, England (Patel and North, 1975). This time a classic open comparison with a crossover design was used. As before, the data suggested that some lasting effect had been produced. The authors described the need to foster rapport between doctor and patients and commented on the development of attachment between patients; they remarked on the importance of these warm relationships for success of the program.

Patients were instructed to practice meditation and relaxation twice every day, reminiscent of daily prayers by the devout.

Patel and North aimed at gradually incorporating new habits into the routine activities of patients while leaving room to tailor the program to suit individual life styles. For example, a busy man had a red disc attached to his watch to remind him to relax whenever he looked at the time; other patients had different mnemonic devices. The results of this later study showed a reduction of mean blood pressure from 168/100 to 141/84 mmHg in patients using relaxation techniques as contrasted with a drop from 169/101 to 160/96 mmHg in patient controls. On training this control group in yoga relaxation techniques, two months later, their mean blood pressure fell to that of the other group.

In a recent review of her work Dr. Patel (1977) points out that the long-term benefits of relaxation training can only be maintained if the patient regularly practices relaxation and integrates this into his daily activities. She discusses how to motivate symptomless hypertensive patients to accept this requirement. Further work incorporating taped cassettes that the patient later takes home raises the question whether this technique, which Patel demonstates can be provided on a group basis, could be used to reduce coronary risk factors. In a preliminary communication she describes reduction of serum cholesterol in hypertensives from 241 ± 39 to $217 \pm 38/100$ milliliters ($p < 0.001$) as a result of six weeks of training (Patel, 1976). In another study, in collaboration with Carruthers, she demonstrates that multiple risk factors are reduced for not only blood pressure and plasma lipids, but also that smoking habits change favorably, i.e., average number of cigarettes smoked per day was reduced from 26 to 10 (Patel and Carruthers, 1977).

In similar work but perhaps with less intensively motivated patients, Benson and his collaborators have reported a decrease of blood pressure in drug-treated hypertensive patients who regularly practiced the relaxation response. Benson used a modified yoga meditation technique without biofeedback to train them, along with the repetitive stimulus of a silently repeated word. Patel's patients practiced the progressive muscle relaxation technique advocated by Jacobson while lying on a couch, whereas, Benson's were in a comfortable seated posture. Patients using both methods practiced 20 minutes each day, before breakfast and before dinner. In Benson's study, the systolic pressure of 14 patients observed over a five-month period fell from a mean pressure of 146 to 135 mmHg, and the diastolic from 92 to 87 mmHg ($p<0.05$) (Benson et al., 1974).

Stone and DeLeo (1976) used a Zen meditation relaxation technique twice a day on patients in a daily six-month trial to determine the effect of psychologic relaxation on blood pressure. They noted a reduction of mean arterial pressure of 12 mmHg in 14 subjects, together with enzymatic evidence of a reduction of peripheral adrenergic activity.

In reviewing clinical studies of behavioral methods to treat hypertension, Shapiro et al. (1977) comment favorably on Patel's work, especially in her controlled comparisons of groups of patients. They believe that research is almost at the point that doctors can begin using behavioral methods in treating hypertension. According to the literature, however, the doctor's attitude is of utmost importance, since his credibility, enthusiasm, authority, empathy, and sympathy all help to create a confident attitude in the patient. Shapiro and his co-workers point out that reassurance combined with a mitigation of social and environmental factors that tend to increase the pressor effects of sympathetic arousal has long been used by psychotherapists. Abboud (1976) commenting on relaxation and autonomic control in hypertensive patients states, "If autonomic functions can be modified and trained in man and if such training is effective in the early phases of hypertension and, more importantly, if it can be maintained over a space of time, the positive feedback mechanisms at the level of both the central

nervous system and the vasculature may be interrupted, and sustained hypertension may be prevented."

Benson and his associates and Stone and DeLeo, nevertheless, had less spectacular results than Patel, and indeed Frankel et al., (1978) reported that the combination of feedback and relaxation therapies had no overall effect in their studies. Possibly in the interest of detached scientific objectivity, Frankel and his co-workers may have failed to maximize the importance of a reassuring therapeutic environment and in communicating with patients may have fallen short of conveying their commitment to the prescribed routine necessary for bringing about altered levels of autonomic activity. In addition, Frankel's sessions were longer than Patel's, possibly exceeding the optimum she used. Be that as it may, Shapiro and his associates consider that the central theme of the new therapies is a direct invitation to the patient to participate in the therapeutic relationship; this, they say, represents a fundamental change in philosophic attitudes toward health care delivery and has far-reaching implications (Shapiro et al., 1977).

Physiologic mechanisms and the relaxation response

Benson and Patel both propose that high blood pressure is lowered during relaxation because of the reduced activity of the sympathetic nervous system. Stone and DeLeo's evidence for this theory is a change in the level of dopamine beta hydroxylase activity and Benson's that oxygen consumption, heart rate, and blood lactate all decrease. Further work will testify whether relaxation, as Benson suggests, is a separate mechanism opposing the fight–flight response (Benson et al., 1974). Relaxation may simply involve a reduction of sympathetic adrenal-medullary activity to below the current resting levels for that individual because of a change in the setting of higher controls, for instance, at the amygdalar level. Certainly other neuroendocrine subsystems can decrease their action and show a reduction of values below control levels. As discussed in Chapters 5 and 7, the gonadotropic system responds to perception of a loss of social status and defeat with a reduction in testosterone, but the flush of successful competition gives subjective perception of a rise in social status and is accompanied by a temporary increase in the hormone (Rose et al., 1975). The pituitary adrenalcortical response develops when the organism perceives itself as helpless and as having lost control (Henry and Ely, 1976). There is a corresponding reduction in adrenal-cortical hormones when the perception is one of social support with the attainment of goals.

Bourne's results with soldiers in Vietnam have already been discussed, but perhaps the most remarkable example of the perception of social approval and attainment of goals was the Gemini astronauts in their 15-day orbit of the earth. While they were in flight, the urinary excretion of the astronauts was so low compared with that of the control values that the results were doubted. It appears probable that their perception of the environment was highly positive and rewarding (Lutwak et al., 1969) and that elated feelings of great control and high accomplishment could have accounted for their remarkable suppression of adrenal-cortical output.

A lengthy study of the parents of children fatally ill with leukemia by Hofer et al. (1972a, b) showed that the sustained high level at which 17-hydroxycorticosteroids (17-OHCS) were set in parents grieving the anticipated loss of a child was gradually lowered during the year as they were slowly convinced it was a false alarm (Fig. 11-6). Often the 17-OHCS setting depended on defensive maneuvers for controlling grief; when these failed and grief broke through, the levels of 17-OHCS would increase. This might occur at certain moments of crisis although the person had had successful

Fig. 11-6. Evidence of chronic elevation of steroid excretion in persons exposed to threat of bereavement. A follow-up of 17 hydroxycorticosteroid (17-OHCS) excretion rates for a husband and wife whose child, at first suspected of suffering from leukemia, eventually proved to have a benign condition *(Hofer et al., 1972a).*

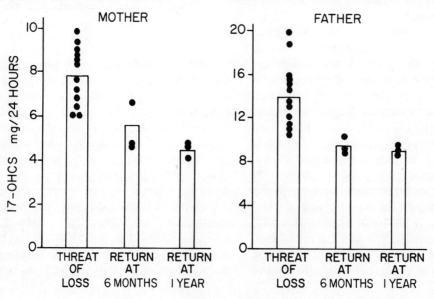

defense with consequent low values on other occasions.

An example of such a pattern was presented in another paper in this series by Friedman et al. (1963). Throughout the interval of a year, one mother's normal level of 17-OHCS excretion was consistently set at a remarkably low value despite the illness of her son. She appeared to accept the diagnosis that her son had leukemia and the chilling prognosis the doctors offered. The mother reacted "realistically" to the situation, could talk quite freely about his illness, and was willing to leave the medical decisions entirely to the doctors. On one occasion she even suggested that they handle a behavior problem, remarking, "I've tried everything and give up, maybe the doctors can do something with him." Seven months later, after her son's death, she made the statement that in actuality throughout his illness she had maintained the hope he would live. Only when his death terminated the hope did she then experience a long and painful period of grieving. Friedman and his associates concluded she had exercised extreme intellectualization as an effective defense with isolation of affect, which failed only after her son actually died; then she experienced maximal distress and with it the excretion of 17-OHCS was reset to a higher level.

The relaxation response in a religious context

Friedman and Rosenman (1974) in looking at our eclectic society have perceived the lack of normative patterns (such as ritual mourning) of a traditional culture which elicits appropriate responses and permits the individual to respond to the drives of his biogrammatic programming. They call for a reengineering of the mode of perception and response to the environment by the person threatened by coronary heart disease in their book *Type A Behavior and Your Heart.* Instead of accepting the thrust toward a behavior pattern which rewards an aggressive life style that is swift, logical, and practical as well as realistic, they propose a cultural shift to permit more attention to intuition, dreams, and fantasy. They urge the rejection of haste in all activities; irritation with delay; aggressive arousal with opposition; and the search for panaceas and money instead of style, beauty, and love. Translated into sociobiologic idiom, one may argue that much of their comment reflects on the insecurity of a would-be achiever living in fear of rivals on all sides.

Their advice to find a place, such as a church or a park or a bookstore, where one may seek peace and tranquillity and the "essence of life" is very close indeed to the practices of the Yogi and of the "intrinsic" Christian. Their suggestion of giving oneself time to think, to meditate, and to philosophize places the same emphasis on nonrational and meditative elements found in religious movements. Furthermore, Friedman and Rosenman recommend that the subject should "subdue whatever degree of hostility he still has," somehow avoiding the development of rage when he is threatened or teased in a way that implies a loss of professional or other social status. This is sound advice to the frustrated would-be achievers threatened by fatal coronary heart disease. It is striking advice from an outstanding, rational, empirically oriented research team, for it is directly in line with the teaching of religions, such as Christianity, Buddhism, and Hinduism. These religions flourished in crowded cities where the control of aggression had become crucial for group survival. Friedman and Rosenman (1974) say that but for the current bias against such matters, they would have mentioned religious belief as the "principal source of things worth having in life."

Benson (1975) makes much the same point in his book *The Relaxation Response.* He reviews a number of religious beliefs, including the contemplation and meditation of Christian mystics, the practices of Eastern religions, such as Yoga of Hinduism and

Buddhism, as well as the mysticism of the Muslim Sufis. They all seek a quiet place where external stimuli can be minimized; often this is a place of worship. They also concentrate on some object that is presented repeatedly and may gaze at a symbol, such as a mandala pattern, or they may repeat a simple prayer or even a single syllable.

In these religious "exercises," as described by their adepts, there is always an attempt to dispel distracting thoughts and to induce passive rather than active attitudes. Thoughts and imagery and feelings drifting into awareness are not actively resisted, but neither are they entertained. The devotee functions as a spectator instead of a participant allowing directed thoughts to drift away—the idea being that there should be no concern with how well things are going. Indeed, Buddhists teach that the attainment of calmness and concentration should involve no clarifying, no explaining, judging, or correcting. The devotee must only observe each state, allowing it to come and go unimpeded, being "mindful only of the mind" (Saddhatissa, 1971). These teachings suggest a downplaying of the logical, analytic processes associated with the left hemisphere. Rossi (1977) has recently proposed that the right hemisphere is involved in this typical religious activity of meditation, and Galin (1976), in the review discussed in Chapter 6, suggests that transcallosal inhibitory pathways may be involved. The contrast with alexithymia, as defined by Sifneos et al. (1978), is also apparent.

The cultural canon as a social asset

Thanks to the huge, newly evolved brain system that gives him a unique conceptual awareness, man, as Reynolds emphasizes, has built up complex social institutions with rules of action and ideas of right and wrong. Unlike other primates, he inhabits a universe perceived in terms of the structures developed during the ancestry not of his species, but of his culture (Reynolds, 1976). The neuroendocrine responses of persons living in a healthy society are determined by this cultural canon which regulates their behavior and serves as an all-embracing, affiliative network facilitating their ability to cope. The primary role of the cultural canon, viewed sociobiologically, is to regulate the persistent and powerful territorial and attachment instincts of individuals as they seek to meet their basic needs; it forces individuals to accept the complex role differentiation within the social hierarchy. Within the framework of its canon, the healthy society successfully protects the mother and infant, and nurtures the bonding going on between them derived from inherited patterns of behavior. As the young mature, it is the task of the culture to broaden their familial attachment to include others, and the attachments formed in childhood and adolescent years include persons and groups to whom the parental figures themselves are strongly attached, thus extending outward to the broader society. Bowlby's (1970, 1973) treatise describes studies showing the importance of the childhood–parental milieu for later adaptation to these broader social roles.

Provided the culture is healthy, these early attachments and acquired values will continue to develop in later life. Neumann has discussed their increasing subtlety and complexity as they extend to country and to social institutions, such as the crafts and professional groups, and to the church, army, university, or business enterprise. The word "canon" refers to the norms or standards of general principles or rules considered by the group as true and valid (Neumann, 1954). These differ, for instance, between a military unit in heavy combat, a scientific research group, and a Trappist monastery. But within any particular culture, any one of a variety of norms will have its proper time and place.

The canon includes the religious and secular ceremonies with which a stable, normal community surrounds the biologically critical events that mark man's progress in the life cycle, from birth, through puberty, betrothal, marriage, childbirth, sickness, injury, to death. In all societies, the rituals of the canon are performed at critical stages of public enterprises, including the laying of cornerstones, the completion of oceangoing vessels, the opening of public buildings, and the initiation of public games and council meetings. Moreover they signify the rites of passage into manhood and womanhood and into specialization of roles, such as hunter, farmer, lawgiver, priest–medicine man, or statesman. These steps through life are the focus of the sacraments and services of the church and of the secular ceremonies of the state.

During religious rituals, litanies are chanted in a specialized sonorous voice and group participation in singing encourages the proper mood in trusting the protective power of a suprahuman deity. Doubts are stilled and confidence inspired by hymns promising support for certain socially desirable types of behavior. In the Protestant canon, the familiar hymn "Onward, Christian Soldiers" encourages defense of the group's beliefs under the banner of a powerful heavenly figure. Nagging doubts are soothed by the encouraging words in another hymn, "Can a mother's tender care cease toward the child she bore? Yes, she may forgetful be, yet will I remember thee." Likewise the admonition, "Who sweeps a room as for Thy laws makes that and the action fine" promises ultimate reward for faithful subordination to the cause, if not in this life, then in the next. The enormously greater effectiveness of the social asset of group faith in comparison with the solitary effort of individual coping is written indelibly on the pages of the history of civilization.

Loss of the cultural canon and social breakdown

If Galin's (1974, 1976) transcallosal hypothesis is correct, as discussed in Chapter 6, the loss of normative ritual and emo-tionally supportive behavior of a healthy culture may be associated with a disturbance of the connection between the two hemispheres: the rational-logical and the intuitive spatiotemporal, and indeed a lack of contact with the instinctively determined archetypes or symbols, extending to the roots of behavior in the limbic system. Anomie, which sociologist Durkheim (1951) described as linked with increased suicide rates, involves a disturbance of the value system; it occurs during social breakdown when the cultural canon has been fragmented and eventually loses all authority. Anomie is prevalent during civil warfare and violence (McClosky and Schaar, 1965) and is associated with the breakdown of the family and the disruption of various attachment bonds.

These disruptions occur after a forced migration. When members of a social group lose access to the sacred symbols of their homeland, such as temples and churches, and mountains, rivers, and walls defining territorial limits, and the ancient monuments and landscapes—an important link between old and young and between male and female is lost. Further, significant religious, professional, and political figures of their cultural group may fail to accompany the emigrants (Neumann, 1954), leaving them bereft of the necessary hierarchic figures to provide tradition and stability. Even without migration, the impact of an alien culture can be devastating, as when Euro–American technology took over in Stone Age Polynesia.

The change leading to anomie can come from within. World society has experienced and is currently disturbed by the industrial, electronic, and intellectual revolutions released at a fierce pace by scientific inquiry. These technologic changes have also invaded non-Western cultural canons the world over (Toffler, 1970). When these changes occur without the tempering influence of appropriate religious and artistic traditions; when the patterns of belief, including prayer and faith, are disrupted; when the social assets of intimate guidance and support provided by both religious and secular customs deteriorate, members of the group are left to their own devices in satisfying their crude, individual, instinctual needs for attachment and territorial protection. It is this gap that the small group movement and the advocates of the relaxation response, which we have discussed, can fill in some measure. These attempts are feeble, however, compared with social man's supreme achievement: a stable culture with a tradition that has persisted relatively unchanged for generations. It is by tradition and culture that man weaves his separate activities into the whole cloth of a great cultural canon—the living fabric of civilization.

The compensatory role of religion in a culture

In a recent summary of his work on the growth and decline of human societies, the historian Toynbee (1972) suggests that religions of the great civilizations originated as compensatory movements, seeking to disengage the individual from the social matrix of the times. The objective, he says, was to escape from a particular civilization's obsessive collective attempt to control the environment. Nowhere is this obsession more clear than in our own culture, whose final climactic achievement has been to escape the earth's gravity in visiting the moon and mechanically exploring Mars. The cultural canon of our society is heavily weighted toward upbuilding a powerful, rational empiric technology which involves the critical analytic information processor of the left hemisphere. Such thinking is quite necessary to achieve control of the social milieu and of the physical environment, but it is primarily cognitive, concerned with facts and figures. We may picture the situation of a successful civilization with technocratic obsessions as sowing the seeds of its own dissolution by risking mental imbalance in many of its members by promoting an "alexithymic" inhibition of neural transmission across the corpus callosum between the left and the right hemispheres.

Activities in religion and art may counter this trend by demanding the interhemispheric transfer of information. It has been suggested that working in conjunction with the limbic system by frontal–limbic pathways, the right hemisphere may play an important role in active imagination (Rossi, 1977). The role of the right hemisphere in dreaming is becoming established (Bakan, 1976), and, in Chapter 6, evidence is presented that dreaming may be critical for the integration of innate behavior patterns of mammals with recently acquired cognitions (Watson and Henry, 1977).

Toynbee (1972) continues his argument by pointing out that man's social hierarchy and stability of role behavior is not automatically enforced by a tightly built-in instinct as it is in social insects. Indeed, the instincts of territoriality and attachment behavior must be modified and expressed by learned processes and integrated by the gradually evolved patterns of cultural canons (Reynolds, 1976).

Previous chapters have outlined the way in which the instinctively determined biogrammar of male–female gender behavior, maternal attachment, dominant and submissive behavior, and the defense of territory may depend on the activation of subcortical structures. The role of the amygdalar complex in attaching emotional values to stimuli has also been proposed; without the motivation it provides, one cannot pursue or avoid desiderata. Three major patterns of this inborn biogrammar (Tiger and Fox, 1972) were differentiated in Chapter 2. Present in all mammals, they include recognition of leadership (dominance and subordination), recognition of gender (males and females), and recognition of differences with age (special treatment for the young and old). Jung has termed them "archetypes of the collective unconscious." The analytic psychology he developed had as a critical concern the function of this innate biogrammar in man and his society, which he described as the anima and the animus (the potential for feminine behavior in the male, and masculine behavior in the female), the mother, the child, the wise old man, the witch, and even the trickster (Jung, 1939, 1959).

Despite their controlling importance in man and their subtle elaboration by the neo-cortical mechanisms of his sociocultural brain, these patterns to which the myths, beliefs, and romance of the various cultural canons pay so much attention, nevertheless, appear to have their roots in the limbic system and the brain stem. The theme that Toynbee pursues may be restated to say that, through the revered symbols of the culture, the archetypal biogrammar of the instinctual drive mechanisms is integrated with man's left hemisphere-dominated technology and language. When society progresses to the point of being obsessed by the cognitive operational mode of thinking and symbolism is neglected, there is a danger of losing what Toynbee (1972) terms "self-mastery" or what Jung (1939) would call "individuation" or what the Christian refers to as "the inner light." It has many names! An approach to this elusive problem can be found in Galin's (1976) review which points to the possibility of functional disturbance in the transfer of information between the hemispheres. Sifneos's related concept of alexithymia also promises to lead to a better understanding of this problem. The fact that Hoppe (1975) found a quantitative as well as a qualitative paucity of dreams, fantasies, and symbolization (i.e., alexithymia) in 10 patients following commissurotomy may indicate that there can indeed be defects in communication between the great brain systems.

The practical implication of such defects is that they lead to difficulties in interpersonal relationships. The alexithymic's ineptitude in communicating his feelings drives him to substitute the endless details of operational thinking for empathic interaction. But thinking is not a substitute for expressing appropriate feelings. His inadequate reactions subject him to tension and feelings of increasing helplessness. Sifneos indicates the alexithymic may be forced to withdraw to conserve himself or that he will resort to impulsive action in an effort to correct a seemingly hopeless state of affairs, and suggests that his physiologic reactions to the stress mobilizes the sympathetic and endocrine systems leading to psychosomatic disease.

Toynbee regarded self-mastery as the goal of religious disengagement. Certainly, the cloister and mysticism involve behavior complementary to operational thinking (Toynbee, 1972), for fasting, prayer, and meditation appear to be concerned with the development of the right-hemisphere function as opposed to that of the left hemisphere. Thus an inner-directed religion, as Benson (1975) has pointed out, encourages the development of an altered state of consciousness. Ornstein (1972) and Rossi (1977) both suggest that meditation and prayer or yoga involve the intuitive gestalt thought of the right hemisphere as opposed to the logic and analysis of the left hemisphere. In Toynbee's (1972) terms, the development of self-mastery by the religions of great civilizations turns the tables on technocracy's obsession with facts and figures by encouraging an affective mode of thought. These religions would thus make a balancing contribution to technocracy by increasing skills in communicating feelings as well as by achieving rituals that control and enormously elaborate the archetypal biogrammar of territorial and attachment instincts. The rituals provide symbols based on the complex patterns of sports, the arts, architecture, music, poetry, literature, and ceremonies of cultural canons.

There are limits, however, to the search for integration and self-mastery and limits to the search for self-realization by prayer and meditation. Bourne (1970) accurately analyzes the needs of the combat soldier for defenses and for that matter, the needs of anyone seeking a place in the sun in a competitive environment. His observation of experienced Special Forces men in Vietnam was that their intense activity, avoidance of relaxation, and lack of introspection were compatible with low corticosteroids and effective protection from subjective distress.

A person wishing to become established even in a narrowly delimited territory must concentrate on practical operational thinking. He must challenge the environment in which he has elected to compete. He must dedicate his energy and attention to achieving status in the social hierarchy. On the one hand, human beings must play roles which demand feelings and fantasy as they are expressed in the parent–child relationship and in attachment behavior that combines with poetry and fantasy, as for example when one "falls in love." But other roles demanded of the same person require a dominant demeanor and technical competence: a paratrooper or a law enforcement officer comes to mind.

The problem is one of balance. We have already described the consequences awaiting a person (Type A personality) with a diffused, poorly focused, aggressive drive who seeks mastery in all situations and those awaiting a chronically depressed or anxious person who is subordinate to the point of ineffectiveness. The physiologic role of prayer, the relaxation response, and the reduced adrenal-cortical secretion accompanying successful attainment of goals are incompatible with the socially disruptive responses of fear and despair. By blocking the arousal of neuroendocrine mechanisms, the deleterious effects of chronic, excessive psychosocial stimulation are avoided. This may be why chronic diseases are rare in stable cultures that revere cultural canons, applaud modest personal goals, and honor traditional forms.

An effective cultural canon protects against disease

The !Kung Bushmen, who have been discussed in Chapter 3, are an example of a people with a highly effective cultural canon well suited to their pattern of evolutionary adaptation. Despite the apparently harsh and difficult conditions for survival, an amazing 110 mmHg casual systolic blood pressure for men in the 60-year-old age group has been demonstrated in two studies more than a decade apart (Kaminer and Lutz, 1960; Truswell et al., 1972). Van der Post's (1961) evaluation of their culture helps to explain their low level of neuroendocrine arousal. Not only do they enjoy the social assets of a closely knit, extended family band living in extraordinarily close physical proximity on their campgrounds, but they are also intense myth-makers who incorporate elaborate rituals and ceremonies into their unchallenged cohesive cultural canon, transmitted for thousands of years.

Lehr et al. (1973) have recently observed the social patterns in a group of men who were subjects of the Western Collaborative Group Study; they followed up on 679 (of the 3411) men 40 to 49 years old. They worked on a sociologic model of possible factors associated with the incidence of coronary heart disease in which the key social–discriminant variables turned out to be the mother's and father's religion, the subject's income and education, and the father's occupation. There was an association between coronary-prone Type A behavior and what Allport calls an "extrinsic" type of religious orientation, which he defined in an interview with Evans (1971) as "using religion for one's own purposes" (i.e., for making friends, influencing people, attaining prestige, or deriving personal comfort). Lehr and his associates contrasted "extrinsic" religion with "intrinsic" religion whose creeds were lived by because they were necessary for the believer's own value system. This data supports that of an earlier study by Wardwell et al. (1968) who worked with a smaller number of subjects. Both teams of investigators found that men of Catholic parentage had half the expected rate of coronary heart disease, whereas those of mixed Catholic–Protestant parentage had over twice as much the expected disease rate. Men of Jewish and Protestant parentage, however, had the approximate rate expected. It was suspected that the success ethic and the Protestant–Jewish sense of personal responsibility for achievement may have played an etiologic role.

Graham et al. (1978) have found a consistent significant association between frequent church attendance and age-adjusted systolic and diastolic blood pressure scores. For systolic pressure the difference was 4.6 mmHg and for diastolic, 2 mmHg. Their study confirms the observations of Medalie who found that Orthodox Jews had an age-adjusted coronary heart disease rate of 29/1000 persons as opposed to traditional Jews with 37/1000 and nonreligious Jews with 56/1000 (Kaplan, 1976). Kaplan and his associates recognize the complex and pervasive effects of a religion constituting a vital part of the individual's cultural pattern. They conclude that these data challenge our present concepts and methodologies to explain how the specific religious processes are related to the etiology and prevention of heart disease.

The monks and nuns of the Catholic Church have provided an example of an "intrinsic" religious movement which operates in a stable social system and has powerful social assets. Their canon includes: the relaxation therapy of devoted prayer and meditation, the social asset of the confessional, a form of encounter-group living, socioeconomic stability, and freedom from family anxieties. In addition, Catholic monks and nuns enjoy a stable, cooperative, hierarchic society, and they share the beliefs and the expressive symbols of their religion. There is quantitative clinical evidence that they enjoy some protection from disease. Kunin and McCormack (1968) contrasted the incidence of bacteriuria and blood pressure elevation in 3300 nuns with that of an equivalent group of women not in holy orders. They sampled over 2700 working women, divided into progressively older age groups, and contrasted them with the nuns. Bacteriuria was nearly 10 times more frequent in the 15–34 year old controls ($p <$ 0.001) and was still threefold in the women 35–54 years old (Fig. 11-7). Bacteriuria was

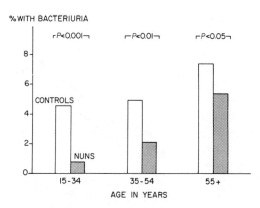

Fig. 11-7. The incidence of urinary tract infections as indicated by bacteriuria is significantly higher in Caucasian working women than in nuns. This difference becomes more marked with decreasing age and extends into childhood. Thus factors in religious life other than celibacy may be responsible. *(From Kunin and McCormack, 1968. Reprinted by permission from the New England Journal of Medicine.)*

more frequent among single Caucasian women in the 15–24 year age group than in nuns of the same age, 2.7 versus 0.4 percent. Bacteriuria was, however, twice as frequent in married women of the same age, i.e., 5.9 versus 2.7 percent. The incidence of bacteriuria did not rise with the number of pregnancies, suggesting that sexual activity was not a critical factor. Furthermore, both systolic and diastolic blood pressures were significantly lower in Negro nuns of all ages ($p <$ 0.01), yet all were active as teachers, nurses, social workers, and missionaries (Fig. 11-8). Perhaps the incidence of bacteriuria can be related to socioenvironmental factors, that is to episodes of arousal of the neuroendocrine system. Renal vasoconstriction is known to occur in response to emotional stimulation, and Shapiro has demonstrated that rats with vasoconstricted kidneys have an enhanced susceptibility to bacterial infection. He has also shown that a hypertensive human population is at risk of renal disease (as described in Chapter 9) (Shapiro, 1963; Shapiro et al., 1971). In our laboratories, we have found a far greater incidence of interstitial nephritis in colonies of highly competitive mice than

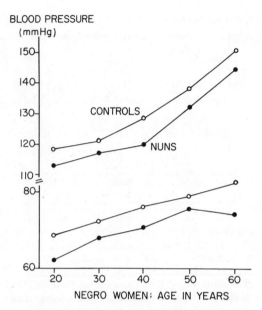

BLOOD PRESSURE (mmHg)

CONTROLS

NUNS

NEGRO WOMEN: AGE IN YEARS

Fig. 11-8. The systolic and diastolic blood pressures of Negro working women are significantly higher at all ages ($p < 0.01$) than in Negro nuns. (The same applies to Caucasian nuns.) As in the incidence of bacteriuria (see Fig. 11-7) analysis suggests that the pattern of living in a cloistered environment may be a factor. *(From Kunin and McCormack, 1968. Reprinted by permission from the New England Journal of Medicine.)*

in colonies with a stable hierarchy (Henry et al., 1971b).

In Chapter 10, we have already pointed out that the incidence of coronary heart disease is much lower in cloistered Benedictine Brothers than in Benedictine Priests eating the same food at refectory tables. The Priests' parochial and teaching duties in a competitive environment had had the effect of producing "Type A persons in a Type A atmosphere" (Caffrey, 1966). Apparently the social assets offered by the church to cloistered monks include protecting them from competitiveness. Nuns enjoy freedom from many confrontations to which lovers, married women, and mothers are exposed. Like the isolated animals in our laboratories, they are protected from the many sources of stressful life changes. Although sacrificing the direct expression of their reproductive instincts, in exchange, they receive the hope of a rewarding and confrontation-free life

both now and after death; furthermore, the noncompetitive highly evolved canon they follow teaches them they are justified in making these sacrifices. This same philosophy of self-sacrifice also sustained the medical corpsmen on rescue missions in Vietnam (Bourne, 1970). Monks and nuns who follow the rule of their order as an "intrinsic" religion are supported by the belief that they are serving a higher cause and that their prayers and dedication assist an entity transcending their personal concerns. They also see themselves as chosen members of an establishment that has the highest possible status: that of identification with the wishes of a supreme being. It is a testable hypothesis that the social assets provided by the church society successfully blunt potential psychosocial stimuli and maintain the intensity of their neuroendocrine responses below the level of pathophysiologic change.

Another group of people for whom these criteria may apply are members of The Church of Jesus Christ of Latter-Day Saints, more popularly known as Mormons. The Mormon Health Code decrees total abstinence from alcohol, tobacco, tea, coffee, and all drinks containing caffeine. Mormons are encouraged to take plenty of exercise, and each congregation has its own gymnasium and basketball court. But what is of overriding importance is that these patterns are all part of the Mormon cultural canon which remains an active living faith. The church keeps a unique record of its faithful—both living and dead—locally and also at the Mormon Headquarters in Salt Lake City. Mormons have assurance that life is eternal and that they will meet their dead loved ones in the hereafter. This decreases the fear of dying and the loneliness of bereavement. In addition, they have no professional clergy in what was at its founding a theocratic state. Thus the experiential factor is strongly emphasized. Boys and girls begin working for the church when they are 12 years old. By the time they are 19 years old, thousands of Mormon youth have become missionaries. At this critical stage of their development, their idealism is challenged and in a warm atmosphere of social support, they leave on a great mission to "search for souls" far away from home. The institution of the family is emphasized as a source of help in times of trouble as Mormons set aside Monday evenings as their "family night." Anecdotal evidence points to an effective cultural canon and data on health suggest that Mormons do indeed enjoy an advantage.

Enstrom (1975) reported that the 1970–1972 cancer mortality rate in the predominantly Mormon state of Utah is two-thirds to

three-fourths that of the rest of the United States (for further details see Fig. 11-9). In addition, the death rate from heart attacks and other cardiovascular disease is two-thirds to one-half the national average (J. E. Enstrom, 1978). Possible reasons for these differences in the incidence of coronary heart disease have been discussed in preceding chapters. The mechanisms that may play a part in the development of cancer are obscure. Yet it is recognized that the age at which a woman has her first child has a direct relationship to the risk of mammary

Fig. 11-9. The overall 1970–1972 mortality rate for cancer among adult Mormons in California is about one-half to three-fourths that of the general population in the state. The figures for the predominantly Mormon state of Utah follow the same trend. Enstrom concluded that it remains to be determined which components of the Mormon lifestyle, including the social and psychologic aspects of their religion, are related to their low mortality rates *(Enstrom, 1975).*

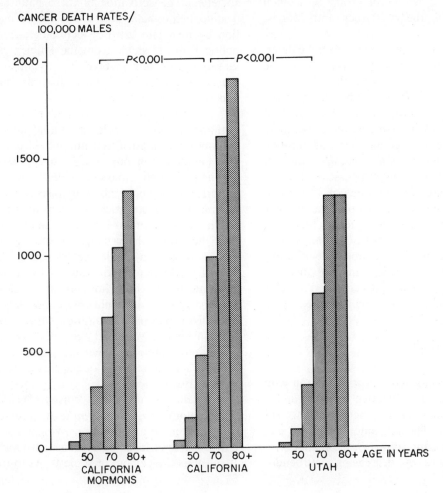

tumor; the older the mother, the greater the risk of tumor. As Cole (1974) recently pointed out, subsequent births have no effect on the formation of tumors, which suggests that some sort of threshold phenomenon is at work. The mechanism underlying the value of early childbirth may be related to a sensitive period for mother–infant bonding in humans (see Chapter 4). Perhaps women who are older than 25 when their first child is born have a limbic system that has matured to the point where attachment bonds are not readily formed; they may not be able to express emotion as well as younger mothers who became attached to their newborn infants while adolescent (Kennell et al., 1975; Klaus et al., 1975). The fact that women with mammary cancer have a greater difficulty in expressing emotions normally than a control group of women supports this theory (Greer and Morris, 1975).

As Enstrom says, it remains to be determined exactly which components of the Mormon lifestyle, including the "Words of Wisdom" issuing from the church, are related to their low mortality rate. Eventually it may be possible to demonstrate experimentally that the average number and duration of limbic system responses per unit time—of an intensity that would put persons at risk—are not as high in Mormons as in persons outside of this stable, supportive, lifetime social system. As a consequence, their neuroendocrine set would rarely assume intense fight–flight arousal or depressive withdrawal patterns, and their immune responses, as well as other physiologic regulatory mechanisms, would tend to remain stable.

Conclusions

A rewarding stable work situation with a strong personal affiliative network and a supportive home environment are powerful social assets. The relaxation response can effect significant downward changes in blood pressure by decreasing neuroendo-

crine arousal. As quantitative studies during actual combat situations have shown, psychosocial defenses can be surprisingly effective; such defenses rely on the support of the group. Bonding between members of the group, group ritual behavior, and shared beliefs will protect against social stimulation; but, the most effective protection historically has come from integrated cultural canons that incorporate an active religion. Toynbee's suggestion that the important religions of the world developed to compensate for the excessive rational empiricism of a secular civilization can be viewed in terms of balancing the activity of the left versus the right hemisphere. The mechanisms are admittedly obscure, but we have argued that attachment and territorial behavior form the warp and woof of the fabric of mammalian societies. The activation of these patterns, despite their unbelievably subtle transformation by man into artistic, technologic, and political forms, stems from the limbic system and ultimately involves the hypothalamus as the effector of the neuroendocrine and autonomic outflow.

In a prescient book, Kropotkin in 1902 outlined the crucial role of mutual aid in evolution. He argued that mutual aid is the real foundation of our ethical conceptions, and he presented a mass of evidence on the importance of cooperation in insect, bird, and mammalian societies as well as in primitive hunter–gatherers. He argued that whatever the cause, the principle of mutual aid has its origins in the lowest stages of the animal world. Kropotkin saw its evolution as uninterrupted throughout human development and believed it could continue to develop still further. His inspiration came from Darwin himself who had seen that mutual aid is more important than the popularized struggle for the survival of the fittest (Kropotkin, 1919).

Seventy years later, Wilson's (1975) *Sociobiology: The New Synthesis* receives much contemporary attention. Weighing the now enormous mass of evidence, he rates altruism as the cement of society. As to the mechanisms, he comments that the biologist realizes that self-knowledge is constrained and shaped by the emotional control centers in the hypothalamus and the limbic system of the brain. These centers flood our consciousness with the emotions of hate, love, guilt, fear, and others that are consulted by ethical philosophers who wish to intuit the standards of good and evil. Wilson asks, what then made the hypothalamus and the limbic system? And his reply is that they evolved by natural selection. This simple biologic statement must be pursued to explain ethics at all depths. Self-existence is not the central question of philosophy. The hypothalamic limbic complex automatically denies such logical reduction by countering it with the feelings of guilt and altruism.

Wilson's critic N. J. Mackintosh is incredulous at such a statement, wondering whether Wilson is not really jesting when he says that ethical philsophers intuit the deontologic canons of morality by consulting the emotive centers of their own hypothalamic limbic systems. The quotation "Summoned or not summoned, God will be there" chosen to open this book, however, implies that there is no escape from the archetypes of the collective unconscious which, subjectively, are aspects of religious experience, yet at the same time can be viewed as biologic functions: patterns of behavior, biogrammar, or instincts. They form a linking network whose symbols project to the peculiarly human interhemispheric world of language, images, and ideas which are nevertheless rooted in the biologic processes of subcortical regions (Jung, 1939, 1959).

For Jung the archetypes also exist in animals, and the theory of archetypes provides a suitable foundation for an overall view of human and animal psychology (Jacobi, 1959; Henry, 1977). As Rossi (1977) recently expressed it: " . . . the archetype is an imprint, image or pattern that exists independently of words and ego consciousness. As such, the archetype and the related concepts of symbol and collective unconscious may be closely associated with the imagery,

gestalt and visuospatial patterns characteristic of right hemispheric functioning." Their autonomy contrasts with the ego-directed, rational, analytic left-hemispheric thought. The symbol is a visible representation that stands for something invisible and intangible. It forms a bridge between the environment and the organism and between the world of words and ideas handled by the left hemisphere and the mystical "not this, not that" component whose locus we guess to be not only in the right hemisphere, but also in the limbic system (Henry, 1977). Mackintosh may have been disturbed by the implication that a location for the Godhead was being found in primitive brain structures. It is true that theologian–psychiatrist Jung saw the archetype of the self, which functions as a union of opposing aspects of the psyche, as constituting the most immediate experience of the Divine psychologically possible to imagine. He also recognized that there were physiologic concomitants of such an experience: "If one could locate such a basic fact as the self at all, the brain stem would be the most likely spot. I am certain that the universally occurring symbols of the self point to a fairly reliable fact of a basic nature, i.e., a structure expressed through an organic pattern." (Jung, personal communication, 1955).

Elsewhere in an essay on the self, he says that a man can have religious experience and individual relation to God if he will take cognizance of the foundations of his consciousness, if he will move toward the unconscious which is the only accessible source. Then to avoid misunderstanding he adds, "This is certainly not to say that what we call the unconscious is identical with God or is set up in his place. It is the medium from which the religious experience seems to flow. As to what the further cause of such an experience may be, the answer to this lies beyond the range of human knowledge. Knowledge of God is a transcendental problem." (Jung, 1958).

Contemporary science is moving toward this problem of the immanence of

God and the moral imperatives. In a Presidential Address to the American Psychological Association, Campbell (1976) has discussed the conflicts between biologic and social evolution and between psychology and moral tradition. Drawing on Wilson's (1975) sociobiologic approach, he contends that the genetic disadvantages of altruistic traits are compensated by moral norms developed during man's social evolution. These norms are handed down as part of the cultural canon. As Burhoe (1976) comments in a discussion of Campbell's paper, religions have provided the motivating mechanisms for overcoming our genetically programmed clannishness. Man's sociocultural brain was selected genetically as the result of living in a social group; it has complex powers for understanding and communicating the adaptive advantages of the individual's services to society.

During the past few centuries, religious myths have lost efficacy because they have become incredible in the light of science, but Burhoe forsees an updating that will restore a credible vision of our ties to society, deliver us from alienation and meaninglessness, and engender the cooperation essential for social harmony. While no group has yet come up with a formulation acceptable to both religious and scientific communities, he argues they now concur that evolution is a self-creating, selective system that moves from the simple to the complex. Thus Fox (1975), a biochemist, specializing in molecular evolution, reflecting on the new views of how life began, states that this concept of self-directed evolution has had to compete with the idea that evolutionary possibilities occur by chance. No view could be further from the truth, however. The potential array of possibilities at each stage is a narrow one, and that narrow range is rigidly determined by what has emerged to the stage in question. The controlling factors are the shapes of the molecules. He says, . . . "the study of cells 'from the inside-out' (constructionism), in addition to 'from the outside-in' (reductionism), yields a new sense of the phenomena of cellular systems. This new feeling has increased our respect for the emergence of a holistic quantum; if I didn't know that life was already here and something of what it is like, I would find it so fantastic that I could not believe in its existence." (Fox, 1975).

Man and his society are products of evolutionary forces; human consciousness has evolved in its present form because man is not only an individual, but also a part of the social organism, and thus a product of the combined action of heredity as represented by the limbic system and the selective force of his culture as acquired by the cerebral hemispheres.

When he spoke of moral imperatives, Wilson had reason to point to the limbic system and the hypothalamus, and Rossi would add the right hemisphere as a further critical brain system. But the left hemisphere's crucial role in technical thinking should not blind us to the importance of the other brains in considering moral and religious experiences. Perhaps it is something to this effect that Jung was saying when he carved the words "Vocatus atque non vocatus, Deus aderit" on his lintel.

Despite their subtlety, the symbols of man's cultural canons, such as cross, flag, president, family, mother, father, land, and nature, are expressions of attachment and territorial instincts whose roots he holds in common with fellow mammals. If you disturb a man by uprooting him from his native land with its cultural influences and place him in an alien culture with other symbols and patterns of behavior, neuroendocrine responses severe enough to leave their mark on his physiologic regulation may ensue. Just before his untimely death, the gifted epidemiologist John Cassel predicted that the results of the collaborative study with Prior, which was then in progress on the Tokelau atolls, and in migrants in New Zealand, would throw light on the question of whether the high blood pressure of migrants was due to modification of their physical or psychosocial environment (Cassel, 1975). Beaglehole et al. (1978) have tested the idea that the subcortical systems of an older person may become inflexible, prohibiting relearning and making it difficult to change the symbols and cultural canon with which he has identified during the sensitive learning period of youth. Their report examines the hypothesis that the stress of life changes would be more evident in persons who experienced incongruity between their personal beliefs and their social situation than in those who experienced no such incongruity, and that this stress would be manifested in measurable physiologic and bodily changes, hence, in effect, that the blood pressure of a group is a measure of its social stability and adaptation.

These observations were made on 900 adult inhabitants of the Tokelau atolls who had migrated to New Zealand. Their densely populated land area, only a few kilometers square, had been swept by a hurricane in 1966 and its diminished resources supported the Christianized but still culturally traditional Polynesians at a subsistence level. A sociocultural as well as a medical evaluation was made in 1968 and 1971 before a number of the subjects had migrated to New Zealand. These immigrants have now been settled in New Zealand for varying periods; some live in well-organized ethnic communities where they maintain close ties with fellow immigrants at home and at work. They worship together in traditional Tokelaun churches and enjoy leisure activities in common. Others, however, through choice, chance, or necessity interact more with non-Tokelaun New Zealanders and thus lack close contact with their own cultural traditions.

As in the Marmot–Syme study of Japanese–Americans (Marmot and Syme, 1976), the Prior-Cassel-Beaglehole project is attempting to determine whether persons who were the most acculturated to the Western way of life would show the most change, as indeed they did. As in the Marmot–Syme study, sociologic interviews and questionnaires measured the subject's degree of interaction with the non-Tokelaun milieu and their commitment to retain the concepts of Tokelaun culture. A partial correlation analysis controlling for body mass and length of residence in New Zealand showed a significant positive association between blood pressure and degree of social interaction with New Zealand society (males, $p<0.005$; females, $p<0.04$).

As part of a series of discussions of the influence of modern life on health, Prior has recently written an article entitled "Civilization and Cardiovascular Changes: A Pacific Viewpoint." Reviewing the implications of the work with Tokelauns, he cites the conclusion of the Marmot–Syme study that "a culture characterized by strong social support, stability, and lack of individual competitiveness may be protective against heart disease." The higher blood pressure in Tokelaun migrants with greater European interaction is consistent with the psychosocial hypothesis and is likely to be modulated through the neuroendocrine system. Thus essential hypertension may represent an exaggeration of the tendency of blood pressure to rise with age due to a repeated sequence in which a small rise in pressure produces changes, which maintain the pressure rise and become the basis for a further rise.

The psychosocial factor is now sufficiently established to warrant more general consideration in the etiology of disease. It has become a necessary concern and must be added to other factors. It is now safe to predict that, in the future, measures to reduce social stress and increase social supports will rank higher than they do now in the thinking of those responsible for the prevention and cure of disease, and that statesmen will view the blood pressure of a group as a measure of its stability and social adjustment.

In the preface, we stated that our Stone Age ancestors living on tiny Pacific atolls for the better part of a thousand years developed cultural practices that avoid the self-destruction and disease that follow the escalation of social disorder. Prior (1976) concludes his article on the former Tokelaun

atoll dwellers as follows: "A greater recognition of the value of coping strategies and
protective factors that derive from a supportive cultural and traditional background and
extended family is certainly the lesson we
are learning from the traditional, small, isolated Polynesian communities, such as Puka
Puka and Tokelau, and studies of their
migration into modern life. The path to
improved health in modern society will
require a greater discipline in lifestyle."

Bibliography

Aars, H. (1968). Aortic baroreceptor activity in normal and hypertensive rabbits. *Acta Physiol. Scand.* **72**, 298–309.

Abboud, F. M. (1976). Relaxation, autonomic control, and hypertension. *N. Engl. J. Med.* **294**, 107–109 (editorial).

Abernethy, V. (1974). Dominance and sexual behavior: A hypothesis. *Am. J. Psychiatry* **131**, 813–817.

Ader, R. (1976). Conditioned elevations in adrenocortical steroid level in the rat. *Psychosom. Med.* **38**, 65 (abstr.).

Ader, R., and Cohen, N. (1975). Behaviorally conditioned immunosuppression. *Psychosom. Med.* **37**, 333–340.

Akiskal, H. S., and McKinney, W. T., Jr. (1975). Overview of recent research in depression: Integration of ten conceptual models into a comprehensive clinical frame. *Arch. Gen. Psychiatry* **32**, 285–305.

Alcock, J. (1975). "Animal Behavior: An Evolutionary Approach," Chapter 16, pp. 466–505. Sinauer Assoc., Sunderland, Massachusetts.

Altman, J. (1966). "Organic Foundations of Animal Behavior." Holt, New York.

Amkraut, A., and Solomon, G. F. (1975). From the symbolic stimulus to the pathophysiologic response: Immune mechanisms. *Int. J. Psychiatry Med* **5**, 541–563.

Anderson, G. E. (1972). College schedule of recent experience. Master's Thesis, Department of Guidance and Counseling, North Dakota State University, Fargo (unpublished).

Andy, O. J., and Stephan, H. (1974). Comparative primate neuroanatomy of structures relating to aggressive behavior. *In* "Primate Aggression, Territoriality, and Xenophobia: A Comparative Perspective" (R. L. Holloway), pp. 305–330. Academic Press, New York.

Antonovsky, A. (1974). Conceptual and methodological problems in the study of resistance resources and stressful life events. *In* "Stressful Life Events: Their Nature and Effects" (B. S. Dohrenwend and B. P. Dohrenwend, eds.), pp. 245–258. Wiley, New York.

Arsenian, J., and Arsenian, J. M. (1948). Tough and easy cultures. A conceptual analysis. *Psychiatry* **11**, 377–385.

Bahnson, C. B. (1969). Dedication. In memory of Dr. David M. Kissen: His work and his thinking. *Ann. N.Y. Acad. Sci.* **164**, 313–318.

Bahnson, C. B., and Bahnson, M. B. (1964).

Denial and repression of primitive impulses and of disturbing emotions in patients with malignant neoplasms. *In* "Psychosomatic Aspects of Neoplastic Disease" (D. M. Kissen and L. L. Leshan, eds.), pp. 42–56. Lippincott, Philadelphia, Pennsylvania.

Bakan, P. (1969). Hypnotizability, laterality of eye movement and functional brain asymmetry. *Percept. Mot. Skills* **28**, 927–932.

Bakan, P. (1976). The right brain is the dreamer. *Psychol. Today* **10**, 66–68.

Ballard, K. (1973). Blood flow in canine adipose tissue during intravenous infusion of norepinephrine. *Am. J. Physiol.* **225**, 1026–1031.

Ballard, K., and Rosell, S. (1971). Adrenergic neurohumoral influences on circulation and lipolysis in canine omental adipose tissue. *Circ. Res.* **28**, 389–396.

Ballard, K., Cobb, C. A., and Rosell, S. (1971). Vascular and lipolytic responses in canine subcutaneous adipose tissue following infusion of catecholamines. *Acta Physiol. Scand.* **81**, 246–253.

Ballard, K., Malmfors, T., and Rosell, S. (1974). Adrenergic innervation and vascular patterns in canine adipose tissue. *Microvasc. Res.* **8**, 164–171.

Barnett, S. A. (1964). Social stress: The concept of stress. *Viewpoints Biol.* **3**, 170–218.

Barnett, S. A., Hocking, W. E., Munro, K. M. H., and Walker, K. Z. (1975). Socially induced renal pathology of captive wild rats *(Rattus villosissimus). Aggressive Behav.* **1**, 123–133.

Beach, F. A. (1974). Human sexuality and evolution. *Adv. Behav. Biol.* **11**, 333–365.

Beaglehole, R., Salmond, C. E., Hooper, A., Huntsman, J., Stanhope, J. M., Cassel, J. C., and Prior, I. A. M. (1978). Blood pressure and social interaction in Tokelauan migrants in New Zealand. *J Chronic Dis.* (in press)

Bellet, S., Roman, L., DeCastro, O., Kin, K. E., and Kershbaum, A. (1969). The effect of coffee ingestion on catecholamine release. *Metab., Clin. Exp.* **18**, 288–291.

Benedict, R. (1946). "The Chrysanthemum and the Sword: Patterns of Japanese Culture," p. 178. Houghton, Boston, Massachusetts.

Benson, H. (1975). "The Relaxation Response." William Morrow, New York.

Benson, H., Rosner, B. A., Marzetta, B. R., and Klemchuk, H. M. (1974). Decreased blood pressure in pharmacologically treated hypertensive patients who regularly elicited the relaxation response. *Lancet* **1**, 289–291.

Benson, H., Kotch, J. B., and Crassweller, K. D. (1976). The usefulness of the relaxation response in the treatment of stress-related cardiovascular disease, *J. S. C. Med. Assoc.* **72**, Suppl., 50–56.

Berger, P. L. (1976). Oh so seductive socialism. *Los Angeles Times* Part IV, Aug. 22, p. 5.

Bernstein, I. S., and Gordon, T. P. (1974). The function of aggression in primate societies. *Am. Sci.* **62**, 304–311.

Bernstein, I. S., Gordon, T. P., and Rose, R. M. (1974). Factors influencing the expression of aggression during introductions to rhesus monkey groups. *In* "Primate Aggression, Territoriality and Xenophobia: A Comparative Perspective" (R. L. Holloway, ed.), pp. 211–240. Academic Press, New York.

Bianco, C. (1974). "The Two Rosetos." Indiana Univ. Press, Bloomington.

Blurton Jones, N. (1972). Categories of child-child interaction. *In* "Ethnological Studies of Child Behaviour" (N. Blurton Jones, ed.), pp. 97–127. Cambridge Univ. Press, London and New York.

Bogen, J. E. (1969). The other side of the brain. II. An appositional mind. *Bull. Los Angeles Neurol. Soc.* **34**, 135–162.

Bogen J. E., and Bogen, G. M. (1969). The other side of the brain. III. The corpus callosum and creativity. *Bull. Los Angeles Neurol. Soc.* **34**, 191–220.

Bohus, B., Nyakas, Cs., and Lissák, K. (1968). Involvement of suprahypothalamic structure in the hormonal feedback action of corticosteroids. *Acta Physiol. Acad. Sci. Hung.* **34**, 1–8.

Borkman, T. (1976). Experiential knowledge: A new concept for the analysis of self-help groups. *Soc. Serv. Rev.* **50**, 445–456.

Bourne, P. G. (1970). "Men, Stress, and Vietnam." Little, Brown, Boston, Massachusetts.

Bourne, P. G. (1971). Altered adrenal function in two combat situations in Viet Nam. *In* "The Physiology of Aggression and Defeat" (B. E. Elefthériou and J. P. Scott, eds.), pp. 265–290. Plenum, New York.

Bowlby, J. (1970). "Attachment and Loss," Vol. 1. Hogarth Press, London.

Bowlby, J. (1973). "Attachment and Loss," Vol. 2. Hogarth Press, London.

Brain, P. F., and Poole, A. E. (1974). The role of

endocrines in isolation-induced intermale fighting in albino laboratory mice. I. Pituitary-adrenocortical influences. *Aggressive Behav.* **1**, 39–69.

Branch, M. H., Olton, D. S., and Best, P. J. (1976). Spatial characteristics of hippocampal unit activity. *Neuroscience,* 2, Part 1, 368 (abstr.).

Brazelton, T. B., Tronick, E., Adamson, L., Als, H., and Weise, S. (1975). Early mother infant reciprocity. *Parent-Infant Interact., Ciba Found. Symp., 1975* No. 33., pp. 137–149.

Bronson, F. H. (1973). Establishment of social rank among grouped male mice: Relative effects on circulating FSH, LH, and corticosterone. *Physiol. Behav.* **10**, 947–951.

Bronson, F. H., and Elefthériou, B. E. (1965). Adrenal response to fighting in mice: Separation of physical and psychological causes. *Science* **147**, 627–628.

Brown, G. W., Bhrolcháin, M. N., and Harris, T. (1975). Social class and psychiatric disturbance among women in an urban population. *Sociology* **9**, 225–254.

Brown, L. E. (1966). Home range and movement of small mammals. *Symp. Zool. Soc. London* **18**, 111–141.

Brown, P. (1972). "The Chimbu. A Study of Change in the New Guinea Highlands." Schenkman Publ. Co., Cambridge, Massachusetts.

Bruhn, J. G., Chandler, B., Miller, M. C., Wolf, S., and Lynn, T. N. (1966). Social aspects of coronary heart disease in two adjacent, ethnically different communities. *Am. J. Public Health* **56**, 1493–1506.

Bruhn, J. G., Paredes, A., Adsett, C. A., and Wolf, S. (1974). Psychological predictors of sudden death in myocardial infarction. *J. Psychosom. Res.* **18**, 187–191.

Burhoe, R. W. (1976). The source of civilization in the natural selection of coadapted information in genes and culture. *Zygon* **11**, 263–303.

Byers, S. O., Friedman, M., Rosenman, R. H., and Freed, S. C. (1962). Excretion of 3-methoxy-4-hydroxymandelic acid in men with behavior pattern associated with high incidence of coronary artery disease. *Fed. Proc., Fed. Am. Soc. Exp. Biol.* **21**, Suppl. 11, 99–101.

Caffrey, C. B. (1966). Behavior patterns and personality characteristics as related to prevalence rates of coronary heart diseases in Trappist and Benedictine monks. Ph.D. Dissertation (Clinical Psychology), Catholic University of America, Washington, D.C. (University Microfilms, Inc., Ann Arbor, Michigan, No. 67-1830, pp. 45–48 coronary heart disease rates).

Calhoun, J. B. (1962). A "behavioral sink." *In* Roots of Behavior: Genetics, Instinct, and Socialization in Animal Behavior (E. L. Bliss, ed.), pp. 295–315. Harper (Hoeber), New York.

Campbell, D. T. (1976). On the conflicts between biological and social evolution and between psychology and moral tradition. *Zygon* **11**, 167–208.

Candland, D. K., and Leshner, A. I. (1974). A model of agonistic behavior: Endocrine and autonomic correlates. *In* "Limbic and Autonomic Nervous Systems Research" (L. V. DiCara, ed.), Chapter 4, pp. 137–163. Plenum, New York.

Cannon, W. B. (1929). "Bodily Changes in Pain, Hunger, Fear and Rage: An Account of Recent Researches into the Function of Emotional Excitement," 2nd ed. Appleton, New York.

Cannon, W. B. (1957). "Voodoo" death. *Psychosom. Med.* **19**, 182–190.

Cannon, W. B., and de La Paz, D. (1911). Emotional stimulation of adrenal secretion. *Am. J. Physiol.* **27**, 64–70.

Carroll, B. J. (1976). Limbic system-adrenal cortex regulation in depression and schizophrenia. *Psychosom. Med.* **38**, 106–121.

Carruthers, M. E. (1969). Aggression and atheroma. *Lancet* **2**, 1170–1171.

Carruthers, M. (1976). Modification of the noradrenaline related effects of smoking by beta-blockade. *Psychol. Med.* **6**, 251–256.

Carruthers, M., and Taggart, P. (1973). Vagotonicity of violence: Biochemical and cardiac responses to violent films and television programmes. *Br. Med. J.* **3**, 384–389.

Cassel, J. (1974). Psychosocial processes and "stress": theoretical formulation. *Int. J. Health Serv.* **4**, 471–482.

Cassel, J. (1975). Studies of hypertension in migrants. *In* "Epidemiology and Control of Hypertension" (P. Oglesby, ed.), pp. 41–58. Stratton Intercontinental Medical Book Corp., New York.

Chagnon, N. A. (1974). "Studying the Yąnoma-mö." Holt, New York.

Chomsky, N. (1972). "Language and Mind" (Enlarged ed.). Harcourt, New York.

Christian, J. J. (1970). Social subordination, population density, and mammalian evolution. *Science* **168**, 84–90.

Christian, J. J. (1971). Population density and reproductive efficiency. *Biol. Reprod.* **4**, 248–294.

Christian, J. J., Lloyd, J. A., and Davis, D. E. (1965). The role of endocrines in the self-regulation of mammalian populations. *Recent Prog. Horm. Res.* **21**, 501–571.

Ciaranello, R. D., Wooten, G. F., and Axelrod, J. (1976). Regulation of rat adrenal dopamine β-hydroxylase. II. Receptor interaction in the regulation of enzyme synthesis and degradation. *Brain Res.* **113**, 349–362.

Cobb, S. (1976). Social support as a moderator of life stress. (Presidential address—1976.) *Psychosom. Med.* **38**, 300–314.

Cohen, B. D., Berent, S., and Silverman, A. J. (1973). Field-dependence and lateralization of function in the human brain. *Arch. Gen. Psychiatry* **28**, 165–167.

Cole, P. (1974). Epidemiology of breast cancer: An overview. *In* "Report to the Profession—Breast Cancer" (B. Levine, E. Tarwater, and E. P. Vollmer, eds.), pp. 11–20. Nat. Inst. Health, Bethesda, Maryland.

Conner, R. L., Vernikos-Danellis, J., and Levine, S. (1971). Stress, fighting and neuroendocrine function. *Nature (London)* **234**, 564–566.

Cooley-Matthews, B. (1977). Studies on force-breeding and social density as they relate to mammary tumor formation in mice. Ph.D. Dissertation (Physiology), University of Southern California, Los Angeles.

Coover, G. D., Ursin, H., and Levine, S. (1973). Plasma-corticosterone levels during active-avoidance learning in rats. *J. Comp. Physiol. Psychol.* **82**, 170–174.

Corley, K. C. (1977). Personal communication.

Corley, K. C., Shiel, F. O'M, Path, M. R. C., Mauck, H. P., and Greenhoot, J. (1973). Electrocardiographic and cardiac morphological changes associated with environmental stress in squirrel monkeys. *Psychosom. Med.* **35**, 361–364.

Corley, K. C., Mauck, H. P., and Shiel, F. O'M. (1975). Cardiac responses associated with

"yoked chair" shock avoidance in squirrel monkeys. *Psychophysiology* **12**, 439–444.

Corley, K. C., Shiel, F. O'M., Mauck, H. P., Clark, L. S., and Barber, J. H. (1977). Myocardial degeneration and cardiac arrest in squirrel monkey: Physiological and psychological correlates. *Psychophysiology* **14**: 322–328.

Craighead, F., Jr., and Craighead, J. (1972). Studying wildlife by satellite. *Nat. Geogr. Mag.* **143**, 120–123.

Crook, J. H. (1970). Social organization and the environment: Aspects of contemporary social ethology. *Anim. Behav.* **18**, 197–209.

Crowcroft, P. (1966). "Mice All Over." G. T. Foulis & Co. Ltd., London.

Cryer, P. E., Haymond, M. W., Santiago, J. V., and Shah, S. D. (1976). Norepinephrine and epinephrine release and adrenergic mediation of smoking-associated hemodynamics and metabolic events. *N. Engl. J. Med.* **295**, 573–577.

Dahl, L. K. (1960). Possible role of salt intake in the development of essential hypertension. *In* "Essential Hypertension" (K. D. Bock and P. T. Cottier, eds.), pp. 53–65. Springer-Verlag, Berlin.

D'Andrade, R. G. (1966). Sex differences and cultural institutions. *In* "The Development of Sex Differences" (E. E. Maccoby, ed.), pp. 174–204. Stanford Univ. Press, Stanford, California.

Davis, D. E., and Christian, J. J. (1957). Relation of adrenal weight to social rank of mice. *Symp. Soc. Exp. Med. Biol.* **94**, 728–731.

Dawber, T. R., Kannel, W. B., Kagan, A., Donabedian, R. K., McNamara, P. M., and Pearson, G. (1967). Environmental factors in hypertension. *In* "The Epidemiology of Hypertension" (J. Stamler, R. Stamler, and T. N. Pullman, eds.), pp. 255–288. Grune & Stratton, New York.

De Chateau, P. (1976). "Neonatal Care Routines: Influences on Maternal and Infant Behaviour and on Breast Feeding," Umeå Univ. Med. Diss. No. 20. University of Umeå, Departments of Paediatrics and Child Psychiatry, Umeå, Switzerland.

De Faire, U., and Theorell, T. (1976). Life changes and myocardial infarction. How useful are life change measurements? *Scand. J. Soc. Med.* **4**, 115–122.

Denenberg, V. H. (1969). Experimental programming of life histories in the rat. *In* "Stimulation in Early Infancy" (A. Ambrose, ed.), pp. 21–43. Academic Press, New York.

DeVore, I., ed. (1965). "Primate Behavior: Field Studies of Monkeys and Apes." Holt, New York.

DeVore, I., and Konner, M. J. (1974). Infancy in hunter-gatherer life: An ethological perspective. *In* "Ethology and Psychiatry" (N. F. White, ed.), Chapter 6, pp. 113–141. Univ. of Toronto Press, Toronto.

Dimond, S. (1972). "The Double Brain." Williams & Wilkins, Baltimore, Maryland.

Dimond, S. J., and Beaumont, J. G. (1974). Experimental studies of hemisphere function in the human brain. *In* "Hemisphere Function in the Human Brain" (S. J. Dimond and J. G. Beaumont, eds.), pp. 48–88. Wiley (Halsted Press), New York.

Donnison, C. P. (1938). "Civilization and Disease." Wood, New York.

Draper, P. (1973): Crowding among hunter-gathers: The !Kung Bushmen. *Science* **182,** 301–303.

Durkheim, E. (1951). "Suicide: A Study in Sociology" (transl. by J. A. Spaulding and G. Simpson). Free Press, Glencoe, Illinois.

Eaton, G. G. (1976). The social order of Japanese macaques. *Sci. Am.* **235,** 97–106.

Edwards, E. A., and Dean, L. M. (1977). Effects of crowding of mice on humoral antibody formation and protection to lethal antigenic challenge. *Psychosom. Med.* **39,** 19–24.

Eibl-Eibesfeldt, I. (1972). "Love and Hate: The Natural History of Behavior Patterns" (transl. by G. Strachan). Holt, New York.

Eibl-Eibesfeldt, I. (1974). The myth of the aggression-free hunter and gatherer society. *In* "Primate Aggression, Territoriality and Xenophobia: A Comparative Perspective" (R. L. Holloway, ed.), pp. 435–457. Academic Press, New York.

Eibl-Eibesfeldt, I. (1975). The ethology of man. *In* "Ethology: The Biology of Behavior" (transl. by E. Klinghammer), 2nd ed., Chapter 18, pp. 442–534. Holt, New York.

Eimas, P. D., Siqueland, E. R., Jusczyk, P., and Vigorito, J. (1971). Speech perception in infants. *Science* **171,** 303–306.

Eimerl, S., DeVore, I., and The Editors of Life. (1965). "The Primates" (Life Nature Library). Time Inc., New York.

Ekman, P. (1972). Universals and cultural differences in facial expressions of emotion. *In* "Nebraska Symposium on Motivation, 1971" (J. K. Cole, ed.), pp. 207–283. Univ. of Nebraska Press, Lincoln.

Ekman, P., and Friesen, W. V. (1969). The repertoire of nonverbal behavior: Categories, origins, usage, and coding. *Semiotica* **1,** 49–98.

Eliasch, H., Lager, C. G., Norrbäck, K., Rosén, A., and Scott, H. (1967). The beta-adrenergic receptor blockade modification of the systemic haemodynamic effects of Link trainer simulated flight. *In* "Emotional Stress: Physiological and Psychological Reactions, Medical, Industrial and Military Implications" (L. Levi, ed.), pp. 120–128. (Försvarsmedicin **3,** Suppl. 2 1967).

Ely, D. L. (1971). Physiological and behavioral differentiation of social roles in a population cage of magnetically tagged CBA mice. Ph.D. Dissertation (Physiology), University of Southern California, Los Angeles.

Ely, D. L., and Henry, J. P. (1974). Effects of prolonged social deprivation on murine behavior patterns, blood pressure, and adrenal weight. *J. Comp. Physiol. Psychol.* **87,** 733–740.

Ely, D. L., Henry, J. A., Henry, J. P., and Rader, R. D. (1972). A monitoring technique providing quantitative rodent behavior analysis. *Physiol. Behav.* **9,** 675–679.

Ely, D. L., Henry, J. P., and Ciaranello, R. D. (1974). Long-term behavioral and biochemical differentiation of dominant and subordinate mice in population cages. *Psychosom. Med.* **36,** 463 (abstr.).

Ely, D. L., Henry, J. P., and Jarosz, C. J. (1975). Effects of marihuana (Δ9-THC) on behavior patterns and social roles in colonies of CBA mice. *Behav. Biol.* **13,** 263–276.

Ely, D. L., Greene, E. G., and Henry, J. P. (1976) Minicomputer monitored social behavior of mice with hippocampus lesions. *Behav. Biol.* **16,** 1–29.

Ely, D. L., Greene, E. G., and Henry, J. P. (1977). Effects of hippocampal lesion on cardiovascular, adrenocortical and behavioral response patterns in mice. *Physiol. Behav.* **18:**1075–1083.

Endröczi, E., and Lissák, K. (1963). Effect of hypothalamic and brain stem structure stimulation on pituitary-adrenocortical function. *Acta Physiol. Acad. Sci. Hung.* **24,** 67–77.

Engel, G. L. (1971). Sudden and rapid death during psychological stress. Folklore or folk wisdom? *Ann. Intern. Med.* **74**, 771–782.

Engel, G. L., and Schmale, A. H. (1972). Conservation-withdrawal: A primary regulatory process for organismic homeostasis. *Physiol., Emotion & Psychosom. Illness, Ciba Found. Symp., 1972* No. 8, pp. 57–76.

Enstrom, J. E. (1975). Cancer mortality among Mormons. *Cancer* **36**, 825–841.

Enstrom, J. E. (1977). Unpublished data.

Evans, R. I. (1971). Gordon Allport—a conversation. *Psychol. Today* **4**, 55–56, 58–59, 84, 86, 90, and 94.

Ewer, R. F. (1968). ''Ethology of Mammals.'' Plenum, New York.

Ferster, C. B., and Skinner, B. F. (1957). ''Schedules of Reinforcement.'' Appleton, New York.

Fishbein, W., Kastaniotis, C., and Chattman, D. (1974). Paradoxical sleep: Prolonged augmentation following learning. *Brain Res.* **79**, 61–75.

Flor-Henry, P. (1976). Lateralized temporal-limbic dysfunction and psychopathology. *Ann. N.Y. Acad. Sci.* **280**, 777–795.

Folkow, B. (1975). Vascular changes in hypertension: Review and recent animal studies. *In* ''Pathophysiology and Management of Arterial Hypertension'' (C. Berglund, L. Hansson, and L. Werkö, eds.), pp. 95–113. A. Lindgren & Söner AB, Mölndal, Sweden.

Folkow, B., and Neil, E. (1971). ''Circulation.'' Oxford Univ. Press, London.

Folkow, B., and Rubinstein, E. H. (1966). Cardiovascular effects of acute and chronic stimulations of the hypothalamic defence area in the rat. *Acta Physiol. Scand.* **68**, 48–57.

Folkow, B., Grimby, G., and Thulesius, O. (1958). Adaptive structural changes of the vascular walls in hypertension and their relation to the control of the peripheral resistance. *Acta Physiol. Scand.* **44**, 255–272.

Folkow, B., Hallbäck, M., Lundgren, Y., and Weiss, L. (1970). Background of increased flow resistance and vascular reactivity in spontaneously hypertensive rats. *Acta Physiol. Scand.* **80**, 93–106.

Folkow, B., Hallbäck, M., Lundgren, Y., Sivertsson, R., and Weiss, L. (1973). Importance of adaptive changes in vascular design for establishment of primary hypertension, studied in man and in spontaneously hypertensive rats. *Circ. Res.* **32/33**, Suppl. 1, 2–13.

Forsyth, R. P. (1969). Blood pressure responses to long-term avoidance schedules in the unrestrained rhesus monkey. *Psychosom. Med.* **31**, 300–309.

Fox, S. W. (1975). The matrix for the protobiological quantum: Cosmic casino or shapes of molecules? *Int. J. Quantum Chem., Symp.* **2**, 307–320.

Frankel, B. L., Patel, D. J., Horwitz, D., Friedewald, W. T., and Gaarder, K. R. (1978). Clinical ineffectiveness of a combination of feedback and relaxation therapies in essential hypertension. *Psychosom. Med.* (in press).

Frankenhaeuser, M., Post, B., Nordheden, B., and Sjoeberg, H. (1969). Physiological and subjective reactions to different physical work loads. *Percept. Mot. Skills* **28**, 343–349.

Frankenhaeuser, M. (1975). Experimental approaches to the study of catecholamines and emotion. *In* ''Emotions: Their Parameters and Measurement'' (L. Levi, ed.), pp. 209–234. Raven, New York.

Frankenhaeuser, M., and Gardell, B. (1976). Underload and overload in working life: Outline of a multidisciplinary approach. *J. Hum. Stress* **2**, 35–46.

Frankenhaeuser, M. (1978). Psychoneuroendocrine Sex Differences in Adaptation to the Psychosocial Environment. Serono Symposia: Clinical Psychoneuroendocrinology in Reproduction, Siena, Italy, December 2–4, 1976. Academic Press, New York. (in press)

Freedman, D. G.: (1974). ''Human Infancy: An Evolutionary Perspective.'' Wiley (Halsted), New York.

Freedman, J. L. (1975). ''Crowding and Behavior.'' Viking Press, New York.

Freis, E. D. (1971). Medical treatment of chronic hypertension. *Med. Concepts Cardiov. Dis.* **40**, 17–22.

Freis, E. D. (1976). Salt, volume and the prevention of hypertension. *Circulation* **53**, 589–594.

Friedman, M., and Rosenman, R. H. (1974). ''Type A Behavior and Your Heart.'' Alfred A. Knopf, New York.

Friedman, M., St. George, S., Byers, S. O., and Rosenman, R. H. (1960). Excretion of catecholamines, 17-ketosteroids, 17-hydroxycorticoids and 5-hydroxyindole in men exhibiting a particular behavior pattern (A) associated with high incidence of clinical coronary artery disease. *J. Clin. Invest.* **39**, 758–764.

Friedman, M., Rosenman, R. H., and St. George, S. (1969). Adrenal response to excess corticotropin in coronary-prone men. *Proc. Soc. Exp. Biol. Med.* **131**, 1305–1307.

Friedman, M., Byers, S. O., Diamant, J., and Rosenman, R. H. (1975). Plasma catecholamine response of coronary-prone subjects (Type A) to a specific challenge. *Metab. Clin. Exp.* **24**, 205–210.

Friedman, R., and Dahl, L. K. (1975). The effect of chronic conflict on the blood pressure of rats with a genetic susceptibility to experimental hypertension. *Psychosom. Med.* **37**, 402–416.

Friedman, S. B., Mason, J. W., and Hamburg, D. A. (1963). Urinary 17-hydroxycorticosteroid levels in parents of children with neoplastic disease: A study of chronic psychological stress. *Psychosom. Med.* **25**, 364–376.

Funkenstein, D. H. (1956). Norepinephrine-like and epinephrine-like substances in relation to human behavior. *J. Ment. Dis.* **123**, 58–68.

Furuyama, M. (1962). Histometrical investigations of arteries in reference to arterial hypertension. *Tohoku J. Exp. Med.* **76**, 388–414.

Galin, D. (1974). Implications for psychiatry of left and right cerebral specialization. *Arch. Gen. Psychiatry* **31**, 572–583.

Galin, D. (1976). Hemispheric specialization: Implications for psychiatry. *In* "Biological Foundations of Psychiatry" (R. G. Grenell and S. Gabay, eds.), Vol. 1, pp. 145–176. Raven, New York.

Gazzaniga, M. S. (1967). The split brain in man. *Sci. Am.* **217**, 24–29.

Gazzaniga, M. S. (1974). Cerebral dominance viewed as a decision system. *In* "Hemisphere Function in the Human Brain" (S. J. Dimond and J. G. Beaumont, eds.), pp. 367–382. Wiley (Halsted), New York.

Geschwind, N. (1974). The anatomical basis of hemispheric differentiation. *In* "Hemisphere Function in the Human Brain" (S. J. Dimond and J. G. Beaumont, eds.), pp. 7–24. Wiley (Halsted), New York.

Getze, J. (1976). Driving Interstate 5: It's 55 or fight. *Los Angeles Times,* II, Aug. 25, p. 7.

Gifford, S., and Gunderson, J. G. (1970). Cushing's disease as a psychosomatic disorder: A selective review of the clinical and experimental literature and a report of ten cases. *Perspect. Biol. Med.* **13**, 169–221.

Gilbert, R. M. (1976). Caffeine as a drug of abuse. *In* "Research Advances in Alcohol and Drug Problems" (R. J. Gibbins *et al.*, eds.), Vol. 3. Wiley, New York. 49–176.

Glass, D. C. (1977). Stress, behavior patterns, and coronary disease. *Am. Sci.* **65**, 177–187.

Goldfien, A., and Ganong, W. F. (1962). Adrenal medullary and adrenal cortical response to stimulation of diencephalon. *Am. J. Physiol.* **202**, 205–211.

Gordon, T. (1967). Further mortality experience among Japanese Americans. *Public Health Rep.* **82**, 973–984.

Graham, T. W., Kaplan, B. H., Cornoni-Huntley, J. C., James, S. A., Becker, C., Hames, C. G., and Heyden, S. (1978). Frequency of church attendance and blood pressure elevation. *Arch. Intern. Med.* (in press).

Greenberg, R., and Pearlman, C. (1974). Cutting the REM nerve: An approach to the adaptive role of REM sleep. *Perspect. Biol. Med.* **17**, 513–521.

Greer, S., and Morris, T. (1975). Psychological attitudes of women who develop breast cancer: A controlled study. *J. Psychosom. Res.* **19**, 147–153.

Grim, C. E. (1973). Demonstration of elevated plasma aldosterone in low renin hypertension. *Clin. Res.* **21**, 493 (abstr.).

Grim, C. E. (1975). Low renin "essential" hypertension. A variant of classic primary aldosteronism? *Arch. Intern. Med.* **135**, 347–350 (editorial).

Groover, M. E., Jr., Seljeskog, E. L., Haglin, J. J., and Hitchcock, C. R. (1963). Myocardial infarction in the Kenya baboon without demonstrable atherosclerosis. *Angiology* **14**, 409–416.

Gunnells, J. C., Jr., McGuffin, W. L., Jr., Robinson, R. R., Grim, C. E., Wells, S., Silver, D., and Glenn, J. F. (1970). Hypertension, adrenal abnormalities, and alterations in plasma renin activity. *Ann. Intern. Med.* **73**, 901–911.

Gur, R. E., Gur, R. C., and Marshalek, B. (1975). Classroom seating and functional brain asymmetry. *J. Educ. Psychol.* **67**, 151–153.

Guthrie, R. D. (1976). "Body Hot Spots: The Anatomy of Human Social Organs and

Behavior." Van Nostrand-Reinhold, Princeton, New Jersey.

Gutmann, D. (1977). The cross-cultural perspective: Notes toward a comparative psychology of aging. *In* "Handbook of the Psychology of Aging (The Handbooks of Aging)" (J. E. Birren *et al.*, eds.), Chapter 14, pp. 302–326. Van Nostrand-Reinhold, Princeton, New Jersey.

Hall, K. R. L., and DeVore, I. (1965). Baboon social behavior. *In* "Primate Behavior: Field Studies of Monkeys and Apes" (I. DeVore, ed.), p. 58. Holt, New York.

Hallbäck, M. (1975). Interaction between central neurogenic mechanisms and changes in cardiovascular design in primary hypertension. Experimental studies in spontaneously hypertensive rats. *Acta Physiol. Scand., Suppl.* **424**.

Hallbäck, M., and Folkow, B. (1974). Cardiovascular responses to acute mental "stress" in spontaneously hypertensive rats. *Acta Physiol. Scand.* **90**, 684–698.

Halliday, J. L. (1949). "Psychosocial Medicine: A Study of the Sick Society." Heinemann, London.

Hamburg, B. A. (1974). The psychobiology of sex differences; an evolutionary perspective. *In* "Sex Differences in Behavior" (R. C. Friedman, R. M. Richart, and R. L. Vande Wiele, eds.), pp. 373–392. Wiley, New York.

Hamburg, B. A. (1978). The biosocial bases of sex difference. *In* "Perspectives on Human Evolution, Vol. 4: Human Evolution: Biosocial Perspectives" (S. L. Washburn and E. R. McCown, eds.). Holt, New York.

Hamburg, D. A. (1968). Evolution of emotional responses: Evidence from recent research on nonhuman primates. *Sci. Psychoanal.* **12**, 39–54.

Hamburg, D. A., and Adams, J. E. (1967). A perspective on coping behavior: Seeking and utilizing information in major transitions. *Arch. Gen. Psychiatry* **17**, 277–284.

Hamburg, D. A., Hamburg, B. A., and Barchas, J. D. (1975). Anger and depression in perspective of behavioral biology. *In* "Emotions: Their Parameters and Measurement" (L. Levi, ed.), pp. 235–278. Raven, New York.

Hanson, J. D., Larson, M. E., and Snowdon, C. T. (1976). The effects of control over high intensity noise on plasma cortisol levels in rhesus monkeys. *Behav. Biol.* **16**, 333–340.

Harlow, H. F., and Harlow, M. K. (1965). The affectional systems. *In* "Behavior of Nonhuman Primates: Modern Research Trends" (A. M. Schrier, H. F. Harlow, and F. Stollnitz, eds.), Vol. 2, Chapter 8, pp. 287–334. Academic Press, New York.

Harlow, H. F., and Harlow, M. K. (1970). Developmental aspects of emotional behavior. *In* "Physiological Correlates of Emotion" (P. Black, ed.), Chapter 3, pp. 37–58. Academic Press, New York.

Harlow, H. F., McGaugh, J. L., and Thompson, R. F. (1971). "Psychology." Albion Publ. Co., San Francisco, California.

Harris, A. H., Gilliam, W. J., Findley, J. D., and Brady, J. V. (1973). Instrumental conditioning of large magnitude, daily 12-hour blood pressure elevations in the baboon. *Science* **182**, 175–177.

Harris, R. E., and Singer, M. T. (1968). Interaction of personality and stress in the pathogenesis of essential hypertension. *In* "Hypertension: Neural Control of Arterial Pressure" (J. E. Wood, ed.), Vol. 16, pp. 104–111. Am. Heart Assoc., New York.

Havel, R. J. (1968). The autonomic nervous system and intermediary carbohydrate and fat metabolism. *Anesthesiology* **29**, 702–713.

Hawkins, N. G., Davies, R., and Holmes, T. H. (1957). Evidence of psychosocial factors in the development of pulmonary tuberculosis. *Am. Rev. Tuber. Pulm. Dis.* **75**, 768–780.

Haymaker, W., Anderson, E., and Nauta, W. J. H., eds. (1969). "The Hypothalamus" Chapter 4, pp. 136–209. Thomas, Springfield, Illinois.

Hennekens, C. H., Drölette, M. E., Jessee, M. J., Davies, J. E., and Hutchison, G. B. (1976). Coffee drinking and death due to coronary heart disease. *N. Engl. J. Med.* **294**, 633–636.

Hennevin, E., Leconte, P., and Bloch, V. (1974). Augmentation du sommeil paradoxal provoquée par l'acquisition, l'extinction et la réacquisition d'un apprentissage à renforcement positif. *Brain Res.* **70**, 43–54.

Henry, J. A., and Jarosz, C. J. (1977). Improved instrumentation for studying social activity in mouse colonies. (Unpublished Manuscript.)

Henry, J. A., Rader, R. D., Ely, D. L., and Henry, J. P. (1974). Instrumentation for studying social activity in mouse colonies. *Biotelemetry* **2**, 223–225.

Henry, J. P. (1976a). Understanding the early pathophysiology of essential hypertension. *Geriatrics* **30**, 59–72.

Henry, J. P. (1976b). Mechanisms of psychosomatic disease in animals. *Adv. Vet. Sci. Comp. Med.* **20**, 115–145.

Henry, J. P. (1977). Comment [on The cerebral hemispheres in analytical psychology by Ernest Rossi]. *J. Anal. Psychol.* **22** 52–57.

Henry, J. P., and Cassel, J. C. (1969). Psychosocial factors in essential hypertension: Recent epidemiologic and animal experimental evidence. *Am. J. Epidemiol.* **90**, 171–200.

Henry, J. P., and Ely, D. L. (1976). Biologic correlates of psychosomatic illness. *In* "Biological Foundations of Psychiatry" (R. G. Grenell and S. Gabay, eds.), Vol. 2, pp. 945–985. Raven, New York.

Henry, J. P., and Stephens, P. M. (1977). The social environment and essential hypertension in mice: Possible role of the innervation of the adrenal cortex. *Prog. Brain Res.* **47**: 263–276.

Henry, J. P., Meehan, J. P., Stephens, P., and Santisteban, G. A. (1965). Arterial pressure in CBA mice as related to age. *J. Gerontol.* **20**, 239–243.

Henry, J. P., Meehan, J. P., and Stephens, P. M. (1967). The use of psychosocial stimuli to induce prolonged systolic hypertension in mice. *Psychosom. Med.* **29**, 408–432.

Henry, J. P., Stephens, P. M., Axelrod, J., and Mueller, R. A. (1971a). Effect of psychosocial stimulation on the enzymes involved in the biosynthesis and metabolism of noradrenaline and adrenaline. *Psychosom. Med.* **33**, 227–237.

Henry, J. P., Ely, D. L., Stephens, P. M., Ratcliffe, H. L., Santisteban, G. A., and Shapiro, A. P. (1971b). The role of psychosocial factors in the development of arteriosclerosis in CBA mice: Observations on the heart, kidney, and aorta. *Atherosclerosis* **14**, 203–218.

Henry, J. P., Ely, D. L., and Stephens, P. M. (1972). Changes in catecholamine-controlling enzymes in response to psychosocial activation of the defence and alarm reactions. *Physiol. Emotion & Psychosom. Illness, Ciba Found. Symp., 1972* No. 8, pp. 225–251.

Henry, J. P., Ely, D. L., and Stephens, P. M. (1974). The role of psychosocial stimulation in the pathogenesis of hypertension. *Verh.*

Dtsch. Ges. Inn. Med. **80**, 107–111 and 1724–1740.

Henry, J. P., Ely, D. L., Watson, F. M. C., and Stephens, P. M. (1975a). Ethological methods as applied to the measurement of emotion. *In* "Emotions: Their Parameters and Measurement" (L. Levi, ed.), pp. 469–497. Raven, New York.

Henry, J. P., Stephens, P. M., and Santisteban, G. A. (1975b). A model of psychosocial hypertension showing reversibility and progression of cardiovascular complications. *Circ. Res.* **36**, 156–164.

Henry, J. P., Stephens, P. M., and Watson, F. M. C. (1975c). Force breeding, social disorder and mammary tumor formation in CBA/USC mouse colonies: A pilot study. *Psychosom. Med.* **37**, 277–283.

Henry, J. P., Kross, M. E., Stephens, P. M., and Watson, F. M. C. (1976). Evidence that differing psychosocial stimuli lead to adrenal cortical stimulation by autonomic or endocrine pathways. *In* "Catecholamines and Stress" (E. Usdin, R. Kvetňanský, and I. J. Kopin, eds.), pp. 457–468. Pergamon, Oxford.

Herd, J. A., Morse, W. H., Kelleher, R. T., and Jones, L. G. (1969). Arterial hypertension in the squirrel monkey during behavioral experiments. *Am. J. Physiol.* **217**, 24–29.

Hinde, R. A. (1974). "Biological Bases of Human Social Behaviour." McGraw-Hill, New York.

Hinde, R. A., and Spencer-Booth, Y. (1971). Effects of brief separation from mother on rhesus monkeys. *Science* **173**, 111–118.

Hines, N. O. (1962). "Proving Ground. An Account of the Radiobiological Studies in the Pacific, 1946–1961," p. 254. Univ. Washington Press, Seattle.

Hinkle, L. E., Jr. (1973). The concept of "stress" in the biological and social sciences. *Sci. Med. Man* **1**, 31–48.

Hinkle, L. E., Jr. (1974). The effect of exposure to culture change, social change, and changes in interpersonal relationships on health. *In* "Stressful Life Events: Their Nature and Effects" (B. S. Dohrenwend and B. P. Dohrenwend, eds.), pp. 9–45. Wiley, New York.

Hofer, M. A. (1976). The organization of sleep and wakefulness after maternal separation in young rats. *Dev. Psychobiol.* **9**, 189–205.

Hofer, M. A., Wolff, C. T., Friedman, S. B., and

Mason, J. W. (1972a). A psychoendocrine study of bereavement. Part I. 17-hydroxy-corticosteroid excretion rates of parents following death of their children from leukemia. *Psychosom. Med.* **34**, 481–491.

Hofer, M. A., Wolff, C. T., Friedman, S. B., and Mason, J. W. (1972b). A psychoendocrine study of bereavement. Part II. Observations on the process of mourning in relation to adrenocortical function. *Psychosom. Med.* **34**, 492–504.

Hoff, E. C., Kell, J. F., Jr., Hastings, N., Sholes, D. M., and Gray, E. H. (1951). Vasomotor, cellular and functional changes produced in kidney by brain stimulation. *J. Neurophysiol.* **14**, 317–332.

Hollender, M. H. (1970). The need or wish to be held. *Arch. Gen. Psychiatry* **22**, 445–453.

Hollender, M. H., and McGehee, J. B. (1974). The wish to be held during pregnancy. *J. Psychosom. Res.* **18**, 193–197.

Holmes, T. H., and Rahe, R. H. (1967). The social readjustment rating scale. *J. Psychosom. Res.* **11**, 213–218.

Hoppe, K. D. (1975). Liaison psychiatry and psychoanalysis. *In* "Liaison Psychiatry" (R. O. Posnau, ed.), pp. 103–109. Grune & Stratton, New York.

Horowitz, M. J. (1976). "Stress Response Syndromes." Jason Aronson, Inc., New York.

Insel, P. M., and Moos, R. H., eds. (1974). "Health and the Social Environment." Heath (Lexington Books), Lexington, Massachusetts.

Isaacson, R. L. (1974). "The Limbic System." Plenum, New York.

Ivens, W. G. (1930). "The Island Builders of the Pacific." Seeley, Service & Co., London.

Jacobi, J. (1959). "Complex/Archetype/Symbol in the Psychology of C. J. Jung" (transl. by R. Manheim), p. 42. Routledge & Kegan Paul, London.

Jacobson, E. (1970). "Modern Treatment of Tense Patients: Including the Neurotic and Depressed with Case Illustrations, Follow-ups, and EMG Measurements." Thomas, Springfield, Illinois.

Jarosz, C. J. (1977). Physiological and social concomitants of dominance in interacting colonies of CBA/USA mice. Ph.D. Dissertation (Physiology), University of Southern California, Los Angeles, California.

Jay, P. (1965). Field studies. *In* "Behavior of Nonhuman Primates: Modern Research Trends" (A. M. Schrier, H. F. Harlow, and F. Stollnitz, eds.), Vol. 2, Chapter 15, pp. 525–591. Academic Press, New York.

Jick, H., Miettinen, O. S., Neff, R. K., Shapiro, S., Heinonen, O. P., and Slone, D. (1973). Coffee and myocardial infarction. *N. Engl. J. Med.* **289**, 63–67.

Jonas, D., and Jonas, D. (1975). "Sex and Status." Stein & Day, New York.

Jones, M. T., Bridges, P. K., and Leak, D. (1970). Correlation between psychic and endocrinological responses to emotional stress. *Prog. Brain Res.* **32**, 325–335.

Jouvet, M. (1975). The function of dreaming: A neurophysiologist's point of view. *In* "Handbook of Psychobiology" (M. S. Gazzaniga and C. Blakemore, eds.), pp. 499–527. Academic Press, New York.

Jung, C. G. (1959). "The Archetypes and the Collective Unconscious" (transl. by R. F. C. Hull). Routledge & Kegan Paul, London.

Jung, C. G. (1961). "Memories, Dreams, Reflections" (A. Jaffe, ed., transl. by R. Winston and C. Winston). Pantheon Books, New York.

Jung, C. G. (1939). "The Integration of the Personality" (transl. by S. Dell). Farrar & Rinehart, New York.

June, C. G. (1958). "The Undiscovered Self" (transl. by R. F. C. Hull). Little, Brown, Boston, Massachusetts.

Jung, C. G. (1955). Personal communication.

Kagan, A. R., and Levi, L. (1974). Health and environment—psychosocial stimuli: A review. *Soc. Sci. Med.* **8**, 225–241.

Kaminer, B., and Lutz, W. P. (1960). Blood pressure in Bushmen of the Kalahari Desert. *Circulation* **22**, 289–295.

Kannel, W. B. (1974). The role of cholesterol in coronary atherogenesis. *Med. Clin. North Am.* **58**, 363–379.

Kannel, W. B., Castelle, W. P., McNamara, P. M., McKee, P. A., and Feinleib, M. (1972). Role of blood pressure in the development of congestive heart failure. *N. Engl. J. Med.* **287**, 781–787.

Kaplan, B. H. (1976). A note on religious beliefs and coronary heart disease. *J.S.C. Med. Assoc.* **72**, Suppl., 60–64.

Kaplan, B. H., Cassel, J. C., and Gore, S. (1977). Social support and health. *Med. Care* **15**, Suppl. 5, 47–58.

Kaplan, N. M. (1973). "Clinical Hypertension." Medcom Press, New York.

Katz, J. L., Gallagher, T., Hellman, L., Sachar, E., and Weiner, H. (1969). Psychoendocrine considerations in cancer of the breast. *Ann. N.Y. Acad. Sci.* **164**, 509–515.

Katz, J. L., Weiner, H., Gallagher, T. F., and Hellman, L. (1970). Stress, distress and ego defenses: Psychoendocrine response to impending breast tumor biopsy. *Arch. Gen. Psychiatry* **23**, 131–142.

Kaufman, I. C. (1974). Mother/infant relations in monkeys and humans: A reply to Professor Hinde. *In* "Ethology and Psychiatry" (N. F. White, ed.), Chapter 2, pp. 47–68. Univ. of Toronto Press, Toronto.

Kaufman, I. C., and Rosenblum, L. A. (1967). The reaction to separation in infant monkeys: Anaclitic depression and conservation-withdrawal. *Psychosom. Med.* **29**, 648–675.

Kawakami, M., Seto, K., Terasawa, E., Yoshida, K., Miyamoto, T., Sekiguchi, M., and Hattori, Y. (1968). Influence of electrical stimulation and lesion in limbic structure upon biosynthesis of adrencorticoid in the rabbit. *Neuroendocrinology* **3**, 337–348.

Kennell, J. H., Jerauld, R., Wolfe, H., Chesler, D., Kreger, N. C., McAlpine, W., Steffa, M., and Klaus, M. H. (1974). Maternal behavior one year after early and extended post-partum contact. *Dev. Med. Child Neurol.* **16**, 172–179.

Kennell, J. H., Trause, M. A., and Klaus, M. H. (1975). Evidence for a sensitive period in the human mother. *Parent-Infant Interact., Ciba Found. Symp., 1975* No. 33, pp. 87–101.

Kent, J. (1972). "The Solomon Islands." Stackpole Books, Harrisburg, Pennsylvania.

Keys, A., Aravanis, C., Blackburn, H., Van Buchem, F. S. P., Buzina, R., Djordjevic, B. S., Fidanza, F., Karvonen, M. J., Menotti, A., Puddu, V., and Taylor, H. L. (1972). Probability of middle-aged men developing coronary heart disease in 5 years. *Circulation* **45**, 815–828.

Kiritz, S., and Moos, R. H. (1974). Physiological effects of social environments. *Psychosom. Med.* **36**, 96–114.

Kissen, D. M. (1958). "Emotional Factors in Pulmonary Tuberculosis. An Evaluation of Psychological Factors in Onset and Relapse and Their Significance in Management, Treatment, and Prevention." Tavistock, London.

Kissen, D. M. (1960). A scientific approach to clinical research in psychosomatic medicine. *Psychosom. Med.* **22**, 118–126.

Kissen, D. M. (1965). Possible contribution of the psychosomatic approach to prevention of lung cancer. *Med. Off.* **114**, 343–345.

Kissen, D. M. (1967). Psychosocial factors, personality and lung cancer in men aged 55–64. *Br. J. Med. Psychol.* **40**, 29–43.

Kissen, D. M., and Eysenck, H. J. (1962). Personality in male lung cancer patients. *J. Psychosom. Res.* **6**, 123–127.

Kissen, D. M., and Rao, L. G. S. (1969). Steroid excretion patterns and personality in lung cancer. *Ann. N.Y. Acad. Sci.* **164**, 476–481.

Kissen, D. M., Brown, R. I. F., and Kissen, M. (1969). A further report on personality and psychosocial factors in lung cancer. *Ann. N.Y. Acad. Sci.* **164**, 535–544.

Kitahama, K., Valatx, J. L., and Jouvet, M. (1975). Action différente de l'a-méthyl DOPA sur le sommeil et l'acquisition d'un labyrinthe chez deux souches consanguines de Souris. *C.R. Hebd. Seance Acad. Sci., Ser. D* **280**, 471–474.

Kittinger, G. W., and Wexler, B. C. (1965). Adrenal gland dehydrogenases and corticosteroid production in normal and arteriosclerotic female rats. *Proc. Soc. Exp. Biol. Med.* **118**, 365–367.

Klaus, M. H., Jerauld, R., Kreger, N. C., McAlpine, W., Steffa, M., and Kennell, J. H. (1972). Maternal attachment: Importance of the first post-partum days. *N. Engl. J. Med.* **286**, 460–463.

Klaus, M. H., Trause, M. A., and Kennell, J. H. (1975). Does human maternal behaviour after delivery show a characteristic pattern? *Parent-Infant Interact., Ciba Found. Symp., 1975* No. 33, pp. 69–85.

Knapp, R., Hollenberg, N. K., Busch, G. J., and Abrams, H. L. (1972). Prolonged unilateral acute renal failure induced by intra-arterial norepinephrine infusion in the dog. *Invest. Radiol.* **7**, 164–173.

Koch, J., and Koch, L. (1976). The urgent drive to make good marriages better. *Psychol. Today* **10**, 33–34, 83, 85, and 95.

Komaroff, A. L., Masuda, M., and Holmes, T. H. (1968). The social readjustment rating scale: A comparative study of Negro, Mexican and white Americans. *J. Psychosom. Res.* **12**, 121–128.

Kropotkin, P. (1919). "Mutual Aid: A Factor of Evolution." Heinemann, London.

Kross, M. E. (1975). Neural modulation of adrenal cortical function in CBA and NZB mice. Ph.D. Dissertation (Physiology), University of Southern California, Los Angeles.

Kummer, H. (1968). "Social Organization of Hamadryas Baboons: A Field Study." Univ. of Chicago Press, Chicago, Illinois.

Kummer, H. (1971). "Primate Societies: Group Techniques of Ecological Adaptation (Worlds of Man Series)." Aldine-Atherton, Chicago, Illinois.

Kunin, C. M., and McCormack, R. C. (1968). An epidemiologic study of bacteriuria and blood pressure among nuns and working women. N. Engl. J. Med. 278, 635–642.

Kurtsin, I. T. (1976). "Theoretical Principles of Psychosomatic Medicine" (E. Lieber, ed., transl. by N. Kaner), Wiley, New York.

Kvetňanský, R., and Mikulaj, L. (1970). Adrenal and urinary catecholamines in rats during adaptation to repeated immobilization stress. Endocrinology 87, 738–743.

Kvetňanský, R., Weise, V. K., and Kopin, I. J. (1970). Elevation of adrenal tyrosine hydroxylase and phenylethanolamine-N-methyltransferase by repeated immobilization of rats. Endocrinology 87, 744–749.

Labarthe, D., Reed, D., Brody, J., and Stallones, R. (1973). Health effects of modernization in Palau. Am. J. Epidemiol. 98, 161–174.

Lang, I. M. (1975). Limbic system involvement in the vagosympathetic arterial pressor response of the rat. M.S. Thesis (Physiology and Biophysics), Temple University, Philadelphia, Pennsylvania.

Lang, I. M., Innes, D. L., and Tansy, M. F. (1975). Areas in the limbic system necessary to the operation of the arterial pressure reflex in the rat. Fed. Proc., Fed. Am. Soc. Exp. Biol. 34, 420. (abstr.).

Lapin, B. A., and Cherkovich, G. M. (1971). Environmental change causing the development of neuroses and corticovisceral pathology in monkeys. In "Society, Stress and Disease" (L. Levi, ed.), Vol. 1, pp. 266–280. Oxford Univ. Press, London and New York.

Lawrence, C. W., and Haynes, J. R. (1970). Epinephrine and nor-epinephrine effects on social dominance behavior. Psychol. Rep. 27, 195–198.

Lea, D. A. M., and Irwin, M. A. (1967). "New Guinea: The Territory and Its People." Oxford Univ. Press, Melbourne, Australia.

Lee, R. B. (1972) The !Kung Bushmen of Botswana. In "Hunters and Gatherers Today: A Socioeconomic Study of Eleven Such Cultures in the Twentieth Century" (M. G. Bicchieri, ed.), Chapter 8, pp. 327–368. Holt, New York.

Lehr, I., Messinger, H. B., and Rosenman, R. H. (1973). A sociobiological approach to the study of coronary heart disease. J. Chronic Dis. 26, 13–30.

LeShan, L. (1966). An emotional life-history pattern associated with neoplastic disease. Ann. N.Y. Acad. Sci. 125, 780–793.

Levi, L. (1967). Sympatho-adrenomedullary responses to emotional stimuli: Methodologic, physiologic, and pathologic considerations. In "An Introduction to Clinical Neuroendocrinology" (E. Bajusz, ed.), pp. 78–105. Karger, Basel.

Levine, S. (1969a). Infantile stimulation: A perspective. In "Stimulation in Early Infancy" (A. Ambrose, ed.), pp. 3–8. Academic Press, New York.

Levine, S. (1969b). An endocrine theory of infantile stimulation. In "Stimulation in Early Infancy" (A. Ambrose, ed.), pp. 45–54. Academic Press, New York.

Levy, J. (1974). Psychobiological implications of bilateral asymmetry. In "Hemisphere Function in the Human Brain" (S. J. Dimond and J. G. Beaumont, eds.), pp. 121–183. Wiley (Halsted Press), New York.

Lewis, J. K., McKinney, W. T., Jr., Young, L. D., and Kraemer, G. W. (1976). Mother-infant separation in rhesus monkeys as a model of human depression: A reconsideration. Arch. Gen. Psychiatry 33, 699–705.

Livingston, R. B. (1976). Sensory processing, perception, and behavior. In "Biological Foundations of Psychiatry" (R. G. Grenell and S. Gabay, eds.), Vol. 1, pp. 47–143. Raven Press, New York.

Louch, C. D., and Higginbotham, M. (1967). The relation between social rank and plasma corticosterone levels in mice. Gen. Comp. Endocrinol. 8, 441–444.

Lowenstein, F. W. (1961). Blood pressure in relation to age and sex in the tropics and subtropics. Lancet 1, 389–392.

Lucero, M. A. (1970). Lengthening of REM sleep duration consecutive to learning in the rat. Brain Res. 20, 319–322.

Lundgren, Y. (1974a). Regression of structural cardiovascular changes after reversal of experimental renal hypertension in rats.

Acta Physiol. Scand. **91**, 275–285.

Lundgren, Y. (1974b). Adaptive changes of cardiovascular design in spontaneous and renal hypertension: Hemodynamic studies in rats. *Acta Physiol. Scand., Suppl.* **408**.

Lutwak, L., Whedon, G. D., Lachance, P. A., Reid, J. M., and Lipscomb, H. S. (1969). Mineral, electrolyte and nitrogen balance studies of the Gemini-VII fourteen-day orbital space flight. *J. Clin. Endocrinol. Metab.* **29**, 1140–1156.

McBroom, P. (1975). Study of disease in MDs clarifies psychic factors. *Med. Trib.* **16**, Aug. 27, 1 and 15.

McClosky, H., and Schaar, J. H. (1965). Psychological dimensions of anomy. *Am. Sociol. Rev.* **30**, 14–40.

McCubbin, J. W., Green, J. H., and Page, I. H. (1956). Baroreceptor function in chronic renal hypertension. *Circ. Res.* **4**, 205–210.

McHugh, P. R., and Smith, G. P. (1967). Plasma 17-OHCS response to amygdaloid stimulation with and without afterdischarges. *Am. J. Physiol.* **212**, 619–622.

Maclay, G., and Knipe, H. (1972). "The Dominant Man: The Pecking Order in Human Society." Delacorte Press, New York.

MacLean, P. D. (1958). Contrasting functions of limbic and neocortical systems of the brain and their relevance to psychophysiological aspects of medicine. *Am. J. Med.* **25**, 611–626.

MacLean, P. D. (1975). Brain mechanisms of primal sexual functions and related behavior. *In* "Sexual Behavior, Pharmacology and Biochemistry" (M. Sandler and G. L. Gessa, eds.), pp. 1–11. Raven, New York.

MacLean, P. D. (1976). Sensory and perceptive factors in emotional functions of the triune brain. *In* "Biological Foundations of Psychiatry" (R. G. Grenell and S. Gabay, eds.), Vol. 1, pp. 177–198. Raven, New York.

Maddocks, I. (1967). Blood pressures in Melanesians. *Med. J. Aust.* **1**, 1123–1126.

Marmot, M. G. (1975). Acculturation and coronary heart disease in Japanese-Americans. Ph.D. Dissertation (Epidemiology), University of California, Berkeley.

Marmot, M. G., and Syme, S. L. (1976). Acculturation and coronary heart disease in Japanese-Americans. *Am. J. Epidemiol.* **104**, 225–247.

Marmot, M. G., Syme, S. L., Kagan, A., Kato, H., Cohen, J. B., and Belsky, J. (1975). Epidemiologic studies of coronary heart disease and stroke in Japanese men living in Japan, Hawaii and California: Prevalence of coronary and hypertensive heart disease and associated risk factors. *Am. J. Epidemiol.* **102**, 514–525.

Marty, P., and M'Uzan, M. de (1963). La "pensée, opératoire." *Rev. Fr. Psychoanal.* **27**, 345–356.

Marx, M. B., Garrity, T. F., and Bowers, F. R. (1975). The influence of recent life experience on the health of college freshmen. *J. Psychosom. Res.* **19**, 87–98.

Mason, J. W. (1968a). A review of psychoendocrine research on the pituitary-adrenal cortical system. *Psychosom. Med.* **30**, 576–607.

Mason, J. W. (1968b). A review of psychoendocrine research on the sympathetic-adrenal medullary system. *Psychosom. Med.* **30**, 631–653.

Mason, J. W., Maher, J. T., Hartley, L. H., Mougey, E. H., Perlow, M. J., and Jones, L. G. (1976). Selectivity of corticosteroid and catecholamine responses to various natural stimuli. *In* "Psychopathology of Human Adaptation" (G. Serban, ed.), pp. 147–171. New York: Plenum Publishing Corp., New York.

Masuda, M. (1976). Life events, life event perceptions, and life style. *Psychosom. Med.* **38**, 66. (abstr.).

Masuda, M., and Holmes, T. H. (1967). The social readjustment rating scale: A cross-cultural study of Japanese and Americans. *J. Psychosom. Res.* **11**, 227–237.

Matsumoto, Y. S. (1970). Social stress and coronary heart disease in Japan. A hypothesis. *Milbank Mem. Fund Q.* **48**, 9–36.

Mikhail, Y., and Amin, F. (1969). Intrinsic innervation of the human adrenal gland. *Acta Anat.* **72**, 25–32.

Mikulaj, L., and Kvetňanský, R. (1966). Changes in adrenocortical activity prior to and following adaptation to trauma in the Noble-Collip drum. *Physiol. Bohemoslov.* **15**, 439–446.

Mikulaj, L., and Mitro, A. (1973). Endocrine functions during adaptation to stress. *Adv. Exp. Med. Biol.* **33**, 631–638.

Mitchell, R. E. (1971). Some social implications of high-density housing. *Am. Sociol. Rev.* **36**, 18–29.

Moberg, G. P., Scapagnini, U., De Groot, J., and Ganong, W. F. (1971). Effect of sectioning the fornix on diurnal fluctuation in plasma corticosterone levels in the rat. *Neuroendocrinology* **7**, 11–15.

Montagu, A. (1971). "Touching: The Human Significance of the Skin." Columbia Univ. Press, New York.

Mühlbock, O. (1956). The hormonal genesis of mammary cancer. *Adv. Cancer Res.* **4**, 371–391.

Murrill, R. I. (1949). A blood pressure study of the natives of Ponape Island, Eastern Carolines. *Hum. Biol.* **21**, 47–59.

Muul, I. (1970). Intra- and inter-familial behaviour of *Glaucomys volans* (rodentia) following parturition. *Anim. Behav.* **18**, 20–25.

Nauta, W. J. H. (1971). The problem of the frontal lobe: A reinterpretation. *J. Psychiatr. Res.* **8**, 167–187.

Nemiah, J. C., and Sifneos, P. E. (1970). Affect and fantasy in patients with psychosomatic disorders. *In* "Modern Trends in Psychosomatic Medicine" (O. W. Hill, ed.), Vol. 2, pp. 26–34. Appleton, New York.

Neumann, E. (1954). "The Origins and History of Consciousness" (transl. by R. F. C. Hull). Routledge & Kegan Paul, London.

Newberry, B. H., Gildow, J., Wogan, J., and Reese, R. L. (1976). Inhibition of Huggins tumors by forced restraint. *Psychosom. Med.* **38**, 155–162.

Noirot, E., and Goyens, J. (1971). Changes in maternal behavior during gestation in the mouse. *Horm. Behav.* **2**, 207–215.

Noirot, E., Goyens, J., and Buhot, M.-C. (1975). Aggressive behavior of pregnant mice toward males. *Horm. Behav.* **6**, 9–17.

Nuckolls, K. B., Cassel, J., and Kaplan, B. H. (1972). Psychosocial assets, life crisis and the prognosis of pregnancy. *Am. J. Epidemiol.* **95**, 431–441.

O'Keefe, J., and Dostrovsky, J. (1971). The hippocampus as a spatial map. Preliminary evidence from unit activity in the freely-moving rat. *Brain Res.* **34**, 171–175.

O'Keefe, J., Nadel, L., Keightley, S., and Kill, D. (1975). Fornix lesions selectively abolish place learning in the rat. *Exp. Neurol.* **48**, 152–166.

Olds, J. (1976). Behavioral studies of hypothalamic functions: Drives and reinforcements. *In* "Biological Foundations of Psychiatry" (R. G. Grenell and S. Gabay, eds.), Vol. 1, pp. 321–447. Raven, New York.

Oliver, W. J., Cohen, E. L., and Neel, J. V. (1975). Blood pressure, sodium intake, and sodium related hormones in the Yanomamö Indians, a "no-salt" culture. *Circulation* **52**, 146–151.

Ornstein, R. E. (1972). "The Psychology of Consciousness." Freeman, San Francisco, California.

Ornstein, R. E. ed. (1973). "The Nature of Human Consciousness: A Book of Readings." Freeman, San Francisco, California.

Page, I. H. (1949). Pathogenesis of arterial hypertension. *J. Am. Med. Assoc.* **140**, 451–458.

Page, I. H., and McCubbin, J. W. (1965). The physiology of arterial hypertension. *Hand. Physiol., Sect. 2: Circ.* **3**, 2163–2208.

Page, L. B. (1976). Epidemiologic evidence on the etiology of human hypertension and its possible prevention. *Am. Heart J.* **91**, 527–534.

Page, L. B., Damon, A., and Moellering, R. C., Jr. (1974). Antecedents of cardiovascular disease in six Solomon Islands societies. *Circulation* **49**, 1132–1146.

Papez, J. W. (1937). A proposed mechanism of emotion. *Arch. Neurol. Psychiatry* **38**, 725–743.

Parkes, C. M., Benjamin, B., and Fitzgerald, R. G. (1969). Broken heart: A statistical study of increased mortality among widowers. *Br. Med. J.* **1**, 740–743.

Patel, C. H. (1973). Yoga and bio-feedback in the management of hypertension. *Lancet* **2**, 1053–1055.

Patel, C. H. (1975a). 12-month follow-up of yoga and bio-feedback in the management of hypertension. *Lancet* **1**, 62–64.

Patel, C. H. (1975b). Yoga and biofeedback in the management of "stress" in hypertensive patients. *Clin. Sci. Mol. Med.* **48**, Suppl. 2, 171–174.

Patel, C. H. (1976). Reduction of serum cholesterol and blood pressure in hypertensive patients by behaviour modification. *J. R. Coll. Gen. Pract.* **26**, 211–215.

Patel, C. H. (1977). Biofeedback-aided relaxation and meditation in the management of hypertension. *Biofeedback Self-Regul.* **2**, 1–41.

Patel, C. H., and Carruthers, M. (1977). Coronary risk factor reduction by biofeedback-aided relaxation and meditation. *J. R. Coll. Gen. Pract.* **27**:401–405.

Patel, C. H., and North, W. R. S. (1975). Randomised controlled trial of yoga and biofeedback in management of hypertension. *Lancet* **2**, 93–95.

Paul, M. I., Kvetňanský, R., Cramer, H., Silbergeld, S., and Kopin, I. J. (1971). Immobilization stress induced changes in adrenocortical and medullary cyclic AMP content in the rat. *Endocrinology* **88**, 338–343.

Pearlman, C., and Becker, M. (1973). Brief post-trial REM sleep deprivation impairs discrimination learning in rats. *Physiol. Psychol.* **1**, 373–376.

Pisa, M. (1976). Impaired incidental place learning in fornicotomized rats. *Neuroscience* **2**, Part 1, 373 (abstr.).

Price, J. (1967). The dominance hierarchy and the evolution of mental illness. *Lancet* **2**, 243–246.

Price, J. S. (1969). The ritualization of agonistic behaviour as a determinant of variation along the neuroticism/stability dimension of personality. *Proc. R. Soc. Med.* **62**, 1107–1110.

Prior, I. (1976). Civilization and cardiovascular changes—a Pacific viewpoint. *Doc. Geigy* pp. 2–3.

Prior, I. A. M., Evans, J. G., Harvey, H. P. B., Davidson, F., and Lindsey, M. (1968). Sodium intake and blood pressure in two Polynesian populations. *N. Engl. J. Med.* **279**, 515–520.

Rabkin, J. G., and Struening, E. L. (1976). Life events, stress, and illness. *Science* **191**, 1013–1020.

Rader, R. D., Stevens, C. M., Meehan, J. P., and Henry, J. P. (1974). Instrumentation for renal hemodynamic studies in unrestrained dogs. *Biotelemetry* **2**, 158–160.

Rahe, R. H. (1972). Subjects' recent life changes and their near-future illness reports. *Ann. Clin. Res.* **4**, 250–265.

Rahe, R. H. (1974). The pathway between subjects' recent life changes and their near-future illness reports: Representative results and methodological issues. *In* "Stressful Life Events: Their Nature and Effects" (B. S. Dohrenwend and B. P. Dohrenwend, eds.), pp. 73–86. Wiley, New York.

Rahe, R. H. (1976). Stress and strain in coronary heart disease. *J. S. C. Med. Assoc.* **72**, Suppl., 7–14.

Rahe, R. H., and Arthur, R. J. (1978). Life change and illness studies: Past history and future directions. *Psychother. Psychosom.* (in press).

Rahe, R. H., Romo, M., Bennett, L., and Siltanen, P. (1974a). Recent life changes, myocar-

dial infarction, and abrupt coronary death. *Arch. Intern. Med.* **133**, 221–228.

Rahe, R. H., Fløistad, I., Bergan, T., Ringdal, R., Gerhardt, R., Gunderson, E. K. E., and Arthur, R. J. (1974b). A model for life changes and illness research: cross-cultural data from the Norwegian navy. *Arch. Gen. Psychiatry* **31**, 172–177.

Rapp, J. P., and Dahl, L. K. (1971). 18-hydroxy-deoxycorticosterone secretion in experimental hypertension in rats. *Circ. Res.* **28/29**, Suppl. 2, 153–159.

Rapp, J. P. Knudsen, K. D., Iwai, J., and Dahl, L. K. (1973). Genetic control of blood pressure and corticosteroid production in rats. *Circ. Res.* **32/33**, Suppl. 1, 139–149.

Ratcliffe, H. L., Luginbühl, H., Schnarr, W. R., and Chacko, K. (1969). Coronary arteriosclerosis in swine: Evidence of a relation to behavior. *J. Comp. Physiol. Psychol.* **68**, 385–392.

Reimer, J. D., and Petras, M. L. (1967). Breeding structure of the house mouse, *Mus, musculus,* in a population cage. *J. Mammal.* **48**, 88–99.

Reite, M., Kaufman, I. C., Pauley, J. D., and Stynes, A. J. (1974). Depression in infant monkeys: Physiological correlates. *Psychosom. Med.* **36**, 363–367.

Reynolds, V. (1976). "The Biology of Human Action." Freeman, San Francisco, California.

Richter, C. P. (1957). On the phenomenon of sudden death in animals and man. *Psychosom. Med.* **19**, 191–198.

Riley, V. (1975). Mouse mammary tumors: Alteration of incidence as apparent function of stress. *Science* **189**, 465–467.

Ringler, N. M., Kennell, J. H., Jarvella, R., Navojosky, B. J., and Klaus, M. H. (1975). Mother-to-child speech at 2 years—effects of early postnatal contact. *Behav. Pediatr.* **86**, 141–144.

Robbins, S. L., and Angell, M. (1976). "Basic Pathology," 2nd ed., p. 440. Saunders, Philadelphia, Pennsylvania.

Roldán, E., Alvarez-Pelaez, R., and Fernandez de Molina, A. (1974). Electrographic study of the amygdaloid defense response. *Physiol. Behav.* **13**, 779–787.

Rolls, E. T. (1975). "The Brain and Reward." Pergamon, Oxford.

Rose, R. M., Bernstein, I. S., and Gordon, T. P. (1975). Consequences of social conflict on plasma testosterone levels in rhesus monkeys. *Psychosom. Med.* **37**, 50–61.

Rosenman, R. H. (1971). The central nervous system and coronary heart disease. *Hosp. Pract.* **6**, 87–97.

Rosenman, R. H. (1976). Personality factors in the pathogenesis of coronary heart disease. *J. S. C. Med. Assoc.* **72**, 38–44.

Rosenman, R. H., Brand, R. J., Jenkins, C. D., Friedman, M., Straus, R., and Wurm, M. (1975). Coronary heart disease in the Western Collaborative Group Study. Final follow-up experience of $8\frac{1}{2}$ years. *J. Am. Med. Assoc.* **233**, 872–877.

Rosenman, R. H., Brand, R. J., Sholtz, R. I., and Friedman, M. (1976). Multivariate prediction of coronary heart disease during 8.5 year follow-up in the Western Collaborative Group Study. *Am. J. Cardiol.* **37**, 903–910.

Rossi, E. (1977). The cerebral hemispheres in analytical psychology. *J. Anal. Psychol.* **22**, 32–51.

Russell, R. P., and Masi, A. T. (1973). Significant associations of adrenal cortical abnormalities with "essential" hypertension. *Am. J. Med.* **54**, 44–51.

Russo, N. J., II, Kapp, B. S., Holmquist, B. K., and Musty, R. E. (1976). Passive avoidance and amygdala lesions: Relationship with pituitary-adrenal system. *Physiol. Behav.* **16**, 191–199.

Sachar, E. J., Fishman, J. R., and Mason, J. W. (1965). Influence of the hypnotic trance on plasma 17-hydroxycorticosteroid concentration. *Psychosom. Med.* **27**, 330–341.

Sachar, E. J. (1976). Neuroendocrine abnormalities in depressive illness. *In* "Topics in Psychoendocrinology" (E. J. Sachar, ed.), pp. 135–156. Greene and Stratton, Inc., New York.

Sackett, G. P. (1968). Abnormal behavior in laboratory-reared rhesus monkeys. *In* "Abnormal Behavior in Animals" (M. W. Fox, ed.), Chapter 18, pp. 293–331. Saunders, Philadelphia, Pennsylvania.

Saddhatissa, H. (1971). "The Buddha's Way," p. 56. Allen & Unwin, London.

Salk, L. (1973). The role of the heartbeat in the relations between mother and infant. *Sci. Am.* **228**, 24–29.

Sassenrath, E. N. (1970). Increased adrenal responsiveness related to social stress in rhesus monkeys. *Horm. Behav.* **1**, 238–298.

Sassenrath, E. N. (1977). Weaning strategies and behavioral sequelae in colony-born rhesus infants (abstract). First Annual Meeting of the American Society of Primatologists, Seattle, Washington, April 16–19, 1977.

Schwartz, G. E., Davidson, R. J., and Maer, F. (1975). Right hemisphere lateralization for emotion in the human brain: Interactions with cognition. *Science* **190**, 286–288.

Scotch, N. A. (1960). Preliminary report on the relation of sociocultural factors to hypertension among the Zulu. *Ann. N.Y. Acad. Sci.* **84**, 1000–10009.

Scotch, N. A. (1963). Sociocultural factors in the epidemiology of Zulu hypertension. *Am. J. Public Health* **53**, 1205–1213.

Seligman, M. E. P. (1975). "Helplessness: On Depression, Development, and Death." Freeman, San Francisco, California.

Selye, H. (1950). "The Physiology and Pathology of Exposure to Stress." Acta, Inc., Montreal.

Selye, H. (1970). The evolution of the stress concept. *Am. J. Cardiol.* **26**, 289–299.

Selye, H. (1974). "Stress Without Distress." Lippincott, Philadelphia, Pennsylvania.

Shaper, A. G. (1972). Cardiovascular disease in the tropics. III. Blood pressure and hypertension. *Br. Med. J.* **3**, 805–807.

Shaper, A. G. (1974). Communities without hypertension. *In* "Cardiovascular Disease in the Tropics" (A. G. Shaper, M. S. R. Hutt, and Z. Fejfar, eds.), pp. 77–83, Br. Med. Assoc., London.

Shapiro, A. P. (1963). Experimental pyelonephritis and hypertension: Implications for the clinical problem. *Ann. Intern. Med.* **59**, 37–52.

Shapiro, A. P., Scheib, E. T., and Crocker, B. (1968). Letter to editor. *Psychosom. Med.* **30**, 347.

Shapiro, A. P., Sapira, J. D., and Scheib, E. T. (1971). Development of bacteriuria in a hypertensive population: A 7-year follow-up study. *Ann. Intern. Med.* **74**, 861–868.

Shapiro, A. P., Schwartz, G. E., Ferguson, D. C. E., Redmond, D. P., and Weiss, S. M. (1977). Behavioral methods in the treatment of hypertension. *Ann. Intern. Med.* **86**, 626–636.

Shepher, J. (1971). Self-imposed incest avoidance and exogamy in second generation kibbutz adults. Ph.D. Thesis (Anthropology), Rutgers University, New Brunswick, New Jersey (University Microfilms, Ann Arbor, Michigan).

Sifneos, P. E., Savitz, R. A., and Frankel, F. H. (1977). The phenomenon of "alexithymia": Observations in neurotic and psychosomatic patients. *Psychother. Psychosom.* (in press).

Silberbauer, G. B. (1972): The G/wi Bushmen. *In* "Hunters and Gatherers Today: A Socioeconomic Study of Eleven Such Cultures in the Twentieth Century" (M. G. Bicchieri, ed.), Chapter 7, pp. 271–326. Holt, New York.

Sivertsson, R. (1970). The hemodynamic importance of structural vascular changes in essential hypertension. *Acta Physiol. Scand, Suppl.* **343**.

Sleight, P. (1975). Baroreceptor function in hypertension. *In* "Pathophysiology and Management of Arterial Hypertension" (C. Berglund, L. Hansson, and L. Werkö, eds.), pp. 45–53. A. Lindgren & Söner AB, Mölndal, Sweden.

Smith, C. I., Kitahama, K., Valatx, J. L., and Jouvet, M. (1974). Increased paradoxical sleep in mice during acquisition of a shock avoidance task. *Brain Res.* **77**, 221–230.

Snyder, R. L. (1968). Reproduction and population pressures. *Prog. Physiol. Psychol.* **2**, 119–160.

Southwick, C. H. (1967). An experimental study of intragroup agonistic behavior in rhesus monkeys *(Macaca mulatta). Behaviour* **28**, 182–209.

Spencer-Booth, Y., and Hinde, R. A. (1971). Effects of 6 days separation from mother on 18- to 32-week old rhesus monkeys. *Anim. Behav.* **19**, 174–191.

Sperry, R. W. (1974). Lateral specialization in the surgically separated hemispheres. *In* "The Neurosciences: Third Study Program" (F. O. Schmitt and F. G. Worden, eds.), pp. 5–19. MIT Press, Cambridge, Massachusetts.

Stevens, S. S. (1966). A metric for the social consensus. *Science* **151**, 530–541.

Stone, R. A., and DeLeo, J. (1976). Psychotherapeutic control of hypertension. *N. Engl. J. Med.* **294**, 80–84.

Stout, C., Morrow, J., Brandt, E. N., Jr., and Wolf, S. (1964). Unusually low incidence of death from myocardial infarction. Study of an Italian American community in Pennsylvania. *J. Am. Med. Assoc.* **188**, 845–849.

Taggart, P., and Carruthers, M. (1971). Endoge-

nous hyperlipidaemia induced by emotional stress of racing driving. *Lancet* **1**, 363–366.

Taggart, P., and Carruthers, M. (1972). Suppression by oxprenolol of adrenergic response to stress. *Lancet* **2**, 256–258.

Theorell, T., and Rahe, R. H. (1975). Life change events, ballistocardiography and coronary death. *J. Hum. Stress* **1**, 18–24.

Thoenen, H., Mueller, R. A., and Axelrod, J. (1969). Trans-synaptic induction of adrenal tyrosine hydroxylase. *J. Pharmacol. Exp. Ther.* **169**, 249–254.

Thomas, C. B. (1973). The relationship of smoking and habits of nervous tension. *In* "Smoking Behavior: Motives and Incentives" (W. L. Dunn, Jr., ed.), pp. 157–170. Wiley, New York.

Thomas, C. B., and Duszynski, K. R. (1974). Closeness to parents and the family constellation in a prospective study of five disease states: Suicide, mental illness, malignant tumor, hypertension and coronary heart disease. *Johns Hopkins Med. J.* **134**, 251–270.

Thomas, C. B., Ross, D. C., and Duszynski, K. R. (1975). Youthful hypercholesteremia: Its associated characteristics and role in premature myocardial infarction. *Johns Hopkins Med. J.* **136**, 193–208.

Thomson, D. S., and the Editors of Time-Life Books. (1975). "Language." Time-Life Books, New York.

Tiger, L. (1969). "Men in Groups." Random House, New York.

Tiger, L., and Fox, R. (1972). "The Imperial Animal." Secker & Warburg, London.

Tiger, L., and Shepher, J. (1975). "Women in the Kibbutz." Harcourt, New York.

Toffler, A. (1970). "Future Shock." Random House, New York.

Toynbee, A. (1972). "A Study of History." London: Oxford Univ. Press.

Trevarthen, C. (1974). Analysis of cerebral activities that generate and regulate consciousness in commissurotomy patients. *In* "Hemisphere Function in the Human Brain" (S. J. Dimond and J. G. Beaumont, eds.), p. 254. Wiley (Halsted Press), New York.

Truswell, A. S., Kennelly, B. M., Hansen, J. D. L., and Lee, R. B. (1972). Blood pressures of !Kung Bushmen in Northern Botswana, *Am. Heart J.* **84**, 5–12.

Turnbull, C. M. (1972). "The Mountain People." Simon & Schuster, New York.

Tyroler, H. A., and Cassel, J. (1964). Health consequences of culture change. II. The effect of urbanization on coronary heart mortality in rural residents. *J. Chronic Dis.* **17**, 167–177.

Unsicker, K. (1971). On the innervation of the rat and pig adrenal cortex. *Z. Zellforsch. Mikrosk. Anat.* **116**, 151–156.

Vander, A. J., Mouw, D. R., Kay, L., Henry, J. P., and Stephens, P. M. (1977). Plasma renin activity in psychosocial hypertension of CBA mice. (In preparation.) Circ. Res.

Van der Post, L. (1961). "The Heart of the Hunter." Hogarth Press, London.

Van Lawick-Goodall, J. (1971). "In the Shadow of Man." Houghton, Boston, Massachusetts.

Van Lawick-Goodall, J. (1973). The behavior of champanzees in their natural habitat. *Am. J. Psychiatry* **130**, 1–12.

Van Loon, G. R., Scapagnini, U., Moberg, G. P., and Ganong, W. F. (1971). Evidence for central adrenergic neural inhibition of ACTH secretion in the rat. *Endocrinology* **89**, 1464–1469.

von Holst, D. (1972). Renal failure as the cause of death in *Tupaia belangeri* (tree shrews) exposed to persistent social stress. *J. Comp. Physiol.* **78**, 236–273.

Wardwell, W. I., Hyman, M., and Bahnson, C. F. (1968). Socio-environmental antecedents to coronary heart disease in 87 white males. *Soc. Sci. Med.* **2**, 165–183.

Washburn, S. L., and Hamburg, D. A. (1968). Aggressive behavior in old world monkeys and apes. *In* "Primates: Studies in Adaptation and Variability" (P. Jay, ed.), pp. 458–468. Holt, New York.

Watson, F. M. C. (1972). Social psychophysiological consequences of early experience in CBA mice. Ph.D. Dissertation (Physiology), University of Southern California, Los Angeles.

Watson, F. M. C., and Henry, J. P. (1977a). Loss of socialized patterns of behavior in mouse colonies following daily sleep disturbance and maturation. *Physiol. Behav.* **18**, 119–123.

Watson, F. M. C., and Henry, J. P. (1977b). The effect of isolation on maternal behavior in mice. *Behav. Biol.* (accepted for publication).

Watson, F. M. C., Henry, J. P., and Haltmeyer,

G. C. (1974). Effects of early experience on emotional and social reactivity in CBA mice. *Physiol. Behav.* **13**, 9–14.

Weber, H. W., and Van der Walt, J. J. (1973). Cardiomyopathy in crowded rabbits: A preliminary report. *S. Afr. Med. J.* **47**, 1591–1595.

Weiland, H., and Sperber, Z. (1970). Patterns of mother-infant contact: The significance of lateral preference. *J. Genet. Psychol.* **117**, 157–165.

Weiner, H. (1975). Are "psychosomatic" diseases, diseases of regulation? *Psychosom. Med.* **37**, 289–291 (editorial).

Weiner, H. (1977). "Psychobiology and Human Disease." Am. Elsevier, New York.

Weiss, J. M. (1971a). Effects of coping behavior in different warning signal conditions on stress pathology in rats. *J. Comp. Physiol. Psychol.* **77**, 1–13.

Weiss, J. M. (1971b). Effects of coping behavior with and without a feedback signal on stress pathology in rats. *J. Comp. Physiol. Psychol.* **77**, 22–30.

Weiss, J. M. (1972a). Psychological factors in stress and disease. *Sci. Am.* **226**, 104–113.

Weiss, J. M. (1972b). Influence of psychological variables on stress-induced pathology. *Physiol., Emotion & Psychosom. Illness, Ciba Found. Symp., 1972* No. 8, pp. 253–265.

Weiss, J. M., Glazer, H. I., Pohorecky, L. A., Brick, J., and Miller, N. E. (1975). Effects of chronic exposure to stressors on avoidance-escape behavior and on brain norepinephrine. *Psychosom. Med.* **37**, 522–534.

Weiss, J. M., Pohorecky, L. A., Salman, S., and Gruenthal, M. (1976). Attenuation of gastric lesions by psychological aspects of aggression in rats. *J. Comp. Physiol. Psychol.* **90**, 252–259.

Weiss, L. (1974). Aspects of the relation between functional and structural cardiovascular factors in primary hypertension: Experimental studies in spontaneously hypertensive rats. *Acta Physiol. Scand. Suppl.* **409**.

Weiss, R. S. (1969). The fund of sociability. Relationships with other people are essential and their loss can be traumatic. *Trans-Action* **6**, 36–43.

Wexler, B. C. (1964a). Spontaneous arteriosclerosis in repeatedly bred male and female rats. *J. Atheroscler. Res.* **4**, 57–80.

Wexler, B. C. (1964b) Correlation of adrenocortical histopathology with arteriosclerosis in breeder rats. *Acta Endocrinol. (Copenhagen)* **46**, 613–631.

White, R. E. C. (1971). WRATS: A computer compatible system for automatically recording and transcribing behavioral data. *Behaviour* **40**, 135–161.

Wilhelmsen, L., Tibblin, G., Elmfeldt, D., Wedel, H., and Werkö, L. (1977). Coffee consumption and coronary heart disease in middle-aged Swedish men. *Acta Med. Scand.* **201**:547–552.

Wilson, E. O. (1975). "Sociobiology: The New Synthesis," pp. 3 and 563. Harvard Univ. Press (Belknap), Cambridge, Massachusetts.

Wolf, S. (1976). Protective social forces that counterbalance stress. *J. S. C. Med. Assoc.* **72**, 57–59.

Wolf, S., and Goodell, H., eds. (1968). "Harold G. Wolff's Stress and Disease," 2nd ed. Thomas, Springfield, Illinois.

Wolinsky, H. (1970). Response of the rat aortic media to hypertension. *Circ. Res.* **26**, 507–522.

Wolinsky, H. (1971). Effects of hypertension and its reversal on the thoracic aorta of male and female rats. *Circ. Res.* **28**, 622–637.

Wolinsky, H. (1972). Long-term effects of hypertension on the rat aortic wall and their relation to concurrent aging changes. *Circ. Res.* **30**, 301–309.

Wynne-Edwards, V. C. (1962a). The role of threat. *In* "Animal Dispersion in Relation to Social Behavior," pp. 129–131. Oliver & Boyd, Edinburgh.

Wynne-Edwards, V. C. (1962b). *In* "Animal Dispersion in Relation to Social Behaviour," Chapter 12, pp. 223–254. Oliver & Boyd, Edinburgh.

Zanchetti, A., and Stella, A. (1975). Neural control of renin release. *Clin. Sci. Mol. Med.* **48**, 215–223.

Zuckerman, S. (1932). "The Social Life of Monkeys and Apes." Harcourt, New York.

Glossary of sociobiologic terms

alexithymia. Alexithymia is a condition in which feelings exist but are denied. Characterized by an absence of fantasy and dreams, action is the predominant way of life. An alexithymic person engages in elaborate descriptions of trivial environmental details and has poor interpersonal relationships (see Type A personality).

anomie. Anomie, which Durkheim, a sociologist, linked to increased suicide rates involves disturbance of the value system. It occurs during dissolution of social order when the cultural canon has been fragmented and has lost its authority. Anomie is prevalent during civil warfare and violence and is associated with a breakdown of the family and disruption of attachment bonds. Lacking social support, individuals are exposed to excessive arousal of the fight–flight and depressive responses and become vulnerable to psychopathology and pathophysiology (see cultural canon).

archetype. Archetype was the term Jung applied to the biologic patterns of behavior whose roots are in what he called "the collective unconscious"; the structures of the limbic system, such as the amygdala and hippocampus, may be involved. This inborn biogrammar of instinctual drive mechanisms finds its normal expression perhaps by way of the right hemisphere in themes of dreams, myths, and symbols and is clothed in technical and dogmatic expression by the rational-empirical left hemisphere. The female's nurturant attachment and the male's territoriality are expressions of archetypal patterns (see instinct; biogrammar).

attachment. Attachment or love or the affectional system is a mechanism whereby members of a social order are bonded together for mutual support. The loving emotion released by their arousal is associated with rewarding behavior involving mutual clasping, grooming, contact comfort, and pleasuring. The related neuroendocrine responses are associated with a reduction of adrenal-cortical hormones. The sociobiologic origin of mother–infant attachment arises from the need to protect the helpless young from predators. The long-term bonding between adult men and women integrates the generations, protects the women and children, and makes a cohesive society whose members share special skills and learned behavior.

biogrammar. Biogrammar represents a programmed preference to learn certain patterns. The human infant's speech is biogrammatically programmed. He learns to speak with great facility at a certain age. Such behavior can be attributed neither to instinct nor to the conditioning of culture but to both. Viewed sociobiologically, our attachment and territorial behavior are at the limbic roots of a biogrammar which is programmed by the cultural canon of the neocortex into the complex fabric of civilization (see archetype; instinct).

conservation–withdrawal.   Conservation–withdrawal is a response of the organism to its failure to control the environment; depression develops with this perception of helplessness. There is avoidance of others and failure to move around; this immobility is typically with a bowed head and flexed stance, and adrenocorticotropic hormone (ACTH) and adrenal-cortical activity increase. This type of stress response has been studied extensively by Selye and differs from Cannon's fight–flight response (see helplessness).

coping behavior.   Various events occurring during social interaction elicit adaptive coping behavior. Effective coping involves a capacity to maintain psychologic equilibrium without experiencing excessive or prolonged neuroendocrine arousal. This depends on the maintenance of self-esteem, and a sense of group support is critical. Coping also involves the rational process of reappraising the possibilities following changes in life situations. The competent individual seeks and utilizes information to deal with these changes. Those who cope successfully value and express their attachment to persons who are important to them and to whom they are also important. Culture and religion are of major importance in providing guidelines.

cultural canon.   Man's complex institutions with their rules of action and ideas of right and wrong develop as the result of an interplay of his biogrammatic roots with his culture. The cultural canon regulates inherited patterns of attachment and territorial behavior and its precepts weave inherited and acquired elements into the complexities of social behavior. Cultural canon refers to the norms and standards: the rules and general principles the group considers to be important, valid, and true. It thus includes a society's religion and the sacraments by which religion is affirmed (see biogrammar; archetype; instinct; anomie).

depression.   Depression is triggered by separation, bereavement, and loss of status. An infant losing maternal support or an animal losing precedence both become depressed as they lose access to desiderata. A perception of helplessness or a loss of control over the environment is central to the emotion. There is a release of the adrenocorticotropic hormone (ACTH) and enhanced acquisition of learned responses. Depression is of value for group survival because the animal that has just acquired higher status is relieved from competitive pressures while the newly subordinated individual rapidly learns appropriate behavior.

dominance.   The dominant animal in a group is the leader, initiating actions in search of food and shelter and controlling sources of disruption. In mice, the dominant has prior access to females and to all aspects of territory. In primates, more complex groupings occur and controlling one function does not necessarily determine control of another. The enormously complex hierarchy of roles seen in a human society is an extension of this intercalation of behavior.

emotion.   Emotion is a heightened state of motivation leading to performance of behavioral patterns critical for species' survival. Typical are the mother–infant relationship and the defense of territory. An emotional state may be deduced if expected behavior is accompanied by appropriate neuroendocrine changes. Thus the solitary withdrawal and flexed posture of a depressed primate infant that has lost its mother are accompanied by increased plasma levels of adrenocortical hormone and an angry cat, besides hissing and spitting, has elevated catecholamines.

fight–flight response.   The fight–flight response is a behavioral pattern under amygdalar control by which an organism responds to the perception that access to a source of valued responses is being challenged. Thus threat to an infant to whom the mother is attached leads to her arousal, and she experiences violent excitation of adrenergic fibers and release of catecholamines from the adrenal medulla. She is then in a state suited for either fight or flight. In the 1900's, Cannon saw this type of stress response as mobilizing resources for reestablishing a threatened control over the environment.

helplessness.   When a mammal is repeatedly

exposed to undesired, uncontrollable events frustrating its approach to desiderata, it learns that responding is futile. As a result, motivation is lost and the victim withdraws from social participation. The ensuing inactivity enhances loss of status and further cuts off access to desired objects. This depressed behavior is characteristic of recent subordination. Biochemically, brain catecholamines decrease and adrenal-cortical secretion increases (see conservation–withdrawal; depression).

instinct. Instinct is behavior highly stereotyped in its eventual end product. In mammals the instincts of attachment and territoriality are modified by environmentally determined neocortical responses. The attachment of a human mother to her child has a genetically determined base that is rapidly strengthened and directed to that individual by learning during a sensitive period soon after delivery. Human behavior has basic instinctual patterns shared with other mammals, originating from genetic endowment, but they are transformed until scarcely recognizable by learning in the cultural milieu (see archetype; biogrammar).

life changes. Life changes are events in the environment that evoke coping behavior. The resulting social readjustments involve various alterations in the accustomed pattern of life. The need to respond by readjustments elicits emotional arousal whose intensity depends on the individual's social support, his expectations, and his capacity to respond effectively to challenge. The intensity and duration of adjustments may or may not exceed a limit critical for the individual. Repeated excesses can result in pathophysiologic changes. The fight or flight response may be evoked with activation of the sympathetic system and elevation of catecholamine levels, or a depressive helpless and hopeless response may occur with adrenal-cortical activation.

psychosocial stress. Psychosocial stress develops when the social environment changes in a way which the organism perceives as demanding an adaptive response. The motivation to behave appropriately is accompanied by hormonal changes of value for the immediate crisis, but if prolonged, they can lead to pathophysiology. The pattern depends on the emotion. Catecholamines rise in response to challenge, evoking the fight or flight response of Cannon. The pituitary gland and the adrenal cortex are aroused by depression and subordination when control of the environment is lost.

relaxation response. The relaxation response is classically exhibited by the nursing mother and is practiced in a religious context, such as in prayer and meditation. Muscles relax, breathing is quiet, and there is a contemplative mental attitude. The fight–flight of defense and the helpless response of the cornered animal seek to deal with external factors, whereas the relaxation response involves the inner imagery of love, poetry, and prayer.

religion. Religion in its inward aspects is seen by Jung as a relationship to the highest or most powerful value the individual perceives—positive or negative. The relationship to this "god" is involuntary as well as voluntary; that is to say, you may or may not be consciously aware of the value system by which you are possessed.

social support. Social support is information leading the subject to believe he is cared for, loved, and esteemed as a member of a sociocultural network with mutual obligations. It is deficient, however, in disrupted social systems that lack a stable hierarchy, well-defined territory, and strong attachment behavior (see anomie; attachment).

territory. In an ethologic sense, territory refers to the exclusive use of a defined area whose boundaries are patrolled and defended against intrusion. This strictly spatial concept is expanded and becomes the abstraction of hierarchic troop structure in nonhuman primates. In man, it includes the realm of ideas and becomes as complex as society itself.

Type A personality. The Type A person is aggressively involved in a chronic struggle to achieve too much and participate in too many events. The trait is not apparent when he is secure and in control, but shows up when he is challenged. It is an expression of the mammalian territorial drive to win a distinct and preferably high-ranking social position. This person, however, does not feel his position is secure in what he perceives as a demanding, competitive, and unstable social environment.

Author index

*Numbers in italic refer to pages on which complete references are listed.

Subject index